An Introduction to Human Ser

THIRD EDITION

An Introduction to Human Services

Marianne Woodside
Tricia McClam

University of Tennessee, Knoxville

Brooks/Cole Publishing Company
ITP® An International Thomson Publishing Company

Pacific Grove • Albany • Belmont • Bonn • Boston • Cincinnati • Detroit • Johannesburg • London
Madrid • Melbourne • Mexico City • New York • Paris • Singapore • Tokyo • Toronto • Washington

Sponsoring Editor: *Lisa Gebo*
Marketing Team: *Jean Vevers Thompson, Deanne Brown, and Romy Taormina*
Editorial Assistants: *Lisa Blanton and Susan Carlson*
Production Editor: *Laurel Jackson*
Manuscript Editor: *Patterson Lamb*
Permissions Editor: *Lillian Campobasso*
Interior and Cover Design: *Terri Wright*
Cover Illustration: *SuperStock*
Art Editor: *Lisa Torri*
Photo Editor: *Terri Wright*
Typesetting: *Carlisle Communications, Inc.*
Cover Printing: *Phoenix Color Corporation*
Printing and Binding: *The Maple-Vail Book Mfg. Group*

For more information, contact:

BROOKS/COLE PUBLISHING COMPANY
511 Forest Lodge Road
Pacific Grove, CA 93950
USA

International Thomson Publishing Europe
Berkshire House 168-173
High Holborn
London WC1V 7AA
England

Thomas Nelson Australia
102 Dodds Street
South Melbourne, 3205
Victoria, Australia

Nelson Canada
1120 Birchmount Road
Scarborough, Ontario
Canada, M1K 5G4

International Thomson Editores
Seneca 53
Col. Polanco
11560 México, D.F., México

International Thomson Publishing GmbH
Königswinterer Strasse 418
53227 Bonn
Germany

International Thomson Publishing Asia
221 Henderson Road
#05-10 Henderson Building
Singapore 0315

International Thomson Publishing Japan
Hirakawacho Kyowa Building, 3F
2-2-1 Hirakawacho
Chiyoda-ku, Tokyo 102
Japan

Printed in the United States of America

10 9 8 7 6 5 4 3 2 1

Library of Congress Cataloging-in-Publication Data

Woodside, Marianne.
An introduction to human services / Marianne Woodside, Tricia McClam. — 3rd ed.
p. cm.
Includes bibliographical references (p.) and index.
ISBN 0-534-34783-5 (alk. paper)
1. Human services. 2. Human services—United States. 3. Social workers—United States. I. McClam, Tricia. II. Title.
HV31.W66 1997
361—dc21 97-15000
CIP

THIS BOOK IS PRINTED ON ACID-FREE RECYCLED PAPER

About the Authors

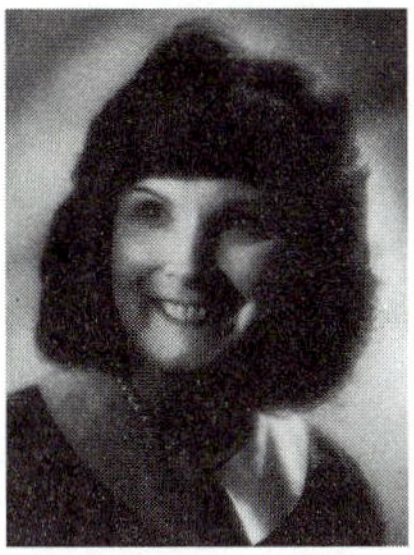

Marianne Woodside

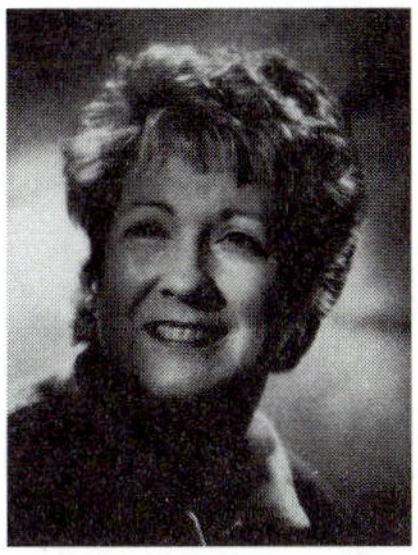

Tricia McClam

Marianne Woodside and Tricia McClam have been involved in human service practice and education for the past 26 years. They are committed to educating students to become knowledgeable about and committed to human service practice. Their primary area of academic focus is human service education and preparing the generalist professional. Interested in human services within the global context, they continue to read and study about human needs and problems as these manifest themselves internationally.

Contents

Preface

In writing the first two editions of this book, our goal was to offer instructors a textbook choice devoted entirely to human services—not psychology, sociology, or social work. We addressed the definition of the term *human services* in its broadest sense and described a variety of clients, the generalist human service professional, and the interaction between helper and client. We approached human services as a profession that, although newly established, continues to grow and develop. Our goal remains the same for this third edition of *An Introduction to Human Services,* but we have revised the text in ways that we believe improve it.

We have completely revised Part One based on the feedback from faculty and students during the review process. Many other revisions resulted from our own research and teaching; they document the changing face of the environment in which human services are delivered. The focus of Chapter 1 continues to be the principles that define human services. Chapter 2 combines a history of helping with a history of the human service movement; this combination allows thoughtful integration of human services into a long-standing historical context and updates developments to the present time. Chapter 3, which is new, offers a look at the current influences on human services: technology, managed care, the international dimension, and resolution-focused therapy. Chapter 4, "Models of Service Delivery," wraps up Part One by introducing three models that contribute to our understanding of human services. We have updated the models to reflect the changes that have occurred during the last decade. Case studies illustrate each model.

Part Two continues to focus on the participants in the delivery of human services—the helper and the client—and includes new information about such client populations as homeless people and the working poor. Part Three explores the world of the beginning professional, including job functions and skills, system considerations, ethical issues, and difficulties encountered in a professional work setting.

FEATURES

Two unique features of the text remain. The first is that this text continues to be introductory rather than encyclopedic. It presents basic information that students need to know about the human service field and encourages the use of other books, electronic materials, media resources, and other sources to enrich students' knowledge of the introductory course content. This knowledge will be more attractive to students when it is applied to case studies, books, current events, and audiovisual materials. In this book, you will find brief case studies, primary sources, and suggested additional readings for each chapter. The instructor's manual that accompanies the text also identifies videotapes, movies, novels, and nonfiction accounts of clients. All these resources can enhance students' understanding of human services. We encourage you to use these resources and to let us know of others that you discover on your own.

A second unique feature of the text is the International Focus sections. As the cultural composition of the United States continues to shift, human service professionals must be prepared to work effectively with culturally diverse clients. At the introductory level, our goal is to expand students' awareness in order to incorporate a global dimension into the human service field. Each International Focus section is related in some way to the content of the chapter and provides an opportunity for thought and discussion about the international dimension of human services. We have also added a broader description of international human services and how it influences practice in the United States.

A WORD ABOUT THE AUTHORS

As practitioners and instructors, we have been involved in human services for the past 26 years. As a result, we have experience both in delivering services and in preparing those who are learning to do so. From our years as practitioners in public schools and in rehabilitation settings, we have gained an understanding of helpers' commitment to their clients, their work, and their professions. In recent years, we have conducted in-depth interviews with practitioners and clients in an effort to better understand the methods of delivering services, the interaction between clients and human service professionals, and the changing context of service delivery. In recognizing the complexity of clients' lives and the complicated problems they sometimes face, we have developed more effective communication skills, a realistic understanding of helping using the human service model, and an appreciation of the problem-solving process that is based on the strengths of clients and their environments. These were valuable skills and understandings for us as practitioners. As instructors, we have discovered the importance of developing them in our students if these new practitioners are to become effective human service professionals.

Our work as educators has also contributed to our understanding of the evolving field of human services. As we developed curriculum with our colleagues, conducted research in human service education, participated in national and regional human service organizations, and traveled and studied internationally, we continued to be students ourselves. Concepts such as serving the whole person, using an interdisciplinary approach, training the generalists, and empowering clients have become basic to our work with beginning students of human services.

ACKNOWLEDGMENTS

Many friends and colleagues have contributed both to our growth as human service educators and to the writing of the third edition of this text. We are particularly grateful to our colleagues in the National Organization for Human Service Education and the Council for Standards in Human Service Education for their support, feedback, and contributions throughout the years. Our colleagues in the Department of Rehabilitation, Deafness, and Human Services at the University of Tennessee, Knoxville, provided daily encouragement throughout this endeavor. The Office of the Chancellor has also been supportive of our efforts.

We would especially like to thank our students and the students in other programs throughout the country who use our text, for we have learned much from them about human services. Introductory students continue to be a favorite group for us to teach because of their enthusiasm and interest in the helping professions. Several students deserve special recognition. They are Charlotte Meyer, Krista Whitesel, Ellen Davidson, and Marj Ferrin.

We also appreciate the willingness of Anthony Florian, Cliff Tennison, Charles Hamilton, and Craig Colvin to provide their assistance. Betsy Johnson and Rhonda Green have been invaluable in helping us type and organize the material for this book. Our families have also encouraged us during this endeavor, and we are grateful for their patience and support.

The reviewers whose constructive comments helped us improve the manuscript include Naydean Blair, Houston Community College; Marilyn Lairsey, Hillsborough Community College; W. Lynn McKinney, University of Rhode Island; and Michael J. Murphy, University of Maine–Augusta.

We would also like to thank the staff at Brooks/Cole for all their work with this manuscript. This includes our editor, Lisa Gebo, as well as Deanne Brown, Laurie Jackson, Karen Morgan, Kelly Shoemaker, Romy Taormina, Jean Thompson, and Lisa Torri. In addition, we would like to thank Lillian Campobasso, Patterson Lamb, and Terri Wright for their work on this book.

Marianne Woodside
Tricia McClam

An Introduction to Human Services

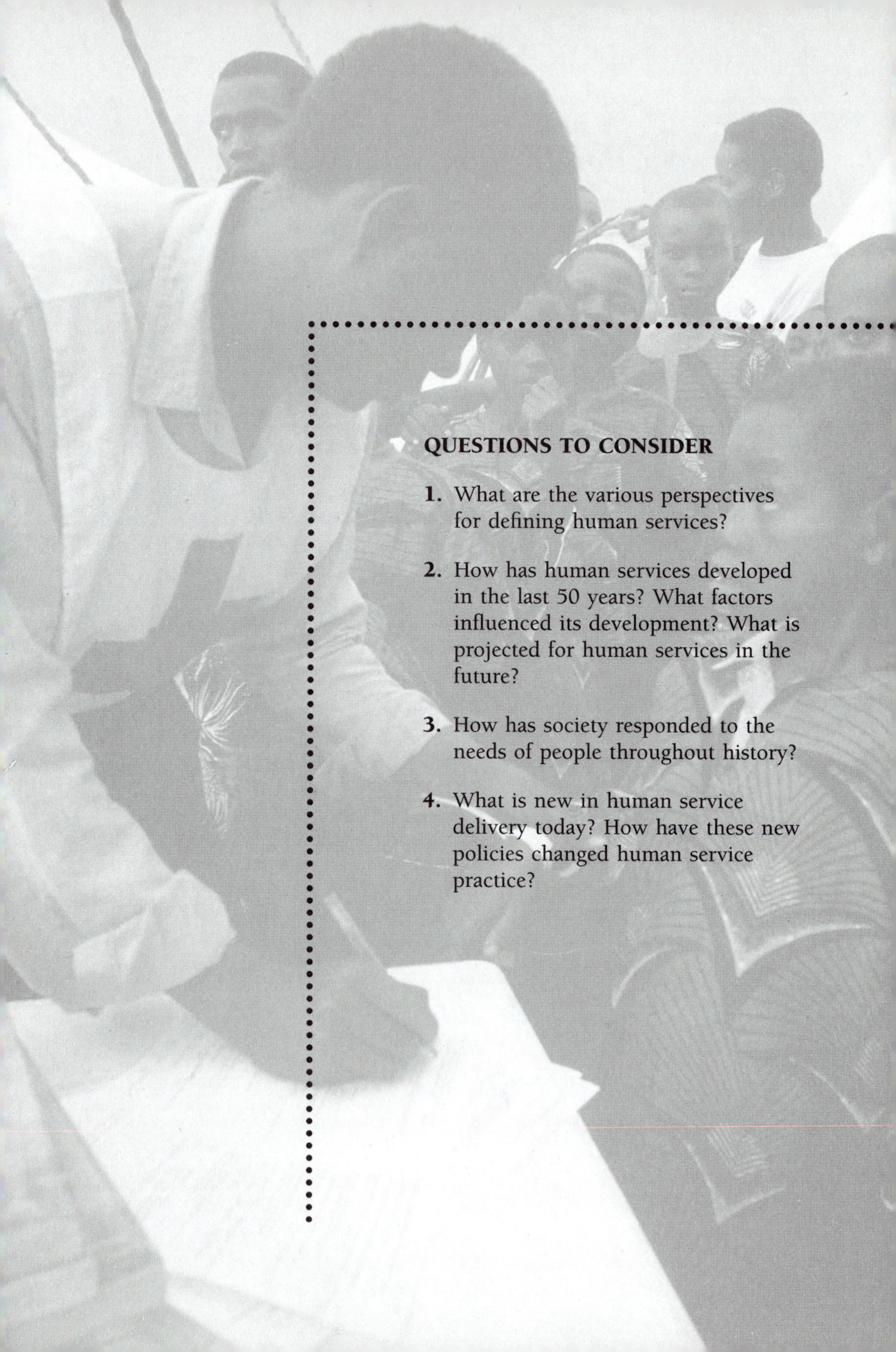

QUESTIONS TO CONSIDER

1. What are the various perspectives for defining human services?

2. How has human services developed in the last 50 years? What factors influenced its development? What is projected for human services in the future?

3. How has society responded to the needs of people throughout history?

4. What is new in human service delivery today? How have these new policies changed human service practice?

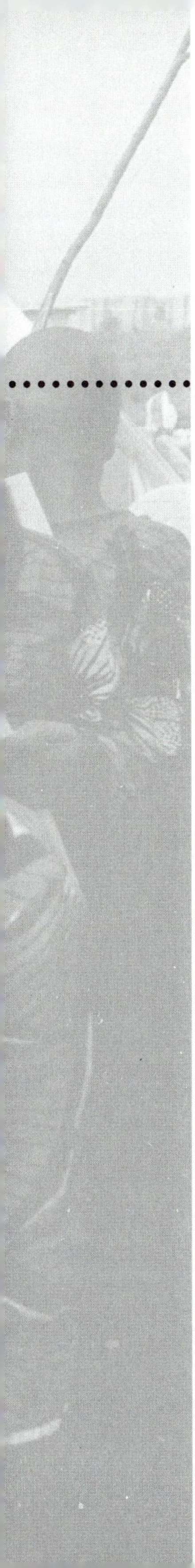

PART ONE

Defining Human Services

Human services may be a question mark to you as you begin this textbook. It is a difficult concept to define. Some think of it as the activities of workers who try to meet the needs of people. Others think of local and state agencies that used to be called departments of welfare or social services; today, many such agencies are departments of human services. Still others consider human services a profession for which a person receives special training.

Part One is titled "Defining Human Services." If you think of human services as a puzzle, the chapters in this part will provide you with the pieces necessary to understand this difficult and complex concept. Each piece will give you a different perspective from which to consider human services. Chapter 1 examines scholarly definitions as well as professional definitions. Chapter 2 provides a historical overview of helping, and a 20th-century perspective on the recent emergence of human services as a profession. Chapter 3 describes current influences on human service delivery and considers the future of human services. Chapter 4 describes three models of service delivery and includes a case study to illustrate each one.

Chapter 1

An Introduction to Human Services

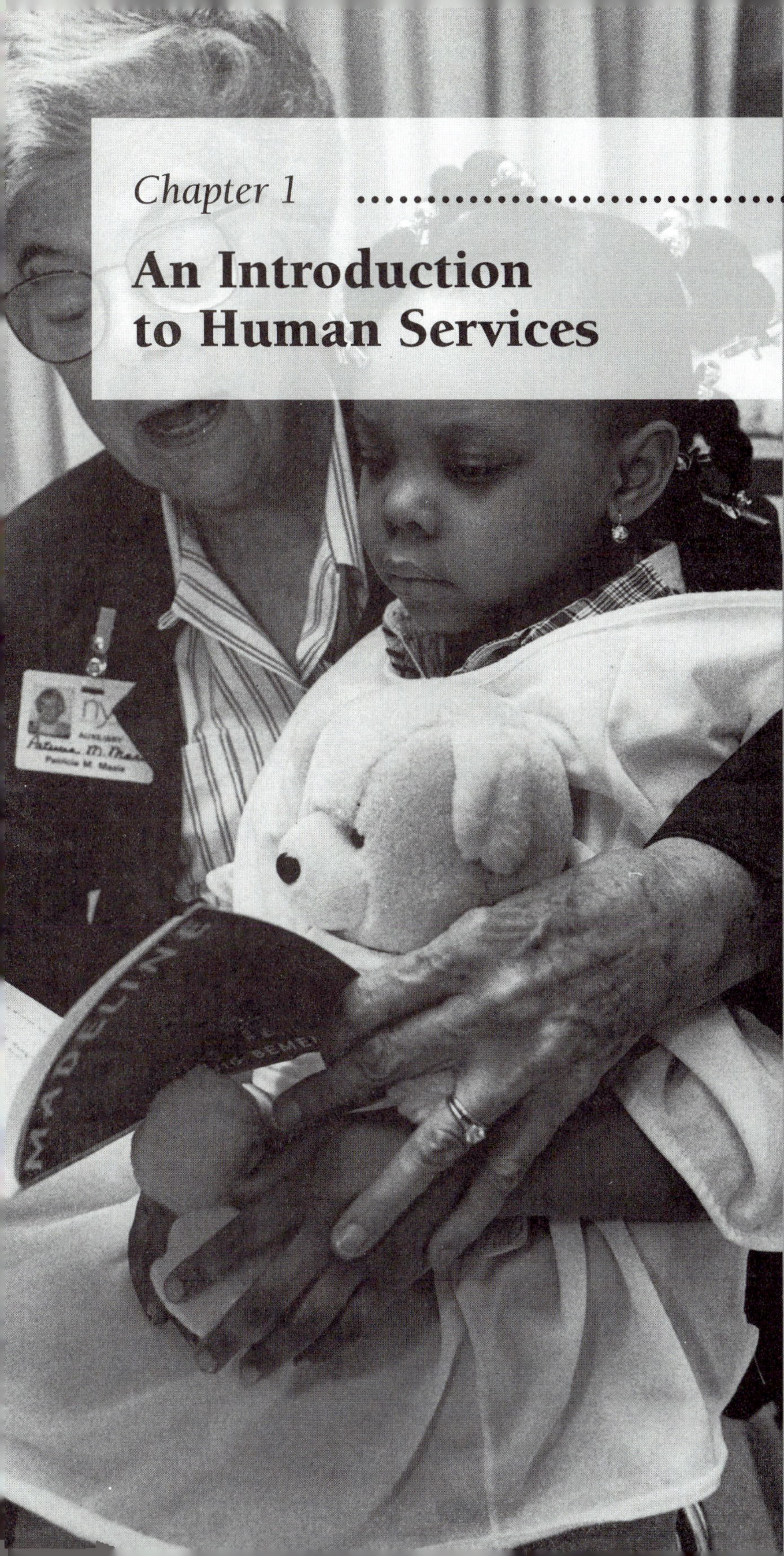

One of the first questions you will probably ask as you pick up this textbook is "What is human services?" This question has come up often in the last several decades as the field has changed and restructured. The purpose of this chapter is to help you gain an understanding of the term; and to accomplish this, we use information from both the formal literature (available in libraries) and "fugitive" literature (documents produced informally by research organizations, institutions, and individual educators and not readily available to the reader).

The definition of human services is derived from five perspectives: (1) the themes and purposes of human services, (2) the dual focus of client and helper, (3) management principles, (4) professional roles, and (5) professional activities. Understanding and integrating these diverse perspectives will help you formulate a definition of human services.

In this chapter, we examine the themes and purposes of human services as described by scholars and prominent leaders in the field. The five themes presented summarize the principles that guide the delivery of human services. They are illustrated by a case study of a young mother living in a large city. We also examine human services from the dual focus of the client and helper. Important ideas to consider here are the nature of the client, the client's environment, and the interaction between the client and the helper.

Another important characteristic of the human service delivery system that helps to define it is the management principles used by human service providers as they continually work to improve services to clients. The fourth perspective on human services introduces roles of professionals and nonprofessionals. Finally, a description of the professional activities of human service helpers illustrates their commitment to helping the client by providing needed services within a supportive environment.

Taken together, the five perspectives presented in this chapter will help clarify what human services is. They will also provide a basic understanding that will serve as a framework for the remainder of the text.

Themes and Purposes of Human Services

The first perspective from which human services can be defined is a scholarly one. Scholars approach the definition of human services by describing the themes and purposes that guide human services; these themes and purposes, have emerged over the past three decades. Those presented in this section represent the thinking of a range of scholars writing in the field today and include concerns with problems in living; the increase in problems in our modern world; the need for self-sufficiency; and the goals of social care, social control, and rehabilitation. A case study of Almeada and her daughter, Anne, illustrates these themes.

Problems in Living

Human beings are not always able to meet their own needs. Human services has developed in response to the need of individuals or groups for assistance to live better lives. Examples of such people are often publicized in the media: the very young, the elderly, people with limited physical or mental capabilities, victims of crimes or national disasters, people with acquired immune deficiency syndrome (AIDS), and many others. Assisting individual clients is an example of the helping interaction; families and groups also receive the attention of human service professionals, as do communities and larger geographic areas.

Anne, a 1-year-old child, lives with her mother, Almeada, in a housing project in Chicago. Their home is a dirty, rat-infested, one-room apartment that offers little beyond protection from the weather. Almeada, 17 years old, works six days a week for a local clothing manufacturer for minimum wage. She spends day after day in a large, hot, noisy workhouse, sewing sleeves in dresses and shirts. This summer, the baby Anne is watched by a 10-year-old neighbor, Andy, from 8 A.M. until 5 P.M. Andy takes Anne to the playground each day and watches her while he plays with his friends. When she needs a nap, he puts her down to sleep on the only grassy spot. He changes her once a day at noon and feeds her a bottle of watered juice, a bottle of watered milk, and cut-up hot dogs. The playground is located in a rough neighborhood and is the hangout for one of the many street gangs in the area. Almeada leaves the house at 6:30 A.M. and does not return until 7:30 P.M. During the hours that Andy is not watching Anne, she is alone in her bed in the apartment. Almeada knows that she needs help for herself and Anne. Before she moved from her old neighborhood, Almeada had been seeing a human service worker, Barbara Bailey. She plans to call Ms. Bailey tomorrow from work and hopes Ms. Bailey will be able to give her some ideas about where to go for help in this new part of the city.

Baby Anne cannot take care of herself. She is one of the many individuals who requires human services just to have the necessities of life. Anne lacks adequate food and housing, and she is in danger because she does not receive appropriate supervision during the day. There is also some question as to whether Almeada can take care of herself properly. She is only 17, works long hours for little pay, and has the major responsibility of raising a child, although she is little more than a child herself.

Human services recognizes problems such as Almeada's as *problems in living.* As part of this recognition, the focus is not on the past but rather on improving the present and changing the future. Doing so involves directing attention to the client, the environment, and the interaction between the two. Individuals grow and develop through the life cycle, encountering problems in living such as adolescent rebellion, becoming a parent, midlife crisis, caring for aging parents, and death and dying. Many difficulties in living arise in connection with families and communities; these may involve relating to children, spouses, and parents; maintaining progress in education; sustaining performance at work; and assuming responsibility for the very young and the very old. An important aspect of problems in living is the difficulty individuals encounter in interacting with their environments. If unemployment is high, finding work is not easy; if friends and relatives abuse drugs and alcohol, abstaining is difficult; if parents and peers do not value education, choosing to stay in school is problematic. Human services addresses problems in living, with a focus on both the individual or group and the situation or event.

Anne's mother, Almeada Smith, was 16 when Anne was born. Almeada received her early schooling in Chicago but quit attending school regularly when she was in the fifth grade. She was held back in the first grade and again in the third grade because she had not mastered basic math and reading skills. Her parents did not think education was important; in fact, they did not require that she attend school at all. They were both alcoholics, continually unemployed and dependent on Almeada to structure their family life. By the time Almeada was 10, she had discovered that life was more pleasant away from home. After school, she would spend long hours playing with her friends on the streets; nights, she would spend with girlfriends. She became sexually active at the age of 12 under pressure from her friends, who ridiculed her until she became "one of the gang." At the time she became sexually active, she knew about AIDS but did not consider it a problem for herself.

Between the ages of 12 and 16, Almeada was in constant turmoil, wondering how and where to live her life. She received advice as well as pressure from parents, friends, and teachers to do what they wanted. From time to time, she was asked to join special programs at school, but her parents would not give their permission. No one was particularly interested in what she wanted to do. Now she is entangled in a troublesome adolescent rebellion in which she rejects parents and teachers and accepts peers as models. Relating to peers brings unwelcome pressure to go along with the gang.

In responding to the needs of clients, human service workers are encountering an increasing number of problems to be solved, a rise that many experts attribute partly to a changing culture and lifestyle. The broad increase in problems is another theme in human services.

The Increase in Problems in the Modern World

Human services has emerged in response to the growth in human problems in our modern world (Mehr, 1995). Life is complicated by several factors new to the last half of this century. A growing number of people feel alienated and isolated from their neighborhoods and communities. No longer can they count on family and neighbors to share everyday joys and sorrows and assist in times of trouble and crisis. Households are in constant transition, as people leave family and friends to seek new job opportunities. Schools, churches, and recreation centers still provide meeting places, but because of the constant turnover, newcomers are welcoming newcomers. Stress is a hallmark of today's world. We worry about how to feed, clothe, and shelter children, families, adults, and the elderly. Illiteracy, a lack of employable skills, and unemployment rates or a low-wage employment add to people's feelings of helplessness and hopelessness, particularly in a technological age. The lifestyles that were once assured with a good education are no longer guaranteed. The world appears smaller as we have increased our capability for global communication. As more information is available, more choices appear possible. At the same time, new sources of worry are the problems of overpopulation, malnutrition, urbanization, and the environment of the planet. There is also threat of nuclear war, terrorism, and religious and social conflict.

For the past two years, Almeada has felt the weight of daily living problems. When she was 16, she discovered she was pregnant, and she received this information with mixed feelings. She was familiar with the problem of pregnancy because many of her friends had been pregnant. They often discussed choices, but to Almeada there was only one choice: to have the baby and take care of it. She tried to seek help from a reproductive health agency but was frightened when she had to walk through a picket line of abortion protesters to get there. Of course, she could not expect much support from her parents, and they were all the family she had ever known. She could not expect help from the father of her unborn baby or any of the other males in her life; most were just passing through the neighborhood. She was not sure where she would live or how she would support herself, but she knew that she would make it.

Almeada lives in a complex world with little support. An effective human service delivery system will teach her to use the skills she needs to manage her own life and survive the complex challenges that face her. This self-sufficiency is another theme of human services.

Self-Sufficiency

For many human service professionals, the key to service delivery is providing clients, or consumers of human services, with the opportunity to be self-sufficient. Economic self-sufficiency strengthens an individual's self-esteem. When a person is able to contribute financially to meeting his or her basic needs for food, clothing, and shelter, that person gains a certain degree of independence, but he or she may still need some assistance. One important facet of moving clients to self-sufficiency is to empower them to make decisions and assume responsibility for their actions. Human services is committed to giving individuals and groups enough assistance to allow them to help themselves. Clients are encouraged to be independent and gain control of their lives as soon as they are able.

It was difficult for Almeada to become economically self-sufficient when she was 16, barely educated, and pregnant. She had little parental guidance or support. She was forced to move back home to live with her parents and seek the little help they could give her. In fact, she began taking care of them again. She got a job as a cashier at the local grocery store. Almeada saved a few dollars a week and bought groceries for the family with the rest. Her parents tried to borrow money from her to buy alcohol; they took her money if she brought it home.

In the early days of her pregnancy, Almeada's life became routine. She worked from 8 A.M. to 5 P.M., walked home, prepared dinner, and visited with her friends later at night. Her advancing pregnancy changed her relationships with some of her friends because she did not have the stamina or the desire to share their evening activities. Even as her life changed, she was determined that no one would interfere with her life; she did not want help. Almeada wanted to make her own decisions. Despite that fiercely independent attitude, she would soon need assistance.

INTERNATIONAL FOCUS
The Sexual Exploitation of Children

The First International Congress was held August 27–31, 1996, in Stockholm, Sweden, to discuss the child sex trade and to begin advocacy for children who are its victims. The conference was organized by UNICEF, the Swedish government, and a Bangkok-based advocacy group called End Child Prostitution in Asian Tourism (ECPAT). Experts report that in Asia, over 1 million children a year are forced into sexual exploitation and that large numbers of children suffer this abuse in other parts of the world. Children are moved from city to city and country to country by sex traders, and many are used by men who believe they have less risk of contracting AIDS from having sex with a younger partner. According to expert Christine Beddoe, "In many developing countries, children are sent into the sex industry to earn money, since prostitution, in the short term, tends to be more lucrative than just about any other type of labor. And all over the world, children who live on the streets often turn to prostitution or are lured into sexual exploitation as a way to survive" (Barr, 1996a, p. 1). In more prosperous countries, many of the children who are exploited are "in flight from sexual abuse that usually began at home" (Daum, 1996, p. 19). For these children, sex for money gives them power that they never had at home.

Advocates believe that the key to attacking the sexual exploitation of children is the recognition that children are individuals who have human rights. In 1989, the United Nations Convention on the Rights of the Child promoted the concept of children's rights by stating that "every child has a right to live a life free of sexual exploitation and other abuses" (Barr, 1996b, p. 9). This idea is frightening to many adults, especially in countries where devotion to the family is considered primary or children are considered the property of their parents. The Convention states that children will not be protected until we believe that we must respect and nurture our children.

SOURCE: Adapted from "World Activists Meet to Combat Child Sex Trade," by C. W. Barr, August 28, 1996a, *The Christian Science Monitor*, pp. 9–11; "Getting Adults to Think in New Ways," by C. W. Barr, September 16, 1996b, *The Christian Science Monitor*, pp. 9–11; "Sexually Exploited Children in Canada: The Law Is Not on Their Side," by K. Daum, September 17,1996, *The Christian Science Monitor*, p. 19.

Almeada was somewhat self-sufficient because she was working and her parents provided housing. As her pregnancy advanced, however, she had to quit work and rely on others. She also needed prenatal care, parenting skills, and an opportunity to assess her decision to keep the baby. Although economic self-sufficiency is a key for many clients, it would clearly be only a beginning for Almeada. The human service delivery system has several functions that help determine the service clients receive. The following section explains three of these.

Social Care, Social Control, and Rehabilitation

Human services serves three distinct functions: social care, social control, and rehabilitation (Neugeboren, 1991). *Social care* is assisting clients in meeting their social needs, with the focus on those who cannot care for themselves. The elderly, children, persons with mental disabilities or mental illness, and victims of crime and crisis are populations who might need social care.

Social control differs from social care in two fundamental ways: who receives the services and under what conditions they receive them. Social care is given to those who cannot provide for themselves (either temporarily or in the long term). In contrast, most recipients of social control are able to care for themselves but have either failed to do so or have done so in a manner that violates society's norms for appropriate behavior. Often, society rather than the individual determines who receives social control services. The purpose of such services is to restrict or monitor clients' independence for a time because the clients have violated rules of the community. Children, youth, and adults in the criminal justice system are clients of social control.

Rehabilitation is the task of returning an individual to a prior state of functioning. What creates the need for rehabilitation? An individual who was once able to live independently becomes unable to function socially, physically, or psychologically. The inability to function can be caused by a crisis, a reversal of economic or social circumstances, an accident, or other circumstances. Rehabilitative services, which are designed to return the individual to his or her original state, can have a short- or a long-term focus. Veterans, persons with physical disabilities, and victims of psychological trauma are among those who receive rehabilitative human services.

In actuality, separating these three functions of human services is often difficult. Many clients have multiple problems, so social care, social control, and rehabilitation may be occurring at the same time.

Almeada finally became involved in the human service system in mid-autumn, when she was seven months pregnant. She refused to go to school. Her parents let her continue to work at the neighborhood store—in fact, they encouraged her to. Her friends often missed school as well, so she saw them every day when they came to the grocery store to do their shopping. Evenings, they all gathered at a shop in the neighborhood.

A new program was started at Almeada's school to provide more comprehensive support to many of its students. This program targeted students who had irregular attendance, low math and reading scores, no discipline record, and positive teacher reports. In the fall, the school officials noted that Almeada, who qualified for this new program, had not returned to school after the summer vacation. The case manager of the program, Barbara Bailey, visited the most recent address on the school records and found Almeada's father at home. He was in a drunken stupor and was unable to give Ms. Bailey information about Almeada. When Ms. Bailey talked to the neighbors, they suggested she try the grocery store where Almeada worked. Ms. Bailey found Almeada in the middle of her daily shift and made an appointment to pick her up after work and take her home.

In the next few months, Ms. Bailey provided social care for Almeada and then for her baby, Anne. The school offered Almeada several options for continuing her education: She could receive homebound instruction until and after the baby was born; she could come back to school; or she could attend a special night school for potential dropouts who work during the day. Ms. Bailey also referred Almeada to a prenatal care class taught by a local teacher one night a week at the school. Because of Almeada's youth and lack of parental support, Ms. Bailey discussed with Almeada the options of keeping the baby or placing it for adoption. She also took Almeada to the family planning clinic to discuss these options further. Almeada remained sure that she wanted to keep her child. Once the baby was born, Almeada needed rehabilitative assistance but, instead, returned to work immediately. She expected her parents to care for Anne while she was gone, but her parents refused to baby-sit. Almeada was afraid that one day they might harm Anne out of their own frustration. Her parents could not stand to have the baby in the home because they had to compete with her for attention. Instead of receiving rehabilitative services, Almeada moved to a new neighborhood, rented a one-room apartment, and found a new job working in a garment factory six days a week. In her new neighborhood, Almeada was without human service support again.

The story of Almeada's struggles and need for assistance is just one of many about individuals who cannot meet their own needs without assistance from others. A common element seen in all human services is that these services help individuals, families, and groups with their problems. There would be little need for these services if people did not need assistance and support from others. The term *human services* encompasses the variety of helping services that addresses the range of problems that people experience.

The themes and purposes of human services—problems in living; increasing problems; self-sufficiency; and social care, social control, and rehabilitation—all contribute to a definition of human services. Examining the interaction between the human service professional and the client also helps define human services.

Dual Focus on Client and Helper

The delivery of human services involves both the client and the helper. The process of helping is client oriented as the helper focuses on assisting clients meet their needs. To do this, the helper performs many roles and assumes a wide variety of responsibilities. Let's look at Almeada and her human service worker, Ms. Bailey, to see the dual focus in action.

When Ms. Bailey first approached Almeada, she talked at length with Almeada about her situation. As her case manager, Ms. Bailey had contacted

Almeada to learn whether she would come back to school and to help her with problems that were barriers to her school attendance. After they talked, it was obvious that Almeada faced many problems. Ms. Bailey planned to work with Almeada, baby Anne, and Almeada's parents if they would accept the help.

Thirty years ago, a worker in Ms. Bailey's position would have focused on school-related issues; she would not have assessed Almeada's needs in other areas or referred her to other services. She might have told Almeada about other human service agencies, but Almeada would have had to contact them on her own. Today, human service professionals assist the whole person and empower clients to help themselves. Ms. Bailey was not able to meet all Almeada's needs, but she did work actively to connect her with other human service agencies in and outside the school. Ms. Bailey was doing what Mehr (1995) defines as human services: providing assistance to those who need help with their social, psychological, and economic problems. And as a case manager, she was coordinating the care that Almeada and Anne received.

As a human service professional, Barbara Bailey has the skills to develop a relationship with Almeada. In this situation, much of Ms. Bailey's success as a case manager is dependent on her personal interaction with Almeada and her ability to establish a relationship. She is also able to apply her problem-solving skills to address the needs of Almeada and Anne. Using the problem-solving process, she initiates human service delivery by considering the relationship of her client with the environment and other professionals in the human service delivery system.

Barbara Bailey, the human service professional who helped Almeada, was a very active helper. First, although she was employed by the school system, she was able to work with other professionals to develop a plan of assistance for Almeada and Anne, using the existing human service organizations for their benefit. Second, Barbara had the ability to engage in problem solving with Almeada and to recommend alternatives. She took a personal interest in Almeada, provided a structure for Almeada's treatment plans, and linked Almeada with other organizations. For Barbara Bailey, Almeada was an important person, and one to be treated with respect and dignity.

The Client and the Client's Environment

Clients do not exist in a vacuum; they are active participants in many different systems that influence their circumstances. Services to the client must be delivered with an understanding of the client's world and with the client's participation. To be effective, the human service professional must ask the client questions about present conditions, current stresses and relationships, and everyday events. Most important, the helper listens to the client, always attempting to see a situation through the client's eyes. Questioning and listening should help the human service professional understand the client's world. The helper must show both a strong commitment to the client and concern for the client's well-being. The helper also assists the client in identifying personal strengths and weaknesses and developing new skills and abilities to enhance personal development.

Human service professionals also function as educators:

> Help is a process, an active process of people thinking together. Often practitioners provide clients with information, observations and suggestions; for if clients are to make a rational choice, they have to be exposed to all available alternatives. Problematic situations are explored in respect to their influence on clients and various social systems. Clients are encouraged to search for solutions as workers present questions concerning who the clients are and what they are doing. (Spicuzza & Spicuzza, 1979, p. 3)

As an educator, the human service professional helps clients develop certain skills to increase their intellectual, emotional, and behavioral options. The client is a complex individual with many intellectual, emotional, and behavioral possibilities. Clients feel better about themselves when human service professionals treat them as thinking, feeling, and acting human beings, capable of change. If the human service professional believes in and promotes change, change will be easier for the client.

Almeada now lives in her new neighborhood with her daughter, Anne, and works six days a week in a garment factory. She knows she needs help. Because her major contact has been with human service professionals in another neighborhood, she does not really know whom to call, so she calls her previous case manager, Barbara Bailey. Ms. Bailey is delighted to hear from Almeada again and is alarmed at her plight. Almeada talks of her current work and child care situation in depressed and hopeless terms. Almeada seems to feel that she has limited options, and Ms. Bailey wants to refer Almeada to a source that can help increase her options. She tells Almeada that she will make a few phone calls and then call her back. Ms. Bailey also wants to bolster Almeada's confidence in herself. As she gathers information about Almeada's move, her new employment, and her care of Anne, she praises Almeada's responsibility and maturity. She helps Almeada see how she has been a successful problem solver. She also praises Almeada's calling her and reaching out for help. Ms. Bailey knows that any positive change Almeada can make will help solve the rest of the problems.

A function of the human service professional is to help clients develop their ability to assess fundamental needs and focus on them early in the helping

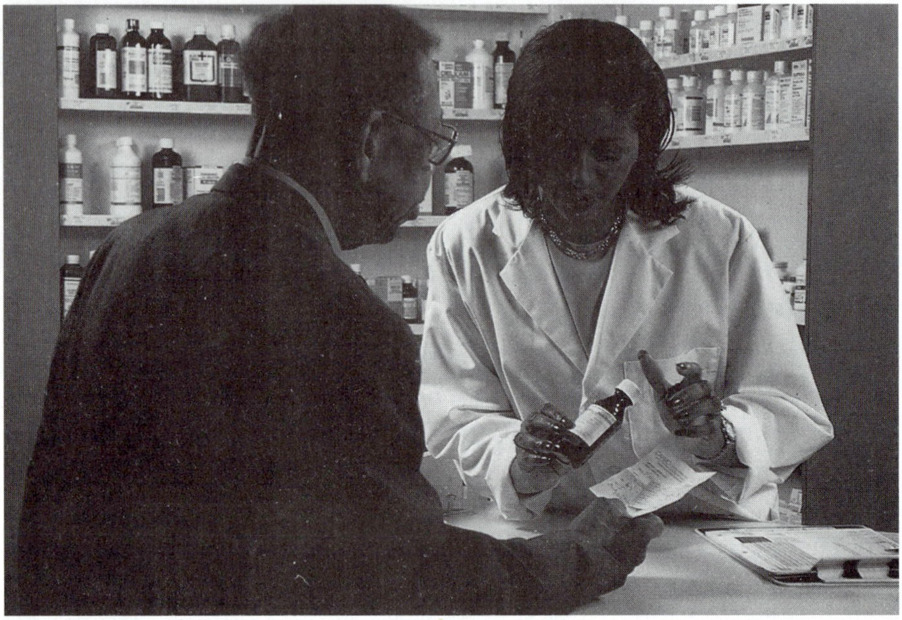

Human services is helping clients meet their needs.

process. Abraham Maslow, a psychologist, described a hierarchy of human needs that begins with basic physical needs and rises through higher levels to address safety and security needs, social belonging needs, self needs, and finally, self-actualization needs at the highest level. He stressed that addressing higher-level needs is difficult unless an individual's basic needs have been met (Maslow, 1971). In other words, if a child is hungry or very tired, or an adult is very scared, that child or that adult will have difficulty focusing on needs related to belonging or self-actualization. Clients are often so overwhelmed by their situations that they do not know how to identify what they need or where to begin to look for help or solutions. A good place to start is with the most basic needs, which are often the simplest to solve and give the client satisfaction early in the helping process.

As an educator, the helper also teaches clients to recognize how their physical and interpersonal environments affect them. Clients are responsible for their own thoughts and behavior. Sometimes, however, clients are unable to make changes because their environments do not support such changes. Clients must be taught to determine the influence their environments have on their lives and to assess when and how their environments can be changed. Sometimes, such changes are impossible.

In summary, an important conception of human services is the dual focus of the helper and the client. The helper is committed to developing a relationship with the client that facilitates problem solving within the client's own environment. Many times the human service professional is also an educator teaching the client skills that can be used long after the potential help has ended.

A Pioneer in Human Services

Dr. Harold McPheeters, a psychiatrist by training, is considered a key figure in the development of human service education. After serving as an administrator in the department of mental health in two states, he joined the Southern Regional Education Board (SREB) in 1965 as director for the Commission on Mental Health and Human Services and director of health programs.

His work began with a planning grant to bring together mental health professionals and community college officials to explore the feasibility of educating mental health practitioners in two-year colleges. That grant provided the groundwork for 20 years of research and training in the mental health and human service field. Defining the concept of the generalist worker, providing support for training mental health/human service professionals, developing a certification program for workers, and beginning an approval process for training programs were efforts completed under Dr. McPheeters's leadership and support. Before his retirement from the SREB in September 1987, Dr. McPheeters wrote (at our request) the following definition of human services, based on his 30 years of experience in the field. His definition integrates many of the ideas that have been presented.

> I never came up with an absolute definition of human services. Originally, our work began with the associate degree programs that were training people to work in some aspect of mental health. However, it soon became apparent that the graduates of those programs and the graduates of other programs that were titled according to other human service fields, such as child care workers, youth services workers, and aging program workers, were all finding employment in a variety of human service fields—not just in the narrow subspecialty areas of mental health, addiction, aging, and so on. So the terminology began to change to "human services" although no very precise definitions were applied. . . . Human services works with those same problems and people, but with a blend of primarily psychological and sociological theories and principles. Human services also has an eclectic approach to collaborating with whatever approaches (for example, medical) are needed to help people solve their problems. I suppose my definition would be something like this: Human services is the occupation/profession that uses a blend of primarily psychological and sociological theories and skills in preventing, detecting, and ameliorating psychosocially dysfunctioning people and in helping them attain the highest level of psychosocial functioning of which they are capable.

Management Principles in Human Service Delivery

Understanding how services are delivered is an important part of defining human services. Three principles of management related to the delivery of services characterize the profession today: networking to develop a human service umbrella, forming teams and partnerships to provide services, and using case management to facilitate client growth. These management strategies help professionals provide more effective and efficient assistance to clients as well as enhance their own work environment.

Networking to Develop a Human Service Umbrella

Human services is not a single service delivery system but a complex web of helping agencies and organizations whose primary goal is to assist people in need. It encompasses a variety of services that include, but are not limited to, child, youth, and family services; corrections; mental health; public health; crisis intervention; and education (see Figure 1-1).

Karin Eriksen (1981) notes that "human services is often called the umbrella for our society's professions which are involved either directly or indirectly in promoting and reinforcing satisfying, healthy living and community cohesiveness" (p. 8). Going beyond the metaphor of the umbrella, Eriksen herself describes human services as a "bridge" between people and systems. One function of bridging is to narrow the gap between the services being offered and the needs of the individuals receiving those services.

Another bridging responsibility is to link human service agencies. Agencies and organizations share the common good of assisting people in need. In the

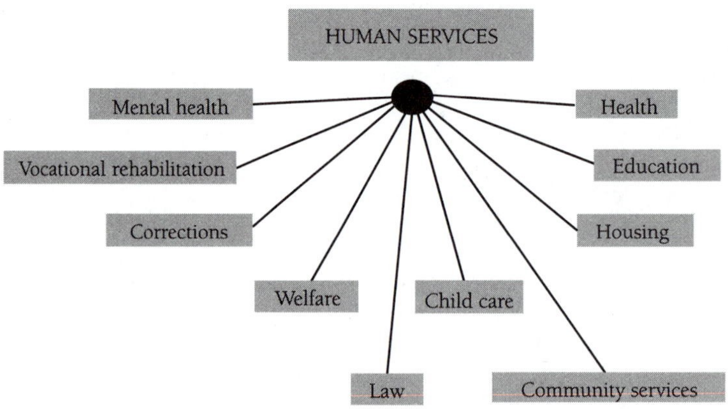

Figure 1-1 ✦ Human services subsystems

SOURCE: Adapted from *Human Services Today*, by K. Eriksen, p. 7. Copyright © 1981 by Reston Publishing.

past, there has been little coordination, and the result has been overlapping worker responsibilities and competition for resources. Today, as service delivery philosophy changes and resources become scarce, agencies are limiting services, tightening eligibility criteria, and focusing on short-term interventions. Only increased communication, cooperation, and collaboration among helpers and agencies can promote effective service delivery. Networking is one way that service providers work together to serve clients.

Barbara Bailey wants to help Almeada in her new neighborhood, and she knows that finding a good entry into the system is critical. Ms. Bailey worries that, without the right help, Almeada will be lost in the human service delivery system. She needs to find another worker who is familiar with Almeada's neighborhood human service system and knows the formal and informal linkages that need to be made to deliver multiple services. She is looking for a worker who will help Almeada move between the many agencies whose services she will require. Almeada needs the support of those who provide child care and teach parenting skills. In addition, she needs assistance in improving her work skills and her health. Vocational development and public health services are rarely offered together. Coordination, monitoring, and evaluation are key services that are needed. Where will Ms. Bailey locate such a professional?

For Almeada or any other client to assume the responsibility of negotiating the network would be difficult; human service professionals must build the bridges between agencies, organizations, and services. Working together to provide services for the good of the client is often called "teaming" and is another management tool used for delivering good-quality services to the client.

Forming Teams and Partnerships to Provide Services

Working as a team to provide services is part of the history of human services. Developers of the human service movement from early in its history stressed the importance of working with other professionals to assist the client in receiving services. More recently, the concept of working as a team has expanded, and "teaming" has become a common approach to organizing the work of an agency or organization.

The advent of teaming follows a progression in management philosophy. In the 1950s, managers were "learning to be friendly." In the 1960s, the trend was to be sensitive to the needs and motivations of one's employees, and in the 1970s, managers began asking employees for help. In the 1980s, managers were initiating meetings to hear from their employees, and in the 1990s, shared ownership between managers and workers was promoted (Scott & Jaffe, 1991). Today, the concept of partnership is being encouraged. Let's look at both teaming and partnership in human services and see how it is applied.

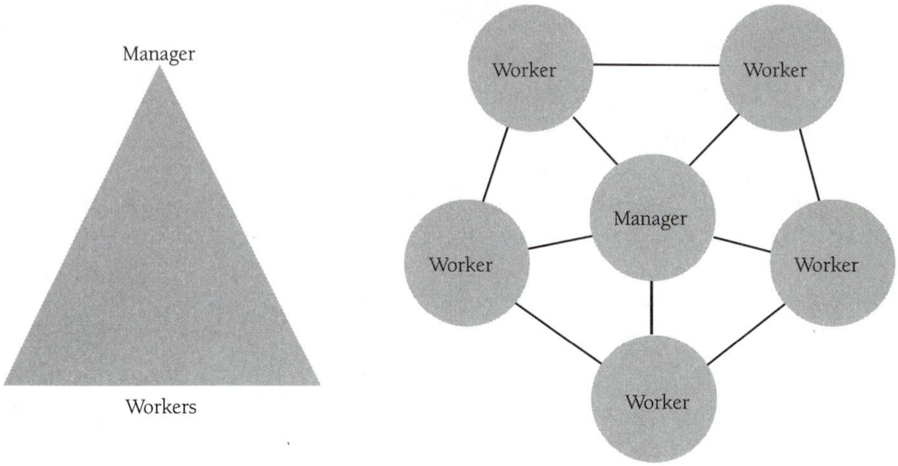

Figure 1-2 ✦ Traditional organizational pyramid and new empowerment circle organization

SOURCE: From *Empowerment: A Practical Guide for Success,* by C. Scott and D. Jaffe, p. 13. Copyright © 1991 by Crisp Publications.

What exactly is the teaming concept? What principles do members of the team follow to deliver quality services? How does teaming improve services to the client or consumer? According to Scott and Jaffe (1991), teaming, or empowerment, is a management concept based primarily on the changing role of the employee. Employees are encouraged to make more decisions and take responsibility with others for serving clients effectively. Responsibility and decision making in a human service context are better represented by a circle than by a pyramid. The circle illustrates the equality of responsibility among the team members (see Figure 1-2).

The following principles underlie the teamwork concept that makes this new management strategy so successful:

1. The customer is central to the planning and delivery of services. This basic principle guides the setting of goals, the intervention, and the evaluation of services. It is not only important in teaming but is also a central philosophical principle of human services.

2. Members of the team must work together cooperatively. The team, not the individual, is the work unit, and all work is considered a joint effort. The successes of each individual are celebrated by the team, and everyone is committed to making the team more effective.

3. There is continual communication between the members of the team. This is a critical component of teamwork. To ensure cooperation and shared problem solving within a challenging environment, each member of the team needs to understand continually the status of other members' work, especially as the work of each is interdependent with that of the others.

4. All team members share responsibility, authority, control, and accountability. This concept is represented by the circle shown in Figure 1-2. The organization's commitment to giving its professionals the skills to assume this type of responsibility is at the heart of the teaming concept (Brown, 1991; Parker, 1991).

After talking to several child and youth services offices, Barbara Bailey contacted Hernando Alvarez, a case manager in the child services division of the state department of human services. He recommended that Almeada call their office and schedule a meeting with an intake worker. Their office, just recently reorganized to be more customer oriented, was open for intake and service from 7 P.M. to 10 P.M. Mondays through Thursdays and on Saturdays from 8 A.M. until noon. Almeada would be assigned to a case manager who would not provide services but would coordinate them. In addition, four other workers would help plan, implement, and evaluate work with Almeada. A backup case manager would also know Almeada's case in detail and be available to support her if her primary case manager was absent. This particular team treats the entire human service delivery system as a larger team. They cooperate with each organization, sharing problems and finding creative solutions that benefit clients. One warning that Mr. Alvarez gave was the uncertainty of upcoming changes in welfare services. Mr. Alvarez hopes that Almeada does not get lost in the changing structure. At the conclusion of her conversation with Mr. Alvarez, Barbara Bailey felt she could make a good referral for Almeada. And she made a promise to herself to contact Mr. Alvarez in two months to check on her client's progress.

As stated in the case of Almeada, one of the major purposes of teaming is to improve the delivery of services to clients or consumers of the services. Teaming also makes the work of the organization more positive for the professionals involved. Teaming is intended to create an atmosphere that encourages creativity and problem solving and lessens tension in the workplace as it increases team spirit and motivation (Career Track, 1991). The following quotation summarizes the team effort.

> When you find yourself part of a group of people who are equally committed to the same mission, when you see that you are appreciated for your special qualities, when you know that your fellow team members care about you and your performance as much as they care about their own . . . it's a team. (Brown, 1992, p. 20)

The primary beneficiary of teaming in a human services setting is the client. The team approach yields more efficient and more effective service. As suggested in the case of Almeada, many professionals, functioning as a group, are working together to provide creative, coordinated services. Such teams are able to evaluate their own performance and make changes to improve their service delivery.

Partnerships are also emerging as a way that organizations in the human service delivery system work together to serve their clients more effectively and efficiently. These partnerships are formed as an agreement is reached between two or more human service organizations that they will work together toward common goals. In addition, partnerships are formed with corporations, businesses, and government entities as those organizations outside the human service delivery system see benefits in supporting the social service sector. The goals of establishing partnerships are several (Snyder, 1996):

- Help promote an understanding of the challenges faced by all involved or concerned with providing human services to those in need
- Provide an opportunity to access talent and expertise beyond each organization
- Provide more cost-effective services
- Increase awareness of broader issues and influence the planning and goal setting for all organizations and agencies involved

Partnering requires many of the same qualities of teaming: a high degree of cooperation, a commitment of time, and a high level of trust. When partnering is successful, there is mutual gain for each of the parties involved.

The concept of partnership has emerged as a way human service organizations relate to each other for several reasons. Many of them are financial. As the cost of service provision increases and available financial resources decrease, many organizations are finding that they can provide services more cost effectively when they work with other agencies. Partnerships have also been encouraged by the increasing pressure to be accountable for resources expended. Agencies find that combining their resources and expertise enables them to provide better services to their clients.

Hernando Alvarez contacted Almeada the day after he talked with Barbara Bailey. Rather than place the burden of contacting the Department of Human Services (DHS) on Almeada, he went to see her at her workplace. He explained that Ms. Bailey had called him and that he was interested in working with Almeada to decide what services she needed and to help her find a way to access those services. Because the Department of Human Services had partnerships with many businesses and industries, he was able to schedule a time that he could meet with Almeada at her business site. Her employer had a small office for DHS workers and encouraged his employees to use the services the agency made available. Mr. Alvarez knew that some services could be provided very quickly; others would evolve more slowly. But he wanted to get some services in place and a relationship with Almeada established before the welfare program completely changed the services available.

Hernando Alvarez and other DHS workers increased their ability to work effectively with clients through their partnership agreements with many local corporations and businesses. For DHS and other agencies, partnerships are usually established at the organizational level and are marked by a general statement of agreement that two or more organizations will work together. The text of the agreement contains language similar to the following: "This statement represents an acknowledgment by Organization A and Organization B of their mutual interest in forming a joint, long-term cooperative relationship whose purpose would be to encourage interaction between the two organizations." Later, the organizations work together to find specific projects and activities that would invite mutual support, and in the case of Almeada's employer, the employer encourages DHS to support their employees.

Just as teaming and partnerships have emerged as powerful tools to improve the delivery of human services, another tool, the role and responsibility of case management, is emerging as a way of increasing our effectiveness in meeting the needs of the multiproblem or long-term client.

Case Management

Several factors make case management a viable alternative for service delivery today (Austin, 1983; Merritt & Neugeboren, 1990). One is the shift from large, state-operated institutions to smaller, community-based facilities. This shift gives special importance to interorganizational coordination, a team approach, and helping professionals with a concern for the whole person because services are not being assessed or delivered in one comprehensive system.

A second factor is the categorical public funding of the past, which resulted in highly complex, redundant, fragmented, and uncoordinated services. The resulting system is burdensome for people with complex problems who are least able to act as advocates for themselves. In many cases, multiproblem clients are assigned a different worker within a given agency for each service and different workers in different agencies. Often there is no central worker who knows and understands the client's total situation or who is responsible for planning and coordinating treatment strategies.

A third factor is the very nature of human service work today. Service providers increasingly find themselves with a dual role: providing direct services and coordinating services from other agencies and/or professionals. Thom Prassa likens having a caseload to being an air traffic controller, coordinating and sometimes juggling many different cases. On a case-by-case basis, he often feels like he is "paratrooping into a fire. We put out fires all the time: suicide attempts, arranging placements, paperwork, talking with parents, and so forth" (personal communication, July 10, 1994). This dual role can create problems in terms of time management, effective and efficient service delivery, and quality assurance.

According to Austin (1983), "Case management is an idea whose time has come" (p. 451). Sullivan, Wolk, and Hartman (1992) see it as "a creative and collaborative process, involving skills in assessment, consulting, teaching, modeling and advocacy that aim to enhance the optimum social functioning of

[the] client served" (p. 198). The goal of case managers is to teach clients how to manage their own lives and to be self-sufficient, returning to the human services system in times of crisis.

What exactly do case managers do? They gather information, make assessments, and monitor services. In addition, they arrange services from other agencies, provide advocacy services, and assume responsibility for allocating scarce resources and providing quality assurance. They also provide direct services. Many human service professionals believe that being a case manager means they will do whatever they must to help their clients.

The case management structure affects both coordination of services and client access to service. Given the fragmented state of service delivery and claims of coordination that are not borne out in practice, what is needed is interorganizational and interagency coordination that does not shuffle clients from one office to another. Exchanging resources rather than clients would ensure that clients do not get lost in the system or become frustrated with service delivery. Another necessary structural change is the establishment of a single point of access rather than entry points at each agency or for each service where, once they have contact with the system, clients are introduced to an array of community services (Merritt & Neugeboren, 1990). True coordination and integration allow clients to proceed through central intake, have their needs assessed, and be assigned to providers.

Part of preparing for case management is learning to be proactive. Problems today call for professionals who understand the need for case management and have the skills to perform effectively in that role. As case manager positions increase, human service professionals will be ready to assume that responsibility; but equally important, those trained as case managers will help develop organizational structures in which case management can work. We need professionals within the human service system who are able to promote these changes. The management principles described in the preceding paragraphs define the emerging context in which human services are being delivered. Equally important to understanding human services is knowing the broad range of agencies and organizations that provide these services.

The Role of the Human Service Professional

The human service professional provides services in a variety of settings. To respond to the many settings and the diversity of clients these settings represent, the helper needs a broad-based education and a willingness to adapt to changing roles and circumstances. There are two principal types of human service providers: the generalist and the nonprofessional.

The Generalist

The concept of the generalist is fundamental to human services. It describes the kinds of skills the professional has and the types of functions the professional performs. The term *generalist* has not always been associated with human services; the concept has evolved over the last few decades. Early in the history of human services, *generalist* referred to a person who worked within a specific discipline, such as psychology or psychiatry. Professionals in these disciplines performed many functions: interviewing, diagnosis, therapy, and follow-up. The term meant that the professional performed all the duties expected of a member of that particular profession.

As the role expanded, the term *generalist* took on a new meaning, connected to a specific client group. Generalists performed duties and had the skills to work with only one group. For example, youth mental health workers specialized in working with children. This would include working with individuals and with groups in educational, recreational, and counseling situations. Such workers would also be familiar with social, biological, and developmental problems of children and adolescents; they would also understand the importance of working with the family.

A third, emerging concept of the generalist is most representative of human services today. The human service generalist has the knowledge, values, and skills to perform a number of job functions in most human service settings. The generalist also understands how these functions fit with client goals and agency goals. For example, a helper trained to conduct interviews, write social histories, and define a treatment plan should be able to perform those responsibilities with the elderly, young children, or persons with mental retardation.

The human service generalist works with the client using both micro- and macroperspectives (Cimmino, 1996). The micro system is represented by the individuals in the client's environment and might include family, friends, teachers, co-workers, and individuals within the human service delivery system. The macro system is represented by the organizations, agencies, communities, and neighborhood locales in which the client interacts. For example, if the human service professional is working with the individual client using the microperspective, then the professional is interviewing the client, establishing rapport, and engaging in planning and problem solving. Using the macroperspective, the human service professional works with the client to understand his or her larger environment. This might include learning how to use the human service bureaucracy to convert needs into political action or to understand how school relates to the neighborhood.

It is interesting to examine follow-up studies of graduates of human service programs to see the development of the generalist concept as well as the broadening definition of human services. Early studies compiled by the Southern Regional Education Board up to 1972 indicated that graduates of human service programs were getting jobs in state hospitals, educational settings, mental health centers, children's agencies, and general hospitals. Three-fourths of the jobs were in mental health agencies. Although these graduates were performing a wide range of services, most were indirect services dealing with patients and other staff members. Their job functions were client advocacy, community consultation, and collecting basic research data—in other words, working from the macroperspective (CSHSE, 1985).

Studies of graduates of human service programs since 1972 differ significantly from the earlier surveys. The results reflect a diversity of employment settings for graduates, including state hospitals, mental health centers, centers for the developmentally disabled, schools, child and family services centers, correctional facilities, nursing homes and other service facilities for the aging, abuse prevention and treatment centers, recreation centers, centers for people with physical disabilities, crisis intervention units, child- and elder-abuse prevention and treatment centers, group homes, and specialized fund-raising organizations. The job functions of these graduates include direct service activities, group and individual counseling, patient advocacy, interviewing, referral, gathering and recording information, treatment planning, discharge, follow-up, grant writing, fund-raising, and administration (Alley & Blanton, 1976; Dunn, 1987; French, 1986; McClam, 1992, 1996; Moorhouse, 1983; Truesdale, 1987; Young, True, & Packard, 1976). These responsibilities reflect work within both the micro- and the macroperspectives.

Job opportunities for human service graduates in the future are expected to be excellent (*Occupational Outlook Handbook*, 1997) and will continue to reflect the generic nature of helping. "The number of human service workers is projected to more than double between 1992 and 2005—making it among the most rapidly growing occupations" (p. 129). In fact, for two years in a row, *U.S. News & World Report* included "human services" as one of 20 hot job tracks in its *1996 Career Guide* and its *1997 Career Guide* ("20 Hot Job Tracks," 1995; "20 Hot Job Tracks," 1996).

Just as the role of the generalist human service worker has evolved over the past four decades, the role of the nonprofessional helper has changed and expanded. This change is described next.

The Nonprofessional

The final report of the Joint Commission on Mental Health recommended broadening the definition of who can legitimately deliver mental health services. Specifically, it suggested that nonmedical personnel, including nonprofessionals, have a role in providing services to clients. This suggestion marked the beginning of a dramatic increase in the use of nonprofessionals. The term *nonprofessional* encompasses community caretakers, natural helpers, and volunteers. Such nonprofessionals provide basic human service functions. You may, in fact, now be receiving services from one or more of the groups discussed in the paragraphs that follow.

Community caretakers, such as police and clergy, provide essential community services. Professionals in their own fields, they are involved in some aspects of mental health work. For example, many of the clergy counsel members of a congregation and others from the community. Police officers work with victims of crime or abuse in many instances.

Hairdressers and bartenders are examples of *natural helpers*. Their primary job function is to cut hair or to mix drinks, but in performing these tasks, they find themselves listening, responding, and discussing alternatives to problem situations in which their customers may find themselves.

A category of nonprofessionals is emerging to assist helpers identify those who need support from the human service delivery system. These *gatekeepers*,

Human Service Jobs for the Late 1990s

RESIDENTIAL COUNSELOR, 1996

Group homes for the developmentally disabled have grown in number by 29% in the past two years, as governments continue to close mental institutions. For troubled or drug-abusing teens and former prisoners, residential services have become a favored way to deliver therapy and ease the transition to a normal life. Counselors supervise residents in housekeeping tasks, provide emotional support and counseling, and lead recreational activities. They also analyze each client's needs by reviewing records, talking with families, and conferring with medical personnel.

Runner-Up Hot Track
Life skills instructor. Developmentally disabled clients learn from these pros to handle tasks such as cooking, using public transportation, and mixing with people.

On the Job
Kathleen Lindner-Taffe, 39, counselor, Pegasus Youth Residence. An associate degree in mental health technology and a certificate in drug counseling allow Lindner-Taffe to help teen residents of the Lawrence, Massachusetts, home work through their addictions.

CASE MANAGER, 1997

An AIDS patient lives alone. Her friends and family visit as often as they can but not often enough to take care of the grocery shopping and trips to and from the doctor. Increasingly, that becomes the province of the social workers, who assess the needs of their clients and line up the necessary counseling, education, medical help, or legal aid. Besides the chronically ill, clients range from the elderly to children with severe emotional disabilities. Insurers, health care organizations, and individuals all see hiring case managers as a way to organize care and thus keep the costs down. Managed care organizations, most of which now have case managers on staff, control over 70% of the group-health insurance market—a 23% jump since 1992.

Runner-Up Hot Track
Residential counselor. Group homes are multiplying to assist persons with mental illness as the government continues to shut down mental institutions.

On the Job
Ana Rebecca Ruiz, 31, AIDS Services of Austin. "The hardest part is seeing people suffer. The relationships I've made are what keep me in the field," says Ruiz, who serves more than 60 HIV-positive clients.

SOURCE: From "20 Hot Job Tracks: Career Guide 1996," 1995, Copyright, October 30, 1995, *U.S. News & World Report, 119*(17), 104, 108; "20 Hot Job Tracks: Career Guide 1997," Copyright, October 28, 1996, *U.S. News & World Report, 121*(17), p. 95.

as they are called by human service professionals, provide referrals for programs that provide services to clients who would not normally access the delivery system. Those who provide the gatekeeping role include superintendents of housing projects or apartment complexes, grocery store managers or clerks, and other natural helpers. These are individuals who come into daily contact with people who may need some assistance (Emlet & Hall, 1991).

Another category of nonprofessionals who are helping human services respond to today's challenges is *self-help groups.* These are laypeople from all walks of life who come together to create a mutual support system to meet their own needs. Members share a common problem; they consider themselves peers; and they organize separately from human service organizations. The purposes of such groups include helping with chronic problems or general problems in living, raising consciousness, securing political rights, and providing support for behavior changes. Over half a million such groups are currently providing support for people with similar problems. Examples include Mothers Against Drunk Driving (MADD) and Alcoholics Anonymous (AA).

Self-help groups have multiplied for several reasons. First, the individual members have needs not met by traditional sources. This situation often arises when fiscal constraints force agencies to trim budgets, personnel, and services. Second, there has been a decline of support from family, church, and neighborhoods as well as a decline in personal involvement with these institutions (Riessman, 1979). A third reason is that self-help groups are very effective in meeting needs. Those involved are able to articulate clearly the needs of the target group and can establish support relatively easy as the others involved have similar experiences and difficulties.

The largest group of nonprofessionals consists of *volunteers.* The United States has a long tradition of volunteerism. Typically, we think of volunteers as people who give their time without any pay, but Ellis and Noyes (1978) maintain that this definition is overly simplistic today. Elements of an accurate definition of volunteer are (1) that people give their time of their own free will, (2) that they do so because of a feeling of social responsibility, and (3) that they show little concern for monetary profit. The third element allows for some form of reward or reimbursement that is much less than the actual value of the service provided. For example, volunteers may be reimbursed for mileage incurred in transporting clients.

People volunteer for various reasons: to work with people, to meet people, to gain job references, or to help others. Whatever the reason, retaining volunteers involves matching the tasks assigned them with their motivations. For example, a person who wants to work with people would probably not be happy if assigned to do filing. Volunteers are valuable resources, particularly in times of decreased funding. They personalize services, can be good advocates, and bring new skills and interests and a high level of enthusiasm to an agency setting. Today, the number of volunteers is growing among young working professionals.

Due to the efforts of networking and outreach, a new model has emerged that simplifies volunteering. Instead of asking for a 2-hour per week commitment

CASA's Kids

Bob Edwards says he'll never forget meeting the 8-year-old boy almost ten years ago. "He was a beautiful child, adorable, with curly black hair, and with two black eyes [acquired in a fight]." Edwards and the boy strolled the grounds of a residential treatment center for emotionally disturbed children outside Austin, Texas, where the boy was living. The boy took pictures of rocks and trees with an instant camera Edwards had brought him. "And he didn't say one word to me."

It was the beginning of what would become a strong bond between a child whose parents had severely abused him and an adult who decided he wanted to try to make a difference in the world—in other words, a CASA volunteer.

CASA (Court Appointed Special Advocates) is a nationwide program of community-based agencies whose caseworkers and volunteers focus on the best interests of children caught in crises of abuse or neglect. The organization aims first at healing and preserving families with state services and resources. Barring that, they work toward permanency for the children, which means adoption, placement with a relative, or placement in a treatment facility or permanent foster home.

The goal is to break the cycle of abuse that can sap ambition and hope from generations of children and can lead to the crime and homelessness and despair that drains society, says Michael S. Piraino, chief executive officer (CEO) of the National CASA Association in Seattle.

The statistics given in a recent CASA orientation video drew gasps from a group of prospective Travis County volunteers: Every day, across the country, 364,000 children are neglected and 1,849 are abused, three fatally. Fortunately, more than 500 CASA chapters have bloomed in the 50 states following the model established by Seattle Judge David Soukup in 1978. Texas has 41 programs covering 75 counties. CASA of Travis County, which counted 159 volunteers serving 350 children in May, celebrates its tenth anniversary this year.

In the ten years since Edwards and Joey met, they've been through nine placements (holding centers, halfway houses, residential treatment facilities, group centers, foster homes), battles about placement in special education classes, differences of opinion with authority figures, and Joey's bouts of antidepressant drug therapy.

"I think he'll look back—and this is the good thing I think I gave him, that CASA has given him—and see that someone stepped up out of the community, without a vested interest at all, and cared about him."

SOURCE: From "CASA's Kids," by E. Eckstein, 1995, *Spirit*, pp. 82, 84, 86, 89, 90, Dallas, TX: American Airlines Magazine Publication. Reprinted by permission.

from an individual, these networks link volunteer and organization on a more impromptu, short-term basis. Calls are made to a central organization a week prior or even the day of the volunteering effort and the volunteer is given a choice of direct service activities such as painting buildings, selling tickets for fund-raising events, or reading to children (Sack, 1995).

The nonprofessionals described here have been welcomed by professionals. Perhaps the most immediate reason for their acceptance is that all agencies face financial constraints at one time or another, and this can lead to a shortage of professionally trained workers. Some agencies may have an uneven distribution of mental health professionals with respect to race, social class, and place of birth; the utilization of nonprofessionals can remedy this. Nonprofessionals have also been willing to work in places and with populations that professionals find unattractive.

The Activities of the Human Service Professional

The professional activities of the human service helper are often discussed in the professional literature and are defined by the helper's relationship with clients and other professionals, academic training, ethical standards, continuing education, and measured competence. Human service professionals often work with individuals with few material possessions and little emotional support and who need many professional services and much professional care. The human service professional is often the first to provide support when the client enters the system. Clients become involved with helpers because they hope for a better existence. They view human service professionals as important people with special information and skills to help them identify and work toward their goals.

The good relationship the human service professional has with other social service professionals is a measure of the status of human services. Other helpers work with human service professionals side by side in a professional setting. For some, the human service professional is the one individual specifically designated to focus on the client's mental health and to coordinate social care. In a nursing home, for example, the human service professional admits the client, takes a social history, monitors and facilitates the client's adjustment, coordinates services with family needs, counsels the client during troubled times, and attends treatment team meetings with the staff to discuss the client's admission, progress, and discharge. Other professionals include physical therapists, physicians, nurses, and pharmacists who focus on the client's physical health. These professionals look to the human service worker to address the client's mental health needs, which may involve support or referral to a specialist. In other settings, the human service worker is one of many mental health professionals. In a mental health institution, for example, psychiatrists, psychiatric nurses, psychiatric social workers, psychologists, human service workers, and psychiatric technicians all focus on the mental health of the client. Each of these workers has a particular function within this setting, and each relies on the others to perform their appropriate tasks effectively. For clients and other social service providers, the work of human service professionals is essential.

A human service professional's activities also include academic training founded on a systematic body of knowledge. Academic preparation for human services takes either two years or four years, depending on the training program. This intense training, academically and experientially based, focuses on the acquisition of knowledge and skills pertinent to human service systems, workers, and clients. The training is also systematic. It begins with the study of introductory concepts of human services, then explores types of clients, problems, and methods of addressing those problems, and culminates in supervised field experience. The body of knowledge on which the training is based is interdisciplinary, drawn from other helping fields including psychology, criminology, rehabilitation, counseling, and social work. Human service field practice is unique in its diversity of settings and populations. However, the basic helping skills and methods of addressing client needs are both unique to human services and borrowed from other helping professions. Trained as generalists, human service professionals are thus taught knowledge and skills that can be transferred to diverse settings and populations. Fullerton (1996) describes it as follows:

> The theories we use in human services vary along many dimensions. They range in scope from comprehensive explanations of human behavior to theories regarding very specific behaviors. They range in perspective from biological to psychological to sociological explanations of the human condition. They vary considerably in the degree to which they have been empirically tested, and they vary in terms of their applicability across age, gender, race, or cultures. (Fullerton, 1996, p. 117)

Practitioners need such flexibility to deal with the complex individuals and environments they encounter.

Ethical standards also define professional human service activities. Human service professionals are committed to the ethical treatment of clients and the development of ethical relationships with co-workers, other professionals, and the system. Ethical standards guide this behavior. Because the client is the central focus in human services, the treatment of the client and the client's rights are of great concern. Introductory texts address issues of confidentiality and respect for the client's values, heritage, beliefs, and self-determination (Mandell & Schram, 1995; Mehr, 1995; Neukrug, 1995; Schmolling, Youkeles, & Burger, 1997). Human service professionals are usually bound by two sets of ethical standards: those developed by human service professionals and educators and those developed specifically for the populations they serve. The Ethical Standards of Human Service Professionals are in Chapter 9 of this book.

Another important professional activity of human service workers is continuing education. A commitment to continue to learn and develop while working in the field is essential for human service professionals. This continuing education takes many forms. According to follow-up studies of human service program graduates, many seek advanced degrees. More than half the graduates of two-year programs seek a bachelor's degree—most often in human services, psychology, sociology, criminal justice, and related fields. Graduates of four-year human service programs seek master's degrees in social work, public health administration, nursing, counseling, educational psychology, rehabilitation, and related fields. Human service professionals also continue their education by belonging to professional organizations. Many of these organizations are related to the specific fields in which their members work or the specific population they serve (Woodside, McClam, & McGarrh, 1993). A final way human service professionals grow and develop is through inservice training. Many agencies sponsor seminars on current social or policy issues, on skill development, or on professional issues. Agencies that do not offer such seminars often encourage their workers to attend seminars sponsored by others.

Competence in human services is certified by the granting of two-year, four-year, or advanced degrees in human services; however, competence is not supervised by a national organization. In 1982, the National Commission for Human Service Workers was incorporated "to provide a national system for voluntary registration and certification of human service workers" (National Commission for Human Service Workers, 1982, p. 1). The commission has disbanded, but there is now some interest in reestablishing registration and certification standards.

In the mid-1990s, a project was undertaken by the federal government to establish standards for a number of emerging professions. The Human Services Research Institute was given the responsibility for researching the current status of human service occupations and describing the contemporary workplace within the human service delivery system. This project developed a standard skill set for human service practitioners that included skill standards, activities the professional assumes, and practical outcomes of the work. The result of this study is a document, *The Community Support Skill Standards: Tools for Managing Change and Achieving Outcomes*, that more clearly defines the work of human service professionals (Taylor, Bradley, & Warren, 1996).

In summary, human service professionals are concerned about and participate actively in training, ethical commitment, continuing education, and registration and certification. It is a relatively new occupation involved in professional activities of value to those who receive its services.

✧ Things to Remember

1. Human services has developed in response to the need of individuals or groups for assistance to live better lives.
2. Because human services recognizes client needs as problems in living, human services does not focus on the past but seeks to improve the present and change the future.
3. Human services has emerged as a response to the increase in human problems in our modern world.

4. Human services provides three distinct functions: social care, social control, and rehabilitation.
5. Human services consists of those services that help people with their problems.
6. There is a dual focus of client and helper that guides the delivery of services.
7. There are management principles that influence delivery and reflect the value of focusing on the client.
8. The interaction between the client and the human service system also defines human services.
9. The services provided are designed to improve an individual's well-being.
10. In the successful delivery of services, the client develops new insights, skills, and competencies.
11. The field of human services is respected by its clients and other helping professions.
12. Human service work is an emerging profession committed to ethical standards and continuing education.

Additional Readings: Focus on Poverty

Gordon, Linda. (1995). *Pitied but not entitled: Single mothers and the history of welfare*. New York: Free Press.

Linda Gordon traces the development of welfare in the United States and the values that drive it today. Of particular interest is AFDC (Aid to Families with Dependent Children), which was designed as a temporary, quick-fix charity program financed by general tax revenues.

Kozol, J. (1991). *Savage inequalities: Children in America's schools*. Scranton, PA: HarperCollins.

Jonathan Kozol demonstrates how public schools perpetrate the inequalities inherent in the rest of their pupils' lives by taking the reader inside a dozen decaying schools in cities like Chicago; Camden, New Jersey; and East St. Louis, Illinois.

Quint, S. (1994). *Schooling homeless children: A working model for America's public schools*. New York: Teachers College Press.

This book is an account of how a school principal helped transform an elementary school and provide needed services to homeless children in Seattle.

Kozol, J. (1995). *Amazing grace: The lives of children and the conscience of a nation*. New York: Crown Publishers.

Jonathan Kozol describes the lives of children who grew up in the South Bronx—the poorest congressional district in the United States. Poverty, racial isolation, violence, and AIDS take a high toll.

Urrea, Luis Alberto. (1993). *Across the wire: Life and hard times on the Mexican border*. New York: Anchor Books.

A series of vignettes organize this account of the underclass, the thousands of Mexicans living just south of the border in unsanitary, dangerous shantytowns. The author worked as a volunteer in an organization that provided food, clothing, and medication to Mexican squatter settlements and relates an inside view of life in the Tijuana trash heaps.

Chapter 2

A History of Helping

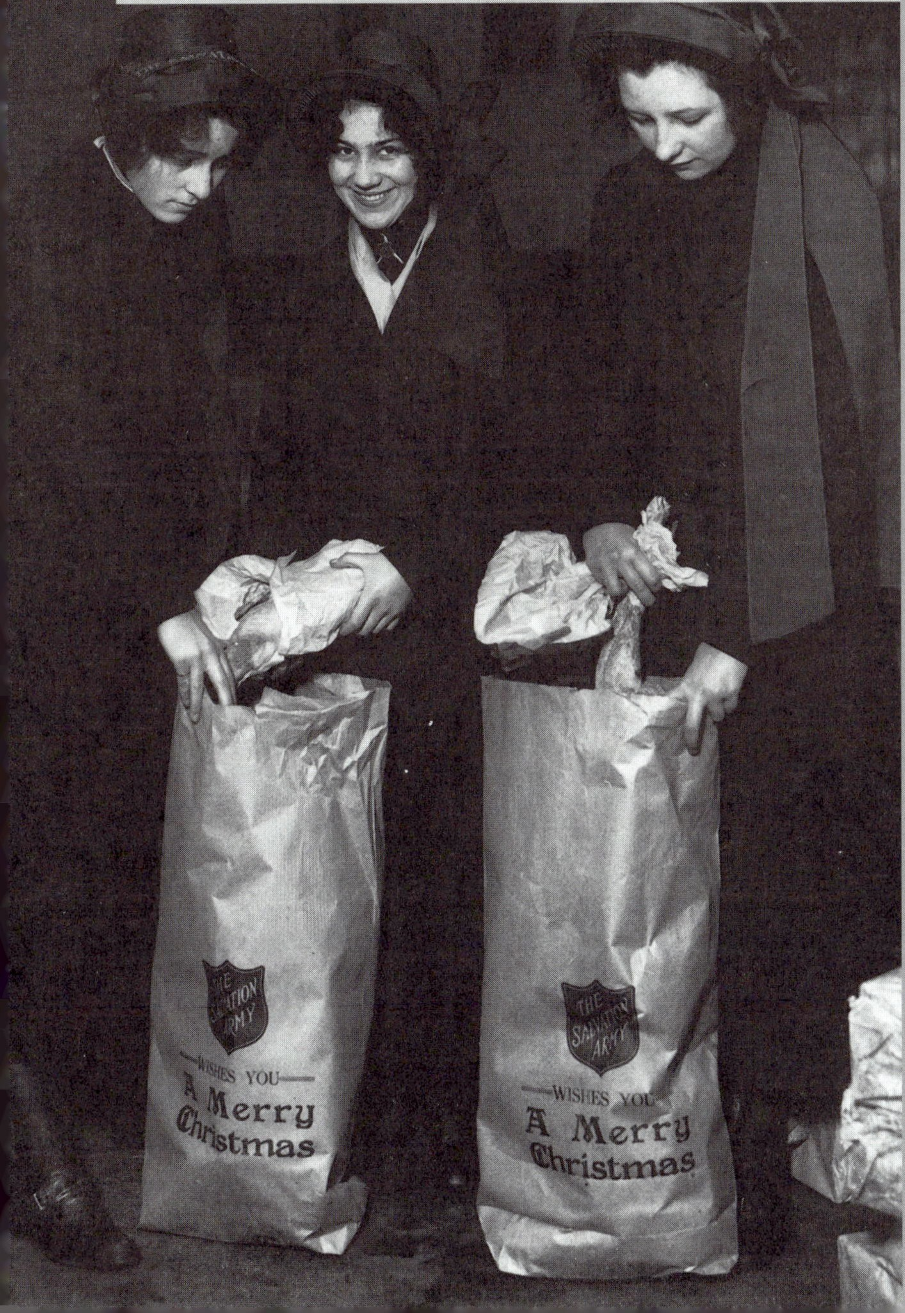

Chapter 2 presents an overview of the history of helping to provide insight into the emergence and growth of services to people in need. This chapter traces the changing beliefs about who is "less fortunate" and examines the different categorizations of less fortunate people throughout history. The categories familiar to us today—the poor, persons with mental impairments, and criminals—have not always been used. What is central to a definition of *less fortunate,* both then and now, is consideration of the "have-nots" in society, who meets their needs, and how those needs are met. In addition, we examine the emergence and growth of the human service movement. This chapter assists us further in defining the human service profession.

Early History

Until the Middle Ages, people believed that mental illness was caused by evil spirits, and early forms of treatment focused on ridding the body of these demons. One treatment used was trephining the skull (using a crude saw to remove circular discs of bone). This hole in the head allowed evil spirits to escape. Another popular method of treatment was exorcising evil spirits through religious rites. Persons with mental illness were feared because their supposed possession by spirits was perceived as a link with the supernatural. Other attempts to control the demons included chaining, beating, starving, and bleeding the unfortunate human host (NIMH, 1971).

Hippocrates, a physician in the third century B.C., was one of the few professionals who used the scientific approach to explain and treat problem behavior and mental illness. He believed that problem behavior was a function of natural illness and that mental disorders had natural causes. In other words, evil spirits were not probable causes of mental illness. He believed that mental illness could be caused by brain disease, heredity, and head injuries. Hippocrates was also able to distinguish between different types of mental problems; among his most significant contributions were labels for illnesses such as *melancholia* and *epilepsy,* which are still used in mental health today. His work marks the beginning of the medical model of service delivery.

Until the 1500s, the church was chiefly responsible for providing human services. Religious figures such as St. Thomas Aquinas and St. Francis of Assisi are considered by some to be the first human service professionals (Eriksen, 1981). Under the church's guidance, many institutions were founded for the poor, orphans, the elderly, and people with disabilities. At this time, deviant behavior was perceived as a sickness, and asylums were established to house those who were so labeled. After A.D. 1500, the power of the church declined and that of government increased, producing conflict between the church and the state.

In addition to services provided by the church, the needy in England also received attention from the government. (In fact, the English Crown's right and duty to protect persons with mental impairments had existed from the 13th century.) For persons with mental impairments, two categories were established: natural fools or idiots, and those who were *non compos mentis. Idiots* became the preferred term for the first category; this included people with retarded intellectual development whose condition was permanent, present at birth, or both. The second category, *non compos mentis,* was the umbrella term for all other mental disabilities. By the 15th century, the term *lunatic* had replaced the phrase *non compos mentis.*

Diagnoses of mental illness were determined by inquisitions (unrelated to those established by the Catholic Church), which were conducted by a government official and a jury of at least 12 men (Neugebauer, 1979). The following questions were asked in the investigation:

Was the person an idiot or a lunatic?
When, how, and in what manner was the individual lucid?
What lands and other property did the individual own?

The Crown's rights and duties were determined by these diagnoses. It was the king's duty to protect an idiot's lands and property and to provide the individual with the necessities of life, and the king was entitled to all the revenues from those lands. More extensive protection was provided for lunatics at no charge to the individual because the revenues of a lunatic's estate were used to support the person and his or her family during the time of the illness. Of course, this system provided no help to the many lunatics who had no estate.

Before the Middle Ages, feudal lords had assumed responsibility for much of the care of poor and sick people who lived on their lands. During the Middle Ages, needy people received aid from three sources. Human service institutions (such as orphanages) continued to assist specific populations. The church also provided services directly to the needy and donations to other service providers. Late in this period, governments began to adopt innovative legislation, which provided the framework for human services for many years to come.

Several types of institutions provided services during the Middle Ages. One important source of aid to the needy was hospitals. Not only did they provide medical assistance to the ill, but they also fed and housed tired travelers, orphans, the elderly, and the poor. These institutions were usually attached to monasteries, and their capacity ranged from a dozen to several hundred patients.

A second type of institution, the insane asylum, was established in Europe during the 15th and 16th centuries. These institutions represented some concern for the care and housing of people with mental illness, but the patients did not receive effective treatment, and their living conditions were poor. The following excerpt (Friedrich, 1976, p. 49) describes the conditions at London's Bethlehem Hospital, an institution typical of the asylums established during that time:

> London's Bethlehem Hospital, better known as Bedlam, founded in the thirteenth century as a priory, converted in the fourteenth century into a hospital, given by Henry VIII to the City of London in 1547 as Britain's first insane asylum, became, within a few decades, little more than a dungeon. Women were chained by the ankles to one long wall. Men were liable to be attached by the neck to a vertical bar. One man was kept that way, even in the eighteenth century, for twelve years.

Relief for the poor was the responsibility of the church during the Middle Ages. Church authorities at the diocese or parish level administered relief to feed and protect the poor within their districts. The money available for their care was sufficient to meet the needs in these local districts (Trattner, 1994). In ministering to the poor, the church served in the capacity of a public institution, and the tithe was considered a public tax. Scholars have suggested that the system run by the church was the model for the secular system established later by the Elizabethan Poor Law of 1601.

The care of the poor by the church altered as the nature and incidence of poverty changed with the socioeconomic conditions. Specifically, the decline of feudalism, the growth of commerce, and the beginning of industrialization made it necessary to find new ways of assisting those in need. The poor, the unemployed, the disabled, widows, dependent children, the elderly, people with mental retardation, and people with mental illness who were previously cared for on the feudal estates by the feudal lords now had no place to go. Most wandered around, often settling in cities that were ill equipped to handle them.

A new type of economy and the employment needs of the incipient industrial revolution also affected a number of poor people. The growth of commerce encouraged the development of a money economy, based on capital investments, credit, interest, rent, and wages. This system was very different from the rural economy, which depended on the bartering of goods and services. As the poor could no longer survive by bartering and had little money, they often could not afford food, housing, and clothing. Compounding their problems was the development of the factory system, which required large groups of people with specialized skills. Employment of these workers was seasonal, cyclical, and beyond their control. To be able to care for oneself, one had to be employed by those who controlled the resources.

The pressures of the poor in the cities created the need for a large-scale attack on poverty and prompted the passage of the Elizabethan Poor Law of 1601. This legislation was critical in the history of human services. It guided social welfare practices in England and the United States for the next 350 years by specifying who was to provide what services to those in need. For example, parents were legally responsible for their children and grandchildren, and children were responsible for the support of parents and grandparents. One of the harsher features was the punishment of vagrants who refused to work by imprisonment, whipping, stoning, or even execution. More significant, however, was the acknowledgment in the legislation that the state had a responsibility to relieve need and suffering and that the disadvantaged not only deserved assistance but also had a legal right to it.

The law included three main features. The first was compulsory taxation to raise funds to help the needy. The administration of this money resembled the church system developed during feudal times. Government representatives, called "overseers of the poor," managed the distribution of money in each parish or county. Second, dependents were classified according to their ability to work: children, the able-bodied, and the "impotent poor" (adults unable to work). Relief was provided to each group: Dependent children were apprenticed or indentured; the able-bodied worked or were punished; and the lame, the blind, and other poor people unable to work received home or institutional relief. Third, the responsibility for the sick, the poor, and others in need rested first with the family. If the family could not provide assistance, the government was responsible for doing so.

An interesting amendment to the Elizabethan Poor Law, added 60 years later, was the Law of Settlement. This law established a residency requirement for determining eligibility for assistance. The requirements of needy people wandering from town to town seeking food and shelter overburdened many towns and districts. This law helped the districts plan for the number they would serve.

The Elizabethan Poor Laws

The Elizabethan Poor Laws were passed as a response to the increasing number of poor in Great Britain. During earlier times the lords were directly responsible for the care of their tenants. But the feudal system began to crumble and the tenant farmers lost their land. Having no source of relief, they drifted to the cities and larger towns. Few of this population had the skills to earn a living wage, and as their numbers increased, pauperism became a national problem. The first attempt to correct this problem was the enactment of voluntary alms to be collected in each parish. When this enactment did not alleviate the problems, an act was passed that required severe punishment for vagabonds and relief for the poor. This act led to an attempt to discriminate between the criminal population and the poor. Finally, the Poor Law of 1601 provided a clear definition of the "poor" and articulated services that they were to receive. This legislation is the foundation for the current social welfare system existing today in Great Britain. The following describes the law.

POOR LAW OF 1601

By this act two or more "substantial householders" were to be yearly nominated by the justices of the peace to serve as overseers of the poor in each parish. The overseers were to raise

> weekly or otherwise, by taxation of every inhabitant, such competent sums of money as they shall think fit, (a) for setting to work the children of all such whose parents shall not be thought able to keep and maintain them; (b) for setting to work all such persons, married and unmarried, having no means to maintain them, and who use no ordinary and daily trade of life to get their living by; (c) for providing a convenient stock of flax, hemp, wool, thread, iron, and other ware and stuff, to set the poor on work; (d) for the necessary relief of the lame, old, impotent, blind, and such other among them being poor and not able to work. Children whose parents cannot maintain them are to be apprenticed till the age of four-and-twenty years in the case of boys and twenty-one years or the time of marriage in the case of girls. The overseers may, with the leave of the Lord of the Manor, erect houses for the impotent poor on any waste or common.

By the end of the 18th century, a dramatic change in the care of persons with mental illness occurred. A move toward more humane treatment of those in mental institutions began in 1792 when Philippe Pinel unchained 50 maniacs at Bicetre Hospital in Paris (see Chapter 4). This period is often called the first revolution in mental health. For those in mental institutions, this period meant

No provision is made for the erection of any house in which work may be done, and it was evidently intended that the flax, hemp, and other raw material should be worked up at the houses of the poor. But an act of 1576 had already empowered the justices of each county to erect "houses of correction" in which "such as be already grown up in idleness and so rogues at this present" should be set to work under strict prison discipline; and the justices were now ordered to commit to these places, or to the common jail, those who refused to work on materials provided by the parish. What they had to expect at the houses of correction may be seen from one of the rules of the Suffolk House for the year 1589:

> Item—it is ordered and agreed upon that every strong or sturdy rogue at his or her first entrance into the said house shall have twelve stripes upon his bare skin with the said whip provided for said house; and every young rogue or idle loiterer six stripes with the said whip in form aforesaid. And that every one of them, without fail, at their first coming into the said house, shall have put upon him, her, or them some clogs, chain, collars of iron, ringle, or manacle, such as the keeper of the said house shall think meet.

The new act was only gradually carried out. In 1622, "A Wellwisher" complained, in a tract called "Grievous Groans for the Poor," that

> tho the number of the poor do daily increase, there hath been no collection for them, no not these seven years, in many parishes of this land, especially in country towns; but many of those parishes turneth forth their poor, yea and their lusty laborers that will not work, or for any misdemeanor want work, to beg, filch, and steal for their maintenance, so that the country is pitifully pestered with them; yea, and the maimed soldiers that have ventured their lives and lost their limbs on our behalf are also thus requited. . . . So they are turned forth to travel in idleness (the highway to hell) . . . until the law bring them unto the fearful end of hanging.

SOURCE: Excerpt from *The New Encyclopedia of Social Reform,* by W. Bliss, pp. 918–920.

improved diets, regular exercise, religious observance, and the development of the mind. As you will read in the next section, in the United States these efforts were led by Amariah Brigham, Samuel B. Woodward, and Benjamin Rush. Unfortunately, the rise in moral treatment lasted only until the mid-19th century because of limited resources, overcrowding, and the passage of time (Macht, 1990).

Human Services in the United States

As we examine the history of human services in the United States, we see the influence of the English developments discussed in the preceding section. During the years of colonization, public relief was supported by individuals and groups, who donated resources and labor to institutions such as schools and hospitals or directly to needy people. Much assistance took the form of neighborly kindness or mutual aid. As the populations of the cities in the colonies grew, so did the number of indigents, idlers, criminals, orphans, and others who needed assistance. The colonists used the Elizabethan Poor Law as a model of how to meet the needs of those individuals.

Colonial America

The four principles that formed the basis of the local practice of poor relief in the colonies can be traced directly to the Elizabethan Poor Law of 1601. The first principle defined poor relief as a public responsibility. The second principle, the question of legal residence, therefore became a practical one, as services were provided at the local or parish level. The third principle spelled out the responsibility family members had to needy individuals; public aid was denied those who had parents, grandparents, adult children, or grandchildren. Finally, legislation combined concerns about children and work by declaring that the children of paupers were to be apprenticed to farmers and artisans who agreed to care for them.

Like England, the colonies responded to the needy by developing institutions. The first almshouse was built in Massachusetts in 1662 for dependents, such as persons with mental illness, the elderly, children, the able-bodied poor, those with physical disabilities, and criminals. Almshouses were not developed systematically, but over the next 150 years, they were established throughout the colonies as the need arose. The numbers of these houses made it increasingly obvious that there were large groups of needy individuals the towns could not support. With this realization began the trend for larger governmental units to accept the responsibility for the "state poor." By the early 1800s, a system of district workhouses had been developed. Besides the almshouses, there were very few specialized formal institutions. Criminals were held in jail until trial and, if found guilty, were fined, whipped, or executed. Poor strangers or vagrants were simply told to leave town. People with mental illness had no special facilities before the American Revolution; their care was the responsibility of their families. Those without relatives to care for them were placed in almshouses. Those with mental illness were often locked up by their families in an attic or cellar or left to wander about the countryside.

Benjamin Franklin was instrumental in establishing one of the few formal institutions for people with mental disturbances, a section of the Pennsylvania Hospital. Another facility devoted exclusively to those with mental disturbances was a state hospital at Williamsburg, Virginia, which opened in 1773. Little attention was given to the treatment of mental disease because it was viewed as an economic and social problem rather than a medical one. Determining insanity was the responsibility of officials, such as governors and church wardens, not members of the medical profession.

The 19th Century: A Time of Change

Large-scale immigration, rapid industrialization, and widespread urbanization led to many societal changes during the colonial years. These changes brought more poverty and more outlays for relief of the poor. During the Middle Ages, need was believed to arise from misfortune, for which society should assume responsibility. Belief in the right to public assistance was established and endorsed by the Elizabethan Poor Law, which placed the responsibility on the government. In the early years in the United States, the colonists used the English system as a model for their philosophy toward and services for the poor and needy. By the early 1800s, however, the philosophy in the United States had changed.

Destitution was viewed as the fault of the individual, and public aid was thought to cause and encourage poverty. This punitive attitude toward the poor—the belief that to be poor was a crime—was manifested in the Poor Law Reform Bill of 1834. Its purpose was to limit the expansion of services provided to the poor or the "have-nots." This bill introduced the concept of "less eligibility," stating that assistance to any person in need must be lower than the lowest working wage paid. The social philosophies of individualism, the work ethic, economic laissez-faire, and Social Darwinism promoted further changes in attitudes toward the poor and the needy.

SOCIAL PHILOSOPHIES

During the 19th century, those espousing the philosophy of individualism viewed America as the land of opportunity. Hard work was the road to success, and that road could be traveled by anyone. The individual was held solely responsible for any failure. Similarly, proponents of the work ethic emphasized the importance of hard work and thrift for financial success and viewed poverty as a sign of spiritual weakness. Wealth was virtuous, and hard work represented the road to salvation.

Laissez-faire was an economic concept that focused on societal rather than individual responsibility. The original French phrase means "leave alone," and this concept encouraged a social attitude of "live and let live." The most desirable government, then, was the one that governed least—negating society's responsibility to help its less fortunate citizens. Those adhering to this philosophy opposed the provision of any human service as a right of the individual.

Social Darwinism, in combination with laissez-faire and the work ethic, created a climate for the reform that was to follow. An outgrowth of Charles Darwin's theory of evolution, it was used to explain social and economic phenomena. According to those who interpreted Darwin in social terms, the natural order of life was that the fittest would survive, creating a society of perfect people. Those who were unfit would not be able to meet their own needs and would not survive. Supporters of Social Darwinism called for the repeal of poor laws and state-supported human services that facilitated the survival of the "unfit," as they believed that all change must be natural. Any attempts to help the less fortunate would be against progress, which depended on "natural selection."

This belief was especially popular between 1870 and 1880. In reality, it often served as a rationalization for unscrupulous business practices. Furthermore, it encouraged the belief that nothing could be done about the situation of the working class and the poor, who faced long work hours, low wages, child labor, and unhealthy working conditions.

These prevailing philosophies discouraged the provision of human services and limited services to those who desperately needed assistance. The private sector became very important in filling the need. Wealthy individuals were instrumental in organizing and reforming institutions. Mental hospitals, almshouses, workhouses, penitentiaries, and institutions for unwed mothers and delinquent youth appeared. Philanthropic societies were formed to support these institutions. By the middle of the 19th century, public and private sectors were working side by side. As welfare problems grew, the private sector was unable to meet increasing needs. In spite of the prevailing philosophies, there was growing demand for public agencies to assume more responsibility for the poor and needy.

By the 1850s, specialized institutions had been established for persons with mental illness, juvenile delinquents, the deaf and blind, and criminals. These institutions were established primarily in the belief that reform, rehabilitation, and education were possible. Institutions could improve society by protecting individuals from negative environmental influences.

In summary, the 19th century was a time of dramatic change in the way society viewed its responsibilities toward the poor and needy. Government relinquished some of its role in providing services, and the private sector assumed more responsibility. Unfortunately, the problems of those in need multiplied, and gradually the government began to increase its assistance again. Institutions also developed in response to the needs of specific populations. Probation, mental health, and child welfare provide examples of how 19th-century attitudes affected the delivery of human services to specific populations.

PROBATION

In the United States, the earliest practice similar to probation as we know it today occurred in 1813, when Judge Peter O. Thatcher of Boston began placing youthful offenders under the supervision of officials such as sheriffs and constables. In 1841, the concept of "friendly supervision" was introduced by John Augustus, a shoemaker. He helped drunks and other unfortunates by bailing them out, sometimes paying their fines, and then providing "friendly supervision" as the individuals adjusted to a new life.

The most well-known organization to provide assistance to ex-convicts was the Salvation Army, created in England in the late 19th century by William Booth. Its members believed in taking a more sympathetic approach to the problems and circumstances of those in need. For example, members of its Prison Gate Brigade met prisoners upon their release and provided whatever assistance they could, including a home, food, and employment (Collier, 1965).

THE TREATMENT OF PERSONS WITH MENTAL ILLNESS

Patients in the early asylums were mostly psychotic or severely retarded. Treatment was medically oriented, and many patients were treated as if they had a physical illness. The beginnings of reform in the late 1700s can be attributed to Dr. Benjamin Rush at the Pennsylvania Hospital in Philadelphia. Dr. Rush, who is considered the father of American psychiatry, fought the superstition and ignorance surrounding mental illness and elevated the study of mental illness to a scientific level. In 1812, he wrote *Medical Inquiries and Observations Upon the Diseases of the Mind,* the first scientific treatise explaining the nature of mental illness. Before his writings, mental patients lived in atrocious conditions and were treated with brutality and cruelty; customary treatment methods were bleeding, restraint, and cold showers. Dr. Rush introduced occupational therapy, amusements, and exercise for patients.

Dorothea Dix was another pioneer who fought to improve conditions and services to people with mental illness during the 19th century. She became involved in social reform when, in 1841, she accepted an offer to teach a Sunday school class of 20 female prisoners in the jail at East Cambridge, Massachusetts. She was appalled at the conditions she found in the jail: overcrowding, filthy quarters, and little or no heat. What alarmed her most was the crowding together of criminals and the insane. She began a personal investigation of all the jails and almshouses in Massachusetts and made careful, systematic records of what she saw. Backed by a group of broad-minded, public-spirited citizens, Dix launched a whole new career as a moral reformer, calling for more enlightened treatment of those with mental illness. Controversy and outrage engulfed her, but those who checked her accounts found them to be factual. Her appeals were based on respect for Christian values and the advancement of civilization (Marshall, 1937).

Throughout the 1840s and 1850s, Dix campaigned before state legislatures to establish asylums for people with mental illness and the developmentally disabled who were housed in jails and almshouses. She encouraged the national government to assume additional responsibility for the care and treatment of people with mental illness. Using methods like fact gathering, preparing memoranda and bills, and rallying public opinion, she began her campaign in Massachusetts, where the number of dependent insane was twice the total capacity of the state's three mental institutions (Trattner, 1994). She won her fight for enlarged facilities for indigent mental patients. The years between 1843 and 1853 are sometimes called her "decade of victory" because she was personally responsible for founding state hospitals in nine states.

In the *Providence Journal* on April 10, 1844, Dix published an article called "Astonishing Tenacity of Life." It is not signed by her but by Thomas G. Hazard. We know from a public document of her own, however, that she provided Hazard with the facts on which his article was based. They concerned her first visit to Little Compton, where she had discovered Abram Simmons, confined in complete darkness, in an unheated cell, seven feet square and six and one-half feet high, built entirely of stone. This dungeon stood in the courtyard of the poorhouse. Simmons had been imprisoned there for over three years. One of his legs was fastened by an ox-chain, shackled to an iron staple in the rock overhead. The article (Hazard, 1844, pp. 252–253) describes Simmons as follows:

> There he stood, near the door, motionless and silent; his tangled hair fell about his shoulders; his bare feet pressed the filthy wet stone floor; he was emaciated to a shadow and more resembled a disinterred corpse than any living creature. Never have I looked upon an object so pitiable, so woe-struck, so imaging despair. Notwithstanding the assertions of the Mistress that he would kill me I took his hands and endeavored to warm them by gentle friction. I spoke to him of release, of liberty, of care and kindness. A tear stole over the hollow cheek, but no words answered my importunities; no other movement indicated consciousness or perception of sensibility.

Dix is also recognized as the founder of St. Elizabeth's Hospital in Washington, D.C. Today we remember her for her tireless work in founding or enlarging 32 mental hospitals in the United States and abroad.

By 1854, the United States Congress had declared the financial care of persons with mental illness the responsibility of the states. This responsibility included paying for construction of proper facilities and needed treatment. In reality, however, the state systems were custodial warehouses, characterized by inadequate doctor-patient ratio, untrained personnel, overcrowding, and lack of public interest.

By the late 19th century, states began to separate persons with mental illness and those with developmental disabilities. There was an attempt to upgrade research, treatment, and physical facilities, and the hospitals eventually provided aftercare and outpatient clinics. The medically oriented approach continued to prevail in institutions, and mental disorders were defined and classified into two groups: those caused by organic brain disturbance and those with no apparent physical cause (psychogenetic).

CHILD WELFARE

Many approaches to child welfare were tried from the mid-19th century to the beginning of the 20th century. One was the removal of dependent, neglected, and delinquent children from almshouses and institutions. Another was the placement of those children in private homes. The first permanent orphanage, Bethesda in Savannah, Georgia, is still in operation today as a modern child care

INTERNATIONAL FOCUS
Mental Health in Developing Countries

All countries have systems of economics, religion, education, and law that have developed over time. Colonization by Western European countries interrupted the evolution of these systems in many developing countries, as Western traditions supplanted earlier systems, including mental health care systems.

Examples of developing countries using European systems of institutionalization or custodial care can be found in Southeast Asia in the early 1800s. In Singapore and Penang, lunatic asylums and hospitals for the insane were modeled after European facilities. No better than warehouses for persons with mental illness, these institutions also housed criminals, vagrants, and other social undesirables. With little hope of better care, many stayed for the remainder of their lives. By the end of the 19th century, the practice of institutionalization had expanded into India and Indonesia. Because such custodial care facilities did little to better the lives of persons with mental illness, a negative perception of institutionalization still influences the attitudes of people in Southeast Asia today.

Based on studies in several parts of the world, the World Health Organization (1975) concluded that there are no fundamental differences among nations with regard to the range or prevalence of mental disorders. In the predominantly rural populations and rapidly growing cities of developing countries, however, a combination of overcrowding, unemployment, limited and outdated health facilities, and rapid social change makes mental disorders a major problem. This problem is compounded when mental disorders take the form of physical complaints or criminal activity.

Mental disorders may be a source of fear, not only to family members and friends but also to administrators, health workers, and politicians. The belief that these conditions are caused by the supernatural continues to be widespread; it can lead to a person's rejection by or isolation from family members and community, skepticism among the public about treatment programs, and regressive attitudes regarding the development of mental health services. Institutionalization remains a dominant form of treatment.

center for emotionally disturbed children (Trattner, 1994). The first juvenile reformatory in America, the House of Refuge for Juvenile Delinquents in New York City, was supported by state funds. Massachusetts and Ohio quickly followed by establishing juvenile facilities. After the 1830s, the number of such institutions multiplied, as the public demanded the removal of children from almshouses. Unfortunately, juvenile institutions were not always an improvement, and overcrowded conditions and poor care prompted the establishment of a system that placed children in private homes.

Other forms of child welfare were the provision of mothers' or widows' pensions, the creation of juvenile courts and probation systems, the passage of compulsory school attendance laws, and crusades against child labor. These actions had several reasons. Many people felt that children seemed to be the most vulnerable and deserving group in society, and it was difficult to argue that the children were responsible for their condition. Children also constituted one of the largest groups of neglected and needy.

Reform Movements

By the latter half of the 19th century, two population shifts were affecting the provision of services to people in need: immigration from abroad and migration from rural to urban areas. In 1860, one-sixth of Americans lived in the cities; by 1900, this figure was one-third; and by 1920, one-half (Trattner, 1994). Between 1860 and 1900, approximately 14 million immigrants from abroad settled in cities, creating an urban population that consisted primarily of former farmers and immigrants. Most were unskilled or semiskilled workers in search of employment. This population explosion in the urban areas created many problems for the urban governments. Two responses to these problems were the organized charity movement and the settlement house movement.

THE ORGANIZED CHARITY MOVEMENT

The goal of the organized charity movement was to eliminate "fraud, inefficiency, and duplicity" in the provision of services (Trattner, 1994, p. 92). According to the movement, the best way to deal with poverty was through personal contact or "friendly visiting" between the rich and the poor. Influenced by laissez-faire, individualism, and Puritanism, the movement soon shifted to reform, seeking better conditions in institutions, promoting better sanitation and health regulations, developing parks and recreation areas, and writing and enforcing housing codes.

The Charity Organization Society, a forerunner of the Community Chest and the United Way, is an example of society's response to the expanding urban population. Members of the Charity Organization Society believed that giving handouts of money and food actually encouraged people to remain poor and to beg for services. They supported the systematic distribution of alms only to the poor who needed them, thus helping the deserving poor while discouraging begging. They hoped to encourage thrift and independence among the poor. Eventually, this group evolved into a clearinghouse for all the city's charitable organizations, similar to the United Way of today.

THE SETTLEMENT HOUSE MOVEMENT

The development of the settlement house movement was in large part a reaction to the inability of the organized charity movement to improve the living and working conditions of the poor. The leaders of the settlement house movement, unlike the leaders of the organized charity movement, did not support the laissez-faire philosophy. They wanted reform that included adequate housing, better schools, the abolition of child labor, and an end to the sweatshops. They thought that the best way to achieve this reform was not through alms or "friendly visiting" but through "social engineering." Human service workers and reformers were "engineers"; they must participate in the system all the time, not only when something was wrong. Individual workers and reformers were perceived as members of an active and attentive movement that intervened at the neighborhood level. The settlement house is an example of social engineering in practice.

Typically, a settlement house was a large house in a slum area. It served as a community center, sponsoring such activities as recreation; classes in English, cooking, and citizenship; vocational training; and child care. Different settlement houses concentrated on different activities, depending on the needs of the neighborhood. Key elements to the success of a settlement house were the commitment of the workers and the location of the house. Social engineering could not be accomplished from afar; workers lived in the house or in the community in which they served. The house was part of the community. Perhaps the best example of a settlement house is Hull House in Chicago, founded by Jane Addams in 1889.

Addams was inspired by Toynbee Hall, a pioneer English settlement house she visited while in England in the 1880s. Upon returning from Europe, she and her college friend Ellen Starr moved to the poor section of Chicago and began raising money to support what was to become Hull House. Because of her upper-middle-class background, she had connections to the wealthy. Friends from college also supported the venture, but the house gathered its greatest support from churches and missions. Hull House was located in the middle of the immigrant section in Chicago. Addams and Starr moved in and invited their immigrant neighbors to read Italian novels and see slides of Italian art. The women came and brought their children; the presence of children necessitated a nursery. Soon a boys' club was established, and then a men's club. Over the years, more than 50 services were available from Hull House.

Walter Lippmann describes the qualities and service of Jane Addams very aptly (Tims, 1961, p. 150):

> Yet if that were all her life has meant, Jane Addams would only stand in a large company of men and women who in every land and under all conditions are persistently kind to their fellow beings. It is not all. There is something else, which was visible in the beauty of her countenance, was audible in her unaffected voice, is in the style of her writings, and was the special element in her influence. It was the quality within her which made it possible for her to descend into the pits of squalor and meanness and cruelty and evil, and yet never to lose, in fact always to hold clearly, the distinctions that are precious to a maturely civilized being. She had compassion without condescension. She had pity without retreat into vulgarity. She had infinite sympathy for common things without forgetfulness of those that are uncommon.
>
> That, I think, is why those who have known her say that she was not only good but great.

These movements are important because they illustrate the continual struggle during the 19th century to assist those in need. Generally, the assistance took two forms: provision of services and advocacy of reform. It was difficult to blame all the problems of urban poverty on the individual. The settlement house movement, in particular, introduced a new philosophy of helping that recognized the impact of societal forces on the lives of individuals. This new philosophy continued to develop in the 20th century.

The 20th Century: New Directions

The early 1900s, sometimes called *the sociological era,* continued the period of social reform. During this time, two significant events or changes affected the history of helping and human services. The first was the development of a new profession. Settlement house and Charity Organization Society workers became known as *social workers.* The basis for the new profession was the belief that such people needed specific skills, knowledge, and understanding to work effectively with the poor. Good intentions were admirable but not sufficient to provide assistance. During this time, social diagnosis, or casework, evolved as the method of practice. Mary Richmond, the author of *Social Diagnosis* (1917), identified this process as one of investigation, diagnosis, prognosis, and treatment. Her book is regarded as the first treatise on social casework theory and method (Zimbalist, 1977). The development of the social work profession is significant; it represents the beginning of the professionalization of human services. Later in this century, the fields of welfare, mental health, child guidance, and probation also became professionalized.

Also during the early 20th century, a reexamination of the causes of poverty took place. A group of writers called muckrakers actively criticized the wealthy, accusing them of moral decay, cheating, and bribery. (The term was first used by President Theodore Roosevelt in criticizing sensationalist, untruthful writers.) Muckrakers such as Lincoln Steffens and Upton Sinclair exposed unfair business, government, and labor practices. They supported the idea that poverty was caused by social and economic conditions, not by the individual, and proposed that poverty was a condition that prevented people from reaching their potential. They claimed that because poverty and need resulted from societal shortcomings, improvements in housing and working conditions could help eliminate poverty.

The Mental Health Movement

Clifford Beers, a victim of mental illness, was confined for three years in public and private mental institutions, where he experienced deprivation and cruelty. To publicize the plight of those with mental illness, he wrote about his collapse and treatment in *A Mind That Found Itself* (1945). In 1908, he founded the Connecticut Society for Mental Hygiene, considered by many to be the beginning of the organized mental health movement in America. By the following year, this pioneer state society had written a prospectus that included the following guidelines (Beers, 1945, p. 395):

> I
> "After all, what the insane most need is a friend!" By coordinating the friendly impulses of those who, if they but knew how, would gladly help the insane, the Society for Mental Hygiene can prove itself that friend.
>
> II
> It is the aim of the Society for Mental Hygiene to become a permanent agency for education and reform in the field of nervous and mental diseases; an agency for education always, for reform as long as radical changes may be needed.
>
> III
> The chief object of the Society for Mental Hygiene shall be the improvement of conditions among those actually insane and confined, and the protection of the mental health of the public at large.

Beers also proposed a national society, the National Committee for Mental Hygiene, which was formed in 1909. This group later changed its name to the National Association for Mental Health and is known today as the Mental Health Association. Its aim is to improve mental hospitals, arouse public concern, and prevent disease. By providing education on causes, diagnosis, prevention, and treatment, this organization furthered the development of the mental health movement.

Services for persons with mental illness improved and expanded. By the 1920s and 1930s, most large cities had free clinics for mental patients, where treatment and social services were provided. By the end of World War II, the profession of clinical psychology was created, in part because the number of veterans hospitalized in Veterans Administration (VA) facilities for psychiatric evaluation had reached more than 40,000 (Cranston, 1986).

Until the 1930s, individual leaders such as Jane Addams, Clifford Beers, and the muckrakers spearheaded the development of services and the reform of conditions for the impoverished. The development of professions that trained workers in social services also began. As important as these contributions were, they had little impact on poverty, mental illness, or other human service concerns on a large scale or at a national level. As a result, the federal government increased its financial commitment to those in need. Presidents of the United States assumed a leadership role in providing services.

Increased Federal Involvement

The Great Depression was marked by vast unemployment, failing business ventures, and the collapse of banks. The economic situation created a wave of panic and long-term psychological and economic depression for individuals

An Asylum in 1902

After fifteen interminable hours the straitjacket was removed. Whereas just prior to its putting on I had been in a vigorous enough condition to offer stout resistance when wantonly assaulted, now, on coming out of it, I was helpless. When my arms were released from their constricted position, the pain was intense. Every joint had been racked. I had no control over the fingers of either hand, and could not have dressed myself had I been promised my freedom for doing so.

For more than the following week I suffered as already described, though of course with gradually decreasing intensity as my racked body became accustomed to the unnatural positions it was forced to take. This first experience occurred on the night of October 18th, 1902. I was subjected to the same unfair, unnecessary, and unscientific ordeal for twenty-one consecutive nights and parts of each of the corresponding twenty-one days. On more than one occasion, indeed, the attendant placed me in the straitjacket during the day for refusing to obey some trivial command. This, too, without an explicit order from the doctor in charge, though perhaps he acted under a general order.

During most of this time I was held also in seclusion in a padded cell. A padded cell is a vile hole. The side walls are padded as high as a man can reach, as is also the inside of the door. One of the worst features of such cells is the lack of ventilation, which deficiency of course aggravates their general unsanitary condition. The cell which I was forced to occupy was practically without heat, and as winter was coming on, I suffered intensely from the cold. Frequently it was so cold I could see my breath. Though my canvas jacket served to protect part of that body which it was at the same time racking, I was seldom comfortably warm; for, once uncovered, my arms being pinioned, I had no way of rearranging the blankets. What little sleep I managed to get I took lying on a hard mattress placed on the bare floor. The condition of the mattress I found in the cell was such that I objected to its further use, and the fact that another was supplied, at a time when few of my requests were being granted, proves its disgusting condition.

For this period of three weeks—from October 18th until November 8th, 1902, when I left this institution and was transferred to a state hospital—I was continuously either under lock and key (in the padded cell or some other room) or under the eye of an attendant. Over half the time I was in the snug, but cruel embrace of a strait-jacket—about three hundred hours in all.

SOURCE: Excerpt from *A Mind That Found Itself*, by Clifford W. Beers, pp. 133–134, 395.

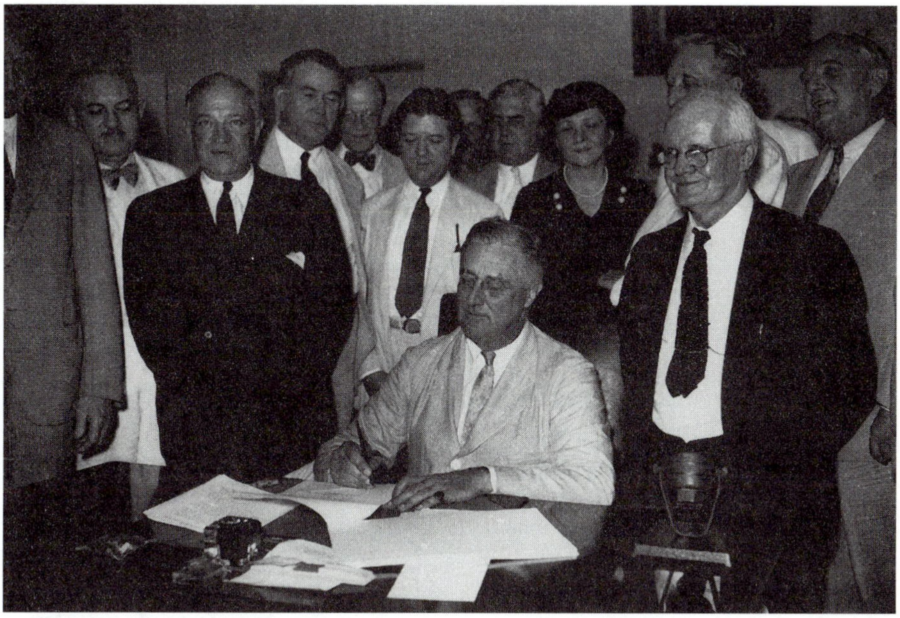

President Franklin D. Roosevelt signing the Social Security Act of 1935.

who could see no end to financial hardship. President Franklin D. Roosevelt introduced New Deal legislation that fundamentally changed the federal government's role in providing human services, focusing on two goals. The first was to provide short-term aid to those who were unemployed. The Works Progress Administration (WPA) and the Civilian Conservation Corps (CCC) were but two of the work relief programs he initiated. The second focus was the enactment of the Social Security Act of 1935 as protection against future economic hardships.

The Social Security Act of 1935, the cornerstone of the present American social welfare system, was passed in response to the need for human services. This landmark piece of legislation was significant for several reasons. First, it translated into action the belief that Americans had the right to protection from economic instability. The federal government assumed responsibility for the economic security of all citizens, and thus began the American welfare state. Second, it expanded welfare activities and improved their standards by establishing a new alignment of responsibility in public welfare. The policy of federal aid or grants to states began, closing the door on three centuries of the "poor law" principle of local responsibility.

What the act actually did was to provide assistance in three areas: social insurance, public assistance, and health and welfare services. Social insurance programs included old-age, survivors', disability, and unemployment insurance, all of which supported an individual's right to benefits regardless of need. Public assistance provided federal funds to states to establish programs such as Aid to the Permanently and Totally Disabled (APTD), Aid to Families with

Dependent Children (AFDC), Aid to the Blind, and Old Age Assistance (OAA). Also available under this category were programs of general assistance to needy people who were not eligible under any other program. The third area, health and welfare services, focused on child welfare, vocational rehabilitation, public health, children with disabilities, and maternal and child health.

Of course, some pieces were missing from these new social welfare efforts. The Social Security Act did not provide for long-term hardships. Unemployment benefits were available for only a limited amount of time, and neither health insurance nor permanent physical disability insurance was provided (Ehrenreich, 1985). In spite of these limitations, the initiatives of the Social Security Act became well-established components of the social welfare system. Few new programs would be developed during the next 20 years.

Under the administration of Harry Truman, the New Deal expanded into the Fair Deal. Most noteworthy were an enlarged Social Security program and public power projects on the Arkansas, Columbia, and Missouri rivers, bringing electricity and employment to these rural areas.

An important step in the provision of services to those with mental illness was the passage of the National Mental Health Act of 1946. This act created a Mental Hygiene Division within the United States Public Health Service and a center for information and research, which later became the National Institute for Mental Health. The Mental Hygiene Division emphasized preventive health measures. Its functions were to assist in the development of state and community health services; to study the causes, prevention, and treatment of mental illness; and to support training of psychiatrists, psychologists, social workers, and nurses.

Presidential Leadership

Presidential leadership combined with these legislative cuts to create a climate in which the human service movement flourished. In 1960, John F. Kennedy was elected president by a slim margin. He ran on a Democratic platform that emphasized the development of social policies to assist the unemployed, persons with mental illness, and persons with mental retardation. During his administration, the Manpower Development and Training Act was passed, funding programs that taught new skills to the unemployed so they could work. Kennedy sponsored aid to underdeveloped rural areas of the country, such as Appalachia, in redevelopment legislation that established special programs in locales with high poverty and unemployment rates. He also responded to the need for changes in the Social Security system. An amendment to the act provided casework to families that were chronically unemployed.

Kennedy renewed the government's commitment to mental health and the treatment of mental illness. He chose to focus on the problems of mental health and mental retardation "because they are of such actual size and tragic impact and because their susceptibility to public action is so much greater than the attention they have received" (Kennedy, 1964b). He called for a national plan to investigate causes, strengthen resources, and improve training and facilities.

Comprehensive community care, commonplace in the 1980s, was also a part of Kennedy's vision for addressing these problems.

Kennedy viewed human services as a comprehensive set of services to assist the needy. In the text of the speech he was to deliver in Austin, Texas, on the day of his assassination, he provided an overall definition of human services that encompasses the range of problems and service activity that characterizes human services today. "From public works to public health, wherever Government programs operate, the past three years we have seen a new burst of action and progress" (Kennedy, 1964a, p. 897). Specifically, he included crime, slums, poverty, pollution, and unemployment. He cited as evidence of his administration's concern and action the hospitals, clinics, and nursing homes being built; the new attack on mental health and mental retardation; the training of more dentists and doctors; and increases in Social Security benefits.

During the years Kennedy served as president, he set the tone for increased emphasis on the eradication of poverty in the United States. His vision brought much hope to populations that had despaired of changing their situations without assistance. Kennedy ignited the support of the nation to help the less fortunate.

Following the assassination of Kennedy in 1963, Lyndon Baines Johnson took the oath of office as president. Johnson assumed the legacy of Kennedy's commitment to the impoverished, but this was not a new role for him. Before his election to the vice presidency, he had spent 23 years as an advocate for those who had little hope for the future and no one to represent them.

Varying estimates are made of the number of poor people in America during the Johnson era. John K. Galbraith's well-known book *The Affluent Society* described a country in which people continuously improved their standard of living and the quality of their lives. Michael Harrington depicted the country very differently in *The Other America.* According to his research, 50 to 60 million Americans lived in poverty, a good many of them in isolated rural regions of the country, especially in the South and the Southeast, and others in large cities on the West and East coasts. These poor people had few skills for employment, lived in substandard housing, and were malnourished and illiterate.

In 1964, Johnson ran for president on a platform addressing the social problems described by Harrington. He proposed a comprehensive network of social policies and program initiatives. His opponent, Republican Senator Barry Goldwater, advocated reducing the government's role in addressing social problems. The public response to positive government social intervention was overwhelming, and Johnson was reelected by a large majority.

In his 1965 State of the Union address, he declared an "unconditional war on poverty" in order to create a "Great Society." Johnson believed the roots of poverty had to be attacked. Programs developed in the War on Poverty and Great Society initiatives included VISTA, the Neighborhood Youth Corps, the Job Corps, College Work Study, and Head Start. Their objective was to eradicate poverty by providing ways for the poor to improve their economic conditions.

The Great Society

The following excerpts are from President Lyndon Johnson's speech at the University of Michigan Commencement, May 22, 1964. The Great Society, a name used in this speech, was to become a watchword for the social programs of the 1960s and early 1970s. Johnson eloquently paints a picture of his dream of eradicating poverty. The social legislation passed during his term to ensure "equality" to every individual was heralded as a step toward the Great Society.

. . . For in your time we have the opportunity to move not only toward the rich society and the powerful society, but upward to the Great Society. The Great Society rests on abundance and liberty for all. It demands an end to poverty and racial injustice, to which we are totally committed in our time. But that is just the beginning.

The Great Society is a place where every child can find knowledge to enrich his mind and to enlarge his talents. It is a place where leisure is a welcome chance to build and reflects not a feared cause of boredom and restlessness. It is a place where the city of man serves not only the needs of the body and the demands of commerce, but the desire for beauty and the hunger for community.

It is a place where man can renew contact with nature. It is a place which honors creation for its own sake and for what it adds to the understanding of the race. It is a place where men are more concerned with the quality of their goals than the quantity of their goods. But most of all, the Great Society is not a safe harbor, a resting place, a final objective, a finished work. It is a challenge constantly renewed, beckoning us toward a destiny where the meaning of our lives matches the marvelous products of our labor. . . .

For better or for worse, your generation has been appointed by history to deal with those problems and to lead America toward a new age. . . .

So will you join in the battle to give every citizen the full equality which God enjoins and the law requires, whatever his belief, or race, or the color of his skin? Will you join in the battle to give every citizen an escape from the crushing weight of poverty? Will you join in the battle to make it possible for all nations to live in enduring peace as neighbors and not as mortal enemies? Will you join in the battle to build the Great Society, to prove that our material progress is only the foundation on which we will build a richer life of mind and Spirit?

SOURCE: Excerpts from "President's Michigan Speech on the 'Great Society,' " by Lyndon Baines Johnson, in *Congressional Quarterly, 20* (1964), p. 874. Reprinted by permission.

Many community action programs encouraged client participation in planning, delivering, and evaluating services.

Johnson also promoted the rights of the poor. For example, the Voting Rights Act of 1965 abolished the literacy tests that had been used to deny uneducated people the vote, and the Affirmative Action Order of 1968 and the Office of Economic Opportunity improved employment opportunities for minorities. Further evidence of the president's commitment were Medicare and Medicaid, amendments to the Social Security Act approved by President Johnson on July 30, 1965. Medicare (Title XVIII) provides health insurance for people over 65. Medicaid (Title XVIX) gives grants to the states to assist them in helping medically indigent citizens receive medical and hospital care.

The Decline in Federal Involvement

The election of Richard Nixon as president in 1968 marked two important changes in the federal government's involvement in social reform: a decline in federal spending and a different way of managing human service programs. Both represented a return to more traditional values and a much more conservative approach to human services. Nixon's New Federalism called for individuals to assume responsibility for their own situations. It started power, resources, and influence flowing back to the states and local communities. The emphasis was on the development of self-help programs and provision of services by the private sector.

President Nixon introduced a new management system, Management by Objective (MBO), in a memo sent to 23 departments in 1973 (Gruber, 1981). The intent of this management system was to correct the problems associated with the vague goals of human service programs and organizations. MBO required specific steps in the administration of programs. First, managers were to establish goals; then each goal was to be translated into specific objectives, with a plan for their achievement; finally, the program would be evaluated, with both the goals and the results assessed.

With regard to human services, Nixon focused on a commitment to the family and a commitment to eradicating poverty. He believed that families were able to determine their own needs and should use aid as they determined best (Bowler, 1974). The Supplemental Security Income program, which provided additional financial support for people needing assistance, translated this theory into practice.

President Gerald Ford's major impact on the human service delivery system was to continue the reduction of the federal government's involvement in human services. Ford supported an increased commitment by the private sector to support assistance to the needy. He had a major impact on human services through his 60 vetoes, which cut more than $9.5 billion that had been appropriated by Congress. Among the programs he vetoed were proposed improvements in federal aid to education, the school lunch program, and health care.

Focus on Mental Health

During his campaign for the presidency, Jimmy Carter discussed reorganizing the federal executive branch. After his election in 1976, he appointed a reorganization team directed by Bert Lance, the director of the Office of Management and the Budget. The Human Resource group directed the study of the human service areas. To prepare the executive department and agencies for this reorganization, Carter sent the following memo:

> I have directed the Reorganization project staff to begin a study on the organization and delivery of human services. These services, ranging from day care to job training, are intended to help people whose special needs are not met by income assistance and health programs. This study will be coordinated with efforts endeavoring to develop welfare and national health insurance proposals.

Five departments (Health, Education, and Welfare; Agriculture; Justice; Labor; and Interior) were involved in the reorganization. Initially, the services had been divided into categories of federal funding rather than sets of human problems. One-third of these programs either overlapped with each other or with programs in other departments. The major problem was in the Department of Health, Education, and Welfare; more than 300 of its programs crossed over into other departments. Another impetus for the reorganization was to fulfill a campaign promise by separating education programs from health and welfare services. The result was the creation of separate departments: the Department of Health and Human Services and the Department of Education. The use of the term *human services* denoted the wide variety of program services addressing human needs. The choice of the term clearly marks the point when *human services* became associated with a wide range of services, not restricted to those associated with mental health.

Carter also attempted to address a problem that had received attention from Kennedy and Johnson: unemployment. He proposed a Better Jobs and Income Program that would have employed 1.4 million people in service positions developed by the government. In addition, more than 32 million people would have received payment for health, Social Security, welfare, and educational services. The program could not generate the political support that was needed because it was too complex to understand and too complicated to administer.

During the Carter administration, the President's Commission on Mental Health, chaired by Rosalyn Carter, found that between 10% and 15% of the population (20–32 million people) needed some form of mental health services at any one time. Unfortunately, the commission also discovered that many people did not have access to good, affordable mental health care. Further, there was a lack of support services for persons with chronic mental illness, which included approximately 1.5 million people in mental hospitals, nursing homes, and other residential facilities. On May 15, 1979, President Carter proposed the Mental Health Systems Act, which promised comprehensiveness, flexibility, and innovation by emphasizing services for persons with chronic mental illness and by emphasizing prevention. It also attempted to address the shortage of mental health personnel in underserved areas, requiring people who received federal money for their training to work in an area with a personnel shortage for a period as long as the time they received financial support. Congress passed the Mental Health Systems Act and authorized funding through 1984.

Dismantling the Welfare System

From the 1930s to the 1980s, the government's social policy was to assume responsibility for citizens who could not provide a reasonable quality of life for themselves. Voters in the 1980s and 1990s elected presidents who advocated substantial reduction of the federal budget and decreased federal government involvement in human services, a stark contrast to the policies of the previous administrations.

President Reagan believed his overwhelming victory in 1980 was a mandate to move the country in a new direction, including the dismantling of the welfare state. To that end, he terminated a number of social programs and drastically cut spending on others. Those affected included "AFDC, childcare, school lunch and other nutrition programs, food stamps, subsidized housing, energy assistance, family planning, public and mental health services, alcohol and drug abuse counseling, legal aid, the Job Corps, and the like" (Trattner, 1994, p. 365).

Reagan's reelection in 1984 was another overwhelming victory. His second term continued to emphasize the economy, defense, and foreign policy (Ginsberg, 1987). The plight of the poor worsened during this period and one result was a welfare reform bill designed to help single parents, particularly women, enter the job market. The Family Support Act was signed into law in 1988. Among the programs authorized was the JOBS program, which required single parents on welfare with children older than 3 years to work or be in training in order to receive assistance. The act also mandated new procedures for collecting child support payments and one year of support for child care and transportation so that single parents could work or participate in training. For the most part, though, both Reagan administrations largely ignored the plight of the poor and disenfranchised, focusing instead on defense spending and tax cuts.

George Bush, Reagan's vice president, won the 1988 presidential election and claimed a mandate to continue many of the policies of the Reagan administrations. Generally, his administration is noted for its emphasis on foreign policy and its lack of attention to domestic issues. The most significant legislation of his four years was the Americans with Disabilities Act (ADA), which was passed in 1990. With little cost to the federal government, ADA was designed to get people into the workforce who otherwise would not be able to enter or who were kept out for other reasons, such as discrimination.

A declining economy, the growing gap between rich and poor, and the need for welfare reform all contributed to the election in 1992 of Democrat Bill Clinton, governor of Arkansas. One of his campaign pledges was to "end welfare as we know it." In 1996, welfare reform legislation was passed to end the federal government's six-decade guarantee of aid to the poor. Major components of the bill turned welfare over to the states, limited the time individuals could receive benefits, and required half of each state's welfare recipients to be working or training for a job by 2002. In addition, the bill reduced the availability of food stamps to poor families and made them completely unavailable to legal immigrants.

Highlights of the New Law

The welfare reform bill signed into law by President Clinton makes the most dramatic changes in federal anti-poverty programs in six decades. Following are highlights:

- Ends a 61-year guarantee of federal aid for poor children. Instead, Aid to Families with Dependent Children, the main federal cash welfare program, and smaller programs are folded into block grants that states will use to operate their own programs.
- Reduces spending by about $55 billion over six years, mainly by cutting food stamps and aid to legal immigrants.
- Imposes a five-year lifetime limit on welfare benefits. States can exempt up to 20% of their caseload for hardship reasons and set shorter time limits.
- Requires recipients to begin working two years after receiving welfare and mandates that 50% of single-parent families work 30 hours a week by 2002. States already running welfare work programs under federally approved waivers can continue the programs until the waivers expire.
- Reduces spending on food stamps, the federal coupons redeemed for food at supermarkets, by $28 billion over six years and allows able-bodied individuals without children to receive food stamps for only three months in any three-year period, unless they are working part time. Individuals can get another three months if they are laid off from work.
- Bars most federal aid, including Medicaid and cash welfare, to future legal immigrants for five years.

Current immigrants cannot receive disability and food stamps during their first five years in the USA, and states have the option to deny other aid. Exceptions include refugees and immigrants who have generally worked for 10 years.

- Makes it more difficult for children to receive federal disability payments due to mental problems—a program that has been widely abused, critics say.

SOURCE: From "Highlights of the New Law," *USA Today,* August 23, 1996, p. 3A. Copyright 1996, *USA Today*. Reprinted with permission.

Many questions surround this new welfare legislation. A primary concern is the ability of welfare recipients to find work. Many experts agree that it actually takes more resources to move women from their welfare aid to jobs because many need education, training, and child care assistance. The following quotes from welfare mothers voice their concerns.

Of California's welfare-to-work program, Jewell Bibs, age 21, says, "They made it sound so good . . . they help you with child care. They help you with bus fare. But they tell you, you can find a good job. And to them, a good job is any job. You can get one of them and you're still going to be poor" (Golden, 1996, p. 9).

Phyllis Martin in Boston has been on a continuous welfare-to-work cycle since 1987. She has twice trained for jobs, worked, and then been part of a large company layoff. She has this to say about her current job as a filing clerk in an architectural firm: "I hope this is it. I mean, I hope this is it" (Nifong, 1996, p. 10).

Manda Seefield of Coal Valley, Illinois, mother of two young children, has been on welfare for the past six years. She says of her ability to find work, "They don't want you unless you have experience . . . but how do you get experience, unless somebody is going to give you a job?" (Johnson, 1996, p. A7).

These mothers express only a few of the problems they see with the new welfare reform. Teena Briton, a welfare mother who attends North Shore Community College in Salem, Massachusetts, summarizes their concerns: "I feel [the state's] going to keep chipping away, chipping away at us until finally it's going to be, like, 'Hey, you've got to get off welfare and that's it.' And that's OK. But let me stay on it long enough to get some hope" (Nifong, 1997, p. 10).

At this writing, the debate continues over the impact of the welfare reform legislation, and there are three major concerns. One is the sufficiency of resources to help people get education, training, and other necessities. A second concern is the consequence of states failing to meet the demand of Congress to move half their welfare recipients into jobs or training programs by 2002 or have their federal grants cut. A third concern is that the $56 billion cuts in AFDC, food stamps, and other programs might throw 1.1 million children into poverty. However these concerns are addressed, this legislation is a significant historical event in the move to dismantle the welfare system in the United States.

The Growth of the Human Service Movement

The beginnings of the human service movement can be found in the impact of the two world wars, the mental health legislation of the postwar period, the initiatives of the Kennedy and Johnson administrations in the 1960s, and the clients' rights movement. The emergence of human service training programs and the development of a human service philosophy mirror the historical events and presidential leadership from the 1960s to the present. This section focuses on the growth of the human service movement.

Legislation

Human services have existed in some form since there have been people on earth, but human services as we know it today began its emergence with the impact of World Wars I and II on the mental health field. During both world wars, many men diagnosed as being in poor mental health were rejected from military service. After each war, many who had experienced combat sought mental health treatment for its aftereffects. Unfortunately, mental health facilities were often inaccessible, inadequate, or overcrowded. Both the high number of

The Mental Health Study Act of 1955

The Mental Health Study Act of 1955 authorized a study to determine the status of mental health treatment in the United States. The joint resolution of the House and Senate that brought about the act is reproduced in part here.

MENTAL HEALTH STUDY ACT: JOINT RESOLUTION

Providing for an objective, thorough, and nationwide analysis and reevaluation of the human and economic problems of mental illness, and for other purposes.

Resolved by the Senate and House of Representatives of the United States of America in Congress assembled, that this joint resolution may be cited as the "Mental Health Study Act of 1955."

Statement of Purposes and Policy

SEC.2.(a) It is the sense of the Congress that there exists a critical need for such an objective, thorough, and nationwide analysis and reevaluation of the human and economic problems of mental illness and of the resources, methods, and practices currently utilized in diagnosing, treating, caring for, and rehabilitating the mentally ill, both within and outside of institutions, as may lead to the development of comprehensive and realistic recommendations for such better utilization of those resources or such improvements on and new developments in methods of diagnosis, treatment, care, and rehabilitation as give promise of resulting in a marked reduction in the incidence and duration of mental illness and, in consequence, a lessening of the appalling emotional and financial drain on the families of those afflicted or on the economic resources of the States of the Nation,

(b) It is declared to be the policy of the Congress to promote mental health and to help solve the complex and the interrelated problems posed by mental illness by encouraging the undertaking of nongovernmental, multidisciplinary research into and reevaluation of all aspects of our resources, methods, and practices for diagnosing, treating, caring for, and rehabilitating the mentally ill, including research aimed at the prevention of mental illness. It is the purpose of this joint resolution to implement that policy.

SOURCE: Public Law 84:182 (1955).

rejected recruits and the poor mental health facilities available to veterans called public attention to the widespread existence of mental illness and the shortage of personnel to treat persons with mental illness effectively.

Recognizing the need for improvements in mental health care, Congress passed the National Mental Health Act (Public Law 79-487) in July 1946. This act created a federal agency, the National Institute of Mental Health (NIMH), to help states develop programs for increased training, research, and practice. As we will see later, this agency played a critical role in the developing human service movement.

A second piece of legislation that helped set the stage for the emergence of human services was the Mental Health Study Act of 1955 (Public Law 84-182), which provided funding for a Joint Commission on Mental Illness and Health. The charge to the commission was "to analyze and evaluate the needs and resources of the mentally ill in the United States and make recommendations for a national mental health program." The commission included representatives of 36 organizations chosen by the National Institute of Mental Health. *Action for Mental Health* by George Albee (1961a) was the final volume of the commission's report, containing recommendations for personnel needs, facilities, and costs. The commission then made recommendations for training, research, facilities, and programs.

Two of the commission's recommendations directly affected the human service movement. First, the commission concluded that the professional sector alone could not meet the health care needs of the majority of people if only traditional mental health professionals were used. According to the commission,

> All mental health professions should recognize that nonmedical mental health workers with aptitude, sound training, practical experience, and demonstrable competence should be permitted to do general, short-term psychotherapy—namely, treating persons by objective, permissive, nondirective techniques of listening to their troubles and helping them resolve these troubles in an individually insightful and socially useful way. Such therapy, combining some elements of psychiatric treatment, client counseling, "someone to tell one's troubles to," and love for one's fellow man, obviously can be carried out in a variety of settings by institutions, groups, and individuals, but in all cases should be undertaken under the auspices of recognized mental health agencies. (Albee, 1961b, p. x)

The commission also recommended that "a national mental health program should set as an objective one fully staffed, full-time mental health clinic available to each 50,000 of population" (Albee, 1961b, p. xiv). A major impact of the Mental Health Study Act on the human service movement was that it acknowledged the personnel shortage that existed, suggested a new type of mental health worker who could be trained in less time, and recommended a setting in which such new workers could be utilized effectively.

The commission's recommendations were well received and quickly became law. The conditions that encouraged this immediate action were an awareness of the increasing numbers of people with mental health problems, the rising costs of institutional care, and the need for more effective use of personnel, treatment facilities, and treatment (James, 1981). A sympathetic administration in the White House also provided impetus for quick action. President Kennedy was especially helpful in renewing the commitment to mental illness and mental health. In a speech on proposed measures to combat mental illness and mental retardation, he stated:

> I have sent to the Congress today a series of proposals to help fight mental illness and mental retardation. These two afflictions have been long neglected. They occur more frequently, affect more people, require more prolonged treatment, cause more individual and family suffering than any other condition in American life.
>
> It has been tolerated too long. It has troubled our national conscience, but only as a problem unpleasant to mention, easy to postpone, and despairing of solution. (Kennedy, 1964b, p. 51)

Funding for the recommendations of the commission was provided by the Community Mental Health Centers Act of 1963, which directed NIMH to set up requirements and regulations for the establishment of community mental health centers. Additionally, grants were to be made available for activities such as staffing, planning, initial operations, consultation, and education services. The idea behind this act was to provide diverse services to the population, including inpatient and outpatient care, emergency services, assistance to the courts, and services for the mental health of children and the elderly. By 1975, Congress had authorized over 609 multiservice centers (James, 1981).

Another response to the personnel shortage was the Scheuer Subprofessional Career Act of 1966, administered by the Department of Labor. The philosophical basis for the act was that poor people and minority group members, if trained appropriately, could provide effective mental health services. Programs were developed to train such people to be teacher aides, child care workers, corrections officers, and mental health workers. Most of the education was essentially inservice training, but some programs had links to vocational schools or community colleges.

Leaders of the Human Service Movement

One of the prime movers of the human service movement was the Southern Regional Education Board. Created by a resolution of the Southern Governors' Conference in 1948 to promote higher education through regional cooperation, SREB added a Mental Health Division in 1954 to focus on mental health workers and training. Dr. Harold McPheeters, director of the Commission on Mental Health and Retardation, was a key figure in the early development of the human service movement. He guided the involvement of SREB in the movement's faculty development, program development and approval, worker certification, and professional scholarship.

As we have already seen, there was ample evidence of a shortage of mental health workers in the United States. In 1966, SREB sponsored a national conference for mental health professionals and community college personnel to discuss the training of new workers at two-year institutions. Based on that conference, SREB applied for and was awarded a five-year grant from NIMH.

The purpose was to assist in the development of mental health programs at the associate or certificate degree level in two-year institutions in the 14-state Southern region.

The conference envisioned a new type of human service worker, a cross between the professional with an advanced degree and the volunteer. A major assumption about the new workers was that their firsthand work experiences, coupled with education and training, would enable them to establish greater rapport and credibility with their clients. In addition, their firsthand knowledge of the problems would give them greater understanding of clients and their difficulties. The initial intent was for these workers to perform innovative roles such as client advocacy and client-community liaison, but in reality they came to perform more traditional roles such as direct caregiving (Southern Regional Education Board, 1979).

The Western Interstate Commission on Higher Education (WICHE) also played a critical role in the development of human service programs. WICHE focused on the development of baccalaureate programs and the creation of job opportunities for graduates. Like SREB, WICHE sponsored regional conferences that brought together individuals from academic institutions and work settings to guide the development of programs and work opportunities (Teague, 1970).

Decade of Growth: The 1970s

EXPANSION

Since the 1960s, the human service movement has experienced unprecedented growth, evidenced by the increase in the number of training programs, the increased size of the mental health delivery system, and the development of the human service administration at the federal level. In 1966, the first human service program was established at Purdue University, a two-year associate degree program that focused on the training of entry-level mental health workers. By 1987, there were approximately 370 certificate, associate, and baccalaureate degree programs (Cogan & Wood, 1987). The students were trained to work in a variety of human services settings. In the 1980s, human service training encompassed a higher level of training, with the development of master's degree programs in the field.

NIMH continued its involvement with the movement during the 1970s. The New Careers branch of NIMH was established in 1970 to provide leadership in the development of entry-level programs for disadvantaged persons. In 1975, this became the Paraprofessional Manpower Branch, which led the way in defining and developing the training for all levels of paraprofessional workers. There was much concern in the existing mental health system about who the new paraprofessionals would be, what jobs they would perform, and whether they would perform adequately. It was the responsibility of the Manpower Branch to address these questions.

In spite of the concern voiced by the other professionals in the mental health system, many of these newly trained human service workers were welcomed. During the 1970s, the number of clients served by the mental health system increased dramatically. New workers were needed, and the traditional ways of providing mental health services were not efficient or effective in meeting the changing needs. Highly skilled professionals with advanced degrees had been serving small numbers of clients. Human service workers could now provide the simpler direct-care services to greater numbers of clients while the highly skilled professionals worked with the more difficult problems and supervised the human service workers. Deinstitutionalization, a movement that began in the 1950s, called for transferring many institutionalized patients to the community for outpatient care. By the 1970s, a major segment of mental health treatment had shifted from the isolation of the institution to the complex environment of the community. As the concept of community mental health developed, different types of professional services were needed.

PROFESSIONAL HUMAN SERVICE ORGANIZATIONS

The establishment of organizations within a discipline or a field signals a move toward professionalism. Such organizations serve many purposes. They may regulate a profession or its workers, facilitate communication among its members, or foster excellence in research or service within the profession. Two organizations in particular were instrumental in the move toward a human service profession. These two influential organizations, the National Organization for Human Service Education (NOHSE) and the Council for Standards in Human Service Education (CSHSE), are still active today.

NOHSE was an outgrowth of the Faculty Development Conferences sponsored by the SREB in the late 1960s and early 1970s. No more funding was available for development conferences, but participants wanted to maintain a network of professional communication. They established NOHSE in 1975 in St. Louis, with the following purposes:

1. To provide a medium for cooperation and communication among human services professionals and faculty
2. To foster excellence in teaching, research, and curriculum planning in the teaching of the human services
3. To serve individual faculty and professional members in their career development and position placement
4. To maintain a registry of members available to serve as consultants and resource individuals qualified in planning, developing, administering, and evaluating education and training programs relating to middle-level human service workers
5. To encourage, support, and assist the development of local, state, and national organizations of students and graduates of human service programs.

At present, NOHSE members include educators, students, and practitioners involved in human service education.

The Council for Standards in Human Service Education emerged from the Program Approval Project at SREB, which was funded by NIMH. It was incorporated in 1979 "to give focus and direction to education and training in mental health and human services throughout the country" (CSHSE, 1985, p. 1). The council works to improve human service education by establishing standards that programs must meet if they are to be approved. The standards are general enough to permit diversity but structured enough to ensure high-quality education. According to Mary Lou Cormier, first president of the council, program approval benefits a variety of individuals: "To the consumer of services, program approval means improving the quality of life; to the service provider, it signifies graduate competence; to the graduate, it denotes a positive educational experience; to the academic institution, it exemplifies quality education" (Cormier, 1979, p. 1).

Retrenchment: The 1980s and 1990s

On June 7, 1978, California voters passed Proposition 13, an amendment to the state constitution (Pilisuk, 1980). The goal of the legislation was to amend the property tax structure. One result was that less money became available to fund a variety of services, including social services. People were beginning to question the effectiveness and efficiency of the government; they did not want to pay for so much government intervention. When the proposition passed, its supporters predicted that there would be substantial reductions in the services offered by government, and an increase in resources available from private sources.

What actually happened was that fewer professionals were employed, but the number of people in need did not decrease. Human service workers, serving larger caseloads, felt overworked, ineffective, and devalued. Their jobs seemed to have lost what little status they had; voters had sent a clear message that the services they provided were not supported. Existing programs were cut back, and fewer new programs were funded, but the needs were as great as ever. Self-care, community support systems, and natural helping networks had to take up the slack. More people in need began to turn to neighborhood groups, churches, friends, and families for assistance.

The passage of Proposition 13 was an early sign of the changing attitude of the American public toward government spending for human services. In 1980, Ronald Reagan was elected president on a platform that called for establishing new priorities in human services, slashing government spending, and reducing the government's involvement in human services. One of Reagan's priorities was to return the administration of human services to the individual states, communities, and private sources. His reasoning was that it is not the government's function to provide such services and that government delivery of such services is not effective or efficient. As a result of Reagan's policy, there has been a shift in service delivery. The number of nonprofit and private agencies in the human services is expanding, and human service institutions and agencies are contracting out for services (Ginsberg, 1987). Reagan also advocated transferring federally owned housing and prisons to the private sector.

Another priority of the Reagan administration was to reassess who receives services and to cut services to those who are not absolutely needy. This change was accomplished with deliberate speed by scaling down the Great Society programs of the Johnson era. Within a matter of months after Reagan's inauguration, there were deep cuts in government spending to support AFDC, food stamps, school lunch programs, and other social programs.

Just as the labor market tends to respond to economic demands, the human service labor market reflects human service demands (Austin, 1983). During the 1960s and 1970s, the human service market was growing, and the number of opportunities for employment and for advancement increased. Today that growth has slowed, and opportunities are developing in the private sector with, for example, the privatization of correctional facilities and the development of employee assistance programs in private industry.

Different levels of academic preparation for human services continue to develop. During the 1970s, the number of baccalaureate degree programs increased. There has also been an increase in the number of master's degree programs in human services. An interesting parallel to master's level work is the development of community agency counseling programs, which evolved in the early 1970s to prepare mental health counselors for work in community and agency settings. They are an outgrowth of counselor education programs designed to prepare counselors for educational settings. When National Defense Education Act funds were no longer available to support school counselor training, the emphasis switched to the preparation of counselors to work in community agencies. The name of these programs changed in 1987 to mental health counseling.

New challenges face human service professionals as we approach the 21st century. Managed care, technological advances, nontraditional service settings, and a shrinking global community are only a few of the changes with which service providers must cope. These challenges will be explored in the next chapter as you begin thinking about human services today.

✧ Things to Remember

1. Before the Middle Ages, people believed that mental illness was caused by evil spirits, and early forms of treatment focused on ridding the body of these spirits.
2. Until the 1500s, the church was chiefly responsible for providing human services. Under the church's guidance, many institutions were founded for the poor, orphans, the elderly, and the handicapped.
3. The decline of feudalism, the growth of commerce, and the beginning of industrialization made it necessary to find new ways of assisting those in need.

4. Pressures caused by the increasing number of poor in the cities created the need for a large-scale attack on poverty and prompted the passage of the Elizabethan Poor Law of 1601, critical legislation that guided social welfare practices in England and the United States for the next 350 years.
5. In the early years, the colonists used the English system as a model for their philosophy toward and services for the poor and needy. By the early 1800s, however, other philosophies prevailed, ones that discouraged and limited the provision of human services.
6. Major reforms during the late 1800s concentrated on improving the treatment of the institutionalized mentally ill and children.
7. The Charity Organization Society, a forerunner of the Community Chest and the United Way, is an example of society's response to the needs of an expanding urban population.
8. A settlement house was a large house in a slum area that served as a community center, sponsoring such activities as recreation; classes in English, cooking, and citizenship; vocational training; and child care.
9. President Franklin D. Roosevelt introduced the Social Security Act of 1935, which fundamentally changed the federal government's role in providing human services.
10. During the years John F. Kennedy served as president, he set the tone for increased emphasis on the eradication of poverty in the United States, bringing hope to populations that had despaired of changing their situations without assistance.
11. In his 1965 State of the Union address, President Lyndon Johnson declared an "unconditional war on poverty." He developed programs that attacked the roots of poverty in order to create a "Great Society."
12. The election of Richard Nixon as president marked two important changes in the federal government's involvement in social reform: a decline in federal spending and a different way of managing human service programs.
13. During the presidency of Ronald Reagan, commitment to human services passed from the federal government to state and local governments, the private sector, and needy individuals themselves.
14. The emergence of human service training programs and the development of a human service philosophy mirror the historical events and presidential leadership from the 1960s to the present.
15. The National Organization for Human Service Education and the Council for Standards in Human Service Education have been instrumental in the development of the human services profession.
16. Several pieces of legislation, such as the National Mental Health Act, have reflected the national recognition of the need for improved mental health care.
17. The concept of a new human service worker was welcomed by a mental health community responding to the mental health care needs created by deinstitutionalization.

Additional Readings: Focus on History

Beers, Clifford W. (1945). A *mind that found itself: An autobiography.* Garden City, NY: Doubleday, Doran.

Clifford Beers writes of his experiences as a three-time patient in mental institutions around the turn of the century.

Johnson, A. B. (1990). *Out of bedlam: The truth about deinstitutionalization.* New York: Basic Books.

The author reviews the history of deinstitutionalization by focusing on the fiscal pressures faced by states and the opportunities to shift costs to the federal government. As a mental health professional herself, she illustrates how bureaucratic complexity and confusion have given deinstitutionalization a bum rap.

Marshall, Helen E. (1937). *The forgotten Samaritan.* Chapel Hill: University of North Carolina Press.

Marshall has produced a well-written biography of Dorothea Dix, humanitarian and reformer.

Trattner, Walter I. (1994). *From poor law to welfare state: A history of social welfare in America.* New York: Free Press.

Trattner gives an overview of social welfare in the United States from the colonial era to the present. He includes highlights of the mental health, child welfare, and public health movements, as well as beginnings of social welfare as a profession.

Chapter 3

Human Services Today

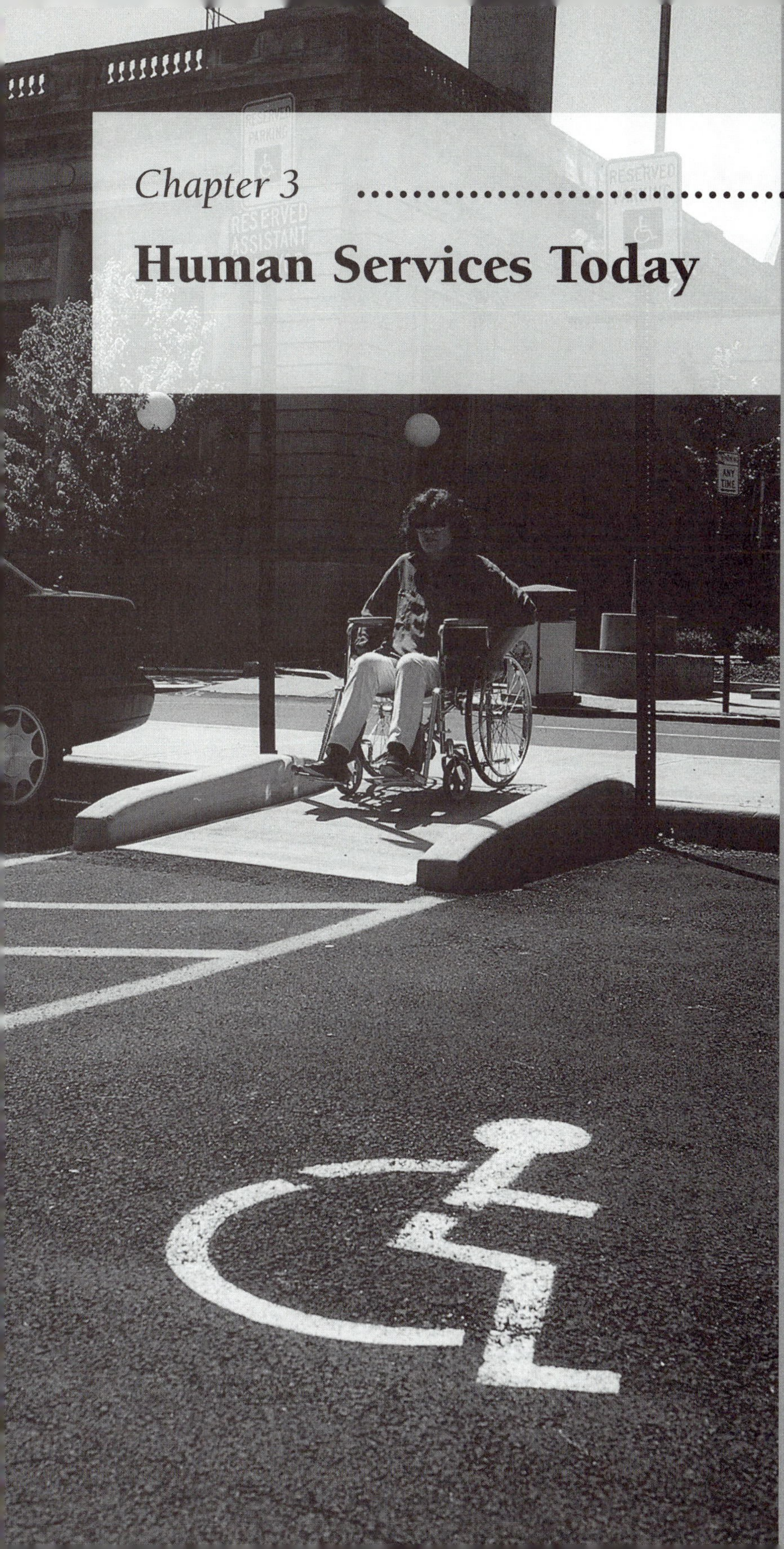

One facet of the definition of human services is how and where services are delivered today. This chapter examines several of these dimensions of human service delivery. As you read about them you will see that human services today has a much broader scope than ever before. It takes place in a variety of settings, addresses global human needs, interfaces with the managed care system, and reflects recent advances in communication and technology. This chapter examines each of these dimensions in more detail to help expand your definition of human services.

New Settings for Service Delivery

One way to describe the broadening scope of human services today is to think about where services are delivered. In many instances, services continue to be delivered in agencies or institutional settings; but with a growing emphasis on making services accessible and comprehensive, service delivery in nontraditional settings has increased.

Human Services in Industry and the Military

Traditionally, human services has been associated with people in financial need, particularly those who are unemployed and those labeled poor. Recently, employers are recognizing that workers who are physically and psychologically well are more productive employees. Industry has learned to identify signals that indicate when an employee needs assistance, such as tardiness, absenteeism, ineffective job performance, and inability to cooperate or communicate with others. Many companies are encouraging their workers to seek help.

Industry's initial interest in human services began when drug and alcohol abuse among employees showed alarming increases. The federal government was instrumental in establishing guidelines for treating this problem. The Federal Comprehensive Alcohol Abuse and Alcohol Prevention, Treatment and Rehabilitation Act (the Hughes Act) was passed in 1970 and created the National Institute on Alcohol Abuse and Alcoholism. The act was significant for the field of human services because it established an approach that was different from the treatment for persons with mental illness. The act required federal agencies to have alcohol abuse and prevention programs available to employees—programs now well known as employee assistance programs (EAPs). EAP services are now offered to employees of most major corporations. Some address broad needs of workers such as counseling for abuse, personal issues, and marital problems; encouraging wellness with diet counseling, exercise, stress management, and personal awareness education; and developing work-related skills through such programs as employee orientation, management development, human relations training, team building, organizational development, and preparation for retirement. The scope of human services has once again expanded beyond the fundamental provision of basic assistance.

Passage of the Americans with Disabilities Act (ADA) has also had a significant impact on business, industry, and other employers. Signed into law by President George Bush on July 26, 1990, ADA was patterned after the 1964 Civil Rights Act. The intent and spirit of ADA was, and continues to be, to enable people with disabilities to have access to goods and services—including employment—that is equal to the access available to citizens without disabilities. ADA is nondiscriminatory legislation, not affirmative action legislation. It makes it unlawful for employers to discriminate against people with disabilities in regard to hiring, firing, compensation, training, and advancement. The act affects almost 50 million Americans with disabilities. The five titles in the act delineate the areas it addresses:

- Employment
- Public Services, including transportation systems (federal, state, and local government)

- Access to Goods and Services in the Public Sector
- Telecommunications
- Miscellaneous Provisions (e.g., insurance issues, limits regarding modifications to historical buildings and other structures, etc.)

The overwhelming majority of the nation's employers openly embrace ADA's equal access and reasonable accommodation tenets. If a candidate is qualified for a particular job and can perform the essential job functions, that person has the same opportunities as anyone else. Through mediation, alternative dispute resolution, arbitration, and litigation, case law is further defining and clarifying ADA's parameters. The integration and acceptance of people with disabilities has increased greatly in the short period since passage of the act, but more remains to be done.

Another nontraditional setting for human service delivery is the military. Meeting basic human needs in the military is different from accomplishing this in a civilian setting, partly because of the atmosphere of discipline and commitment to the organization. In 1881, the American Red Cross began providing social services to the military out of a concern for the health and welfare of the individuals in uniform. A medical orientation characterized military social service until 1976, when the Service to Armed Forces (SAF) was developed to help the military better serve the families of military personnel. Field offices were established in military hospitals and military installations to assist communication between service personnel and families. The field offices provide a team of professionals, including a human service worker to counsel military personnel (Masi, 1982).

Schools as a Part of the Human Service Delivery System

Schools are becoming a site for human service delivery. The following observations by public school teachers illustrate the challenges they are encountering in schools today and the need for expanded services in educational settings.

> *Jill Robbins, a 1991 Teacher of the Year in Knox County, Tennessee:* "We are seeing more and more students who need more kinds of social services. . . . I think I spend more of my time in guidance counselor-related activities than ever before." (Powell, 1991, p. 4)
>
> *Donna Viveiros, a teacher from Fall River, Massachusetts:* "Children come to school with all kinds of problems from home. Students can't sit still; they're hungry; their home life is just upside down." (Vreeland, 1991, p. B1)
>
> *Joy G. Dryfoos, an elementary education teacher:* "Schools are being called on to be those 'surrogate parents' that can increase the 'teachability' of children who arrive on their doorsteps in poor shape." (Hornblower, 1996, p. 37)

Collaboration and Cooperation

The LINK Project matches Western Washington University students with at-risk youth in the Bellingham School District in a variety of situations. Western volunteers work with English as a second language students, special education students, after school tutorial centers, and students in small group and one/one settings. The LINK Project is active in five schools, as well as maintaining a small presence in two elementary schools.

The LINK Project staff is responsible for recruiting, training, and evaluating volunteers throughout the year. The LINK Project is also responsible for managing the fiscal component, providing opportunities for reflection, and providing infrastructure for growth. The LINK Project has served as a catalyst and incubator to the creation and support of programs which serve the needs of Native American students, an eighth-grade service learning project, and a mentoring program for students in the highly capable program who are at risk in a variety of ways.

SOURCE: From "Community-Based Schools: Collaboration Between Human Services and Schools as Radical Educational Reform," by R. Lawson and P. Anderson, 1996, in H. S. Harris and D. C. Maloney (Eds.), *Human Services: Contemporary Issues and Trends* (p. 167), Boston: Allyn & Bacon.

Teachers such as these encounter the problems of children and youth each time they enter the classroom. The rate of poverty is high and the results of educational tests are troubling. Can learning occur in an environment characterized by gangs, dropouts, teenage pregnancy, substance abuse, AIDS, and violence? Predictions for the future do not offer much hope. By the year 2000, one child in four will be poor and almost one-third of all school-age children will be from minority populations whose primary language is not English (DeVita, 1989).

The challenge to human service professionals is to build on the commonalities they share with educational professionals to coordinate comprehensive services that assist the whole person. Because human service and educational professionals share the same clients, a team approach ensures that those clients receive services with little duplication but much reinforcement. Another commonality is their role as service deliverers. Whether interacting with clients in a school classroom, an agency office, or an institutional setting, every helping professional plays many roles: teacher/educator, caregiver, advocate, and broker.

A partnership between human services and education is essential to meet the complex needs of children and families. In the past year, several colleges of education, human service education programs, and public schools have begun cooperative efforts that recognize common goals and the importance of coming together. Services delivered within the context of a unified system are coordinated and comprehensive.

Institutional and Community-Based Services

There has been a change in philosophy regarding the delivery of services in institutional settings and in the community. The difference in settings is an obvious factor. Earlier, institutions were located in out-of-the-way places because pastoral settings were believed to be peaceful and calming. These settings may also have been chosen because members of society did not like to be reminded of the existence of people with mental illness. Correctional facilities have been built in rural areas because the criminal population is considered dangerous to others. Again, people who were not incarcerated did not like to be reminded of this population. Now, however, in both mental health and corrections, there is a trend toward community-based care. In the past, many people who were institutionalized could have functioned in the community with some professional support. The goal of community-based mental health care is to enable clients to interact with their environments in the least restrictive setting in which they can function.

Community-based mental health has changed the nature of service delivery. The focus of treatment has become health and wellness instead of illness. The process involves other social institutions such as schools, recreation facilities, and churches. In addition, the psychological and medical treatment received by clients has been adapted for community-based care. Much of the human service work is in case management; the human service worker acts as planner, consultant, and liaison between the mental health agency, the client, and the other institutions. Human service professionals also provide support for the families of persons with mental illness.

Community-based care in corrections is designed to take individuals from prisons and local jails and place them in the community with supervision and a planned program. These programs link educational services, counseling, substance abuse treatment, and employment assistance. In these programs, much of the responsibility falls to the client to take the initiative in using available services.

Another area of community-based care has developed between human service professionals and families who have children with problems. In the earlier model, the family and the child were seen as clients; now the parents are considered part of the helping network. According to Cohen and Lavach (1995), in the parents-as-helpers model, parents are seen as

- Experts on and teachers of their own children
- Advocates for their children
- Change agents in improving the environment in which their children live

In this model, families are empowered to assume responsibility for their own care and the care of their children but are still eligible for support when it is appropriate.

As described in this section, human services occur in an increasing diversity of settings; the challenge for the generalist helper is to use skills, knowledge, and values to serve clients effectively across these varied settings. From these nontraditional settings, we describe human services in its broadest terms, that of the international dimension.

The International Dimension

Talking about human services today without discussing its international dimension would be difficult. All people and societies on the planet are drawing closer together as a result of technological advances in transportation and communication. Today, people travel the world in a matter of hours rather than days or weeks. Advances in communication keep us instantly informed about developments throughout the world by satellite, electronic mail, and faxes. The Internet, the world's largest computer network, had over 25 million users in 1995 and the number is expected to double every year (DeWitt, 1994). The "information superhighway" has no borders, with users in most countries on the globe.

We have also become increasingly interdependent. The United Nations recognizes 226 nations in the world. In 1996, there were 37,000 transnational corporations (Harris & Moran, 1996). One out of six U.S. manufacturing jobs is dependent on foreign trade, and four out of five new manufacturing jobs result from international commerce. These few facts demonstrate clearly that the world is becoming a smaller place when we consider factors other than physical distance. Because we know this is true, we need to know what is happening internationally in terms of human services—the recent changes that have occurred, and the challenges that remain.

Challenges in International Human Services

During 1995, the world's population grew by 100 million people to 5.75 billion, the largest increase ever. Ninety percent of the growth is in poor countries "already terribly torn by civil strife and social unrest and where all too many people live in brutal poverty," according to Werner Fornos of the Population Institute ("Poor Nations," 1995, p. A10). Although this information may seem discouraging, there are positive changes. Since the devastation of World War II occurred, vast improvements have come about in the health care and living conditions of the world. Average life expectancy, even in low-income nations such as Zaire, Egypt, and India, has risen from 40 to 66 years (Desjarlais, Eisenberg, Good, & Kleinman, 1995). Diseases such as smallpox have been eradicated whereas others such as leprosy and epilepsy have been lessened by medical interventions. Infant mortality rates have fallen and literacy rates have risen.

At the same time, mental, behavioral, and social health problems are an increasing part of the health burden on all parts of the globe (see Figure 3-1). A recent World Bank study (1993) found mental health problems to be a major cause of lost years of good-quality life. Behavior-related illnesses (34%) include

INTERNATIONAL FOCUS
The Streets of Bombay

Vikki, 17, has lived on Bombay's streets for a decade, since he ran away from his impoverished village and alcoholic father. He joined a population of homeless children that is larger than many cities.

Most of the estimated 100,000 street children in Bombay live in tarpaper shanties, at railway stations, or on the pavement. Most are doomed to lives of menial labor or petty crime.

But Vikki may have found an escape. He is one of 400 youths who have attended workshops run by a humanitarian group to teach street children the basics of good business.

Called Project Mainstream, the two-day workshops began in February to train teenagers how to be good salespeople; run profitable vegetable, betel nut, or snack stands; make incense sticks; or become florists.

Taking a pragmatic approach to the problems of small-time business, the courses also teach how to handle municipal officials who demand bribes, varying from 20 rupees (75 cents) to 200 rupees ($7.50), to overlook violations such as selling without a license. That usually means paying them.

Helped by a loan of $45, Vikki sells toasted vegetable sandwiches from his stand outside Crawford Market, the city's wholesale fruit market. At 5 rupees a serving, he's been turning a profit of about 100 rupees ($1.80), enough to buy two flimsy T-shirts or a meager meal for two at a roadside kiosk.

The pressure of life on the street is enormous. At least five street children attempt suicide every month in Bombay, says the Coordinating Committee for Vulnerable Children, a volunteer group.

About three-fourths of the street youngsters are substance abusers, usually of hashish or an adulterated form of heroin known as brown sugar, the committee says.

Project Mainstream is financed mainly by Indian and Canadian Rotary Clubs. "Any honest, money-making endeavor must be supported by the community," said Mahendra Mehta, of the Bombay Rotary Club.

In Bombay, as in many of India's megacities, the government cannot provide basic services such as health care and education to the influx of rural poor. Community and volunteer organizations take up some of that slack.

The Coordinating Committee directs 22 grass-roots organizations that reach an estimated 4,000 children. They run centers where children can bathe and receive counseling. They also conduct informal schools and try to reunite children with families and select children for Project Mainstream.

SOURCE: From "Bombay Street Kids Become Entrepreneurs," by Naresh Fernandes, October 15, 1995, *Seattle Times*, p. A4. Reprinted by permission of Associated Press.

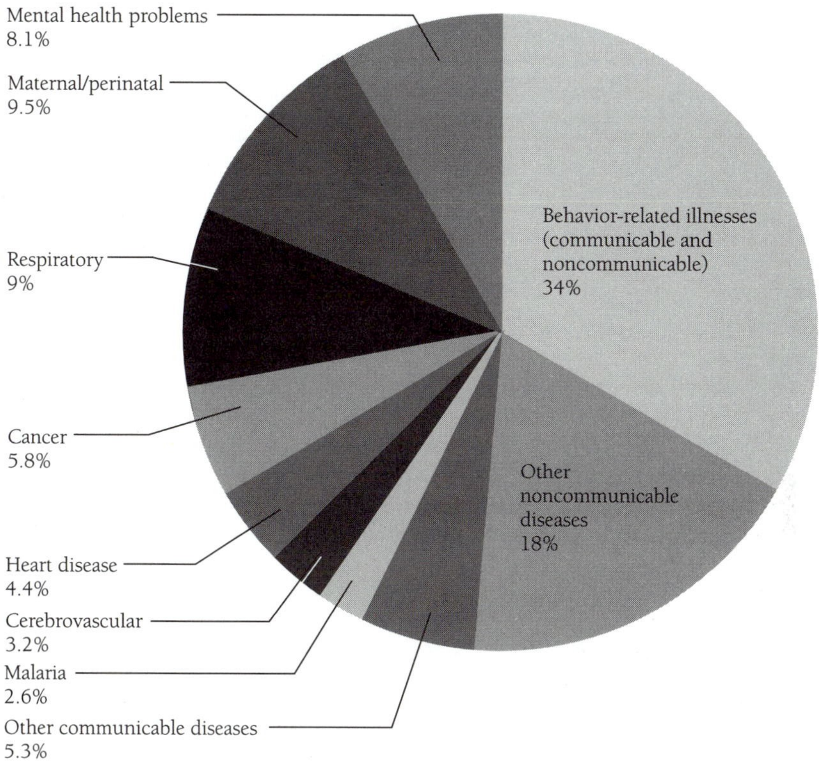

Figure 3-1 ✦ Global distribution of health burdens: Percentage of disability adjusted life years lost

SOURCE: From "Global Distribution of Health Burdens, 1990," by World Bank, 1993. *World Development Report 1993: Investing in Health.* New York: Oxford University Press.

violence, diarrheal diseases, malnutrition, tuberculosis, sexually transmitted diseases, and unintentional injuries such as those sustained in motor vehicle accidents. Mental illness, violence, dislocation, poverty, exploitation, substance abuse, and other behavioral problems affect hundreds of millions of people of all ages. A closer look at poverty and its related problems can help us understand their very serious nature.

A logical place to start is with urbanization and its consequences. Urbanization is a long-term global trend. Two-thirds of the world's population are expected to live in cities by 2025. There will soon be more people living in cities than in rural areas. The number of cities in the world with a million or more people will have increased from 83 in 1950 to more than 560 in 2015 (Lederer, 1996). Paris, London, and New York will no longer come to mind when people talk about the great metropolises of the world. Instead, congested Dhaka, Jakarta, Lagos, and other Asian, African, and Latin American urban centers will become the "megacities."

Urbanization is most pronounced in poor countries that are least able to cope with its pressures. Today, a third of the world's population—about 600

TABLE 3-1 ✦ MATERNAL DEATHS (Women who die each year in pregnancy or childbirth)

Area	*Number of deaths*
Europe	3,000
Central Asia	14,000
Americas	23,000
Mideast and North Africa	35,000
Sub-Saharan Africa	219,000
Asia and Pacific	291,000
World Total	**585,000**

SOURCE: From "A World in Need," Copyright, June 24, 1996, *U.S. News & World Report,* p. 20.

million people—do not have the means to meet their basic needs, such as clean water and sewage disposal. Bombay, the largest city in India, has a population of 15.1 million. By 2015, it will be the second largest metropolis in the world—with 27.4 million people. In Bombay, between 200 and 250 families arrive each day, hoping for a better life in the city. Many begin their lives in Bombay as pavement dwellers because there is no other place to live. Land is scarce, and rooms and apartments are full. The newcomers may remain on the sidewalks for the rest of their lives, or they may move to a slum dwelling. In either case, clean water, electricity, paved paths/roads, and working community toilets are often nonexistent. Although slum living represents upward mobility in many developing countries, slum dwellers complain about the gangs, high rent, drugs, violence, sewage, and floods.

Another widespread problem is the abuse and neglect suffered by women and children throughout the world. Over 18 million suffer debilitating illnesses or injuries that often disable them. A 1996 UNICEF report estimates that 585,000 women die each year in pregnancy and childbirth (Crossette, 1996) (see Table 3-1). To get a perspective on the problem, consider these figures: Roughly 1 in 13 women in sub-Saharan Africa and 1 in 35 in South Asia die of causes related to pregnancy and childbirth whereas the numbers are 1 in 3,200 in Europe, 1 in 3,300 in the United States, and 1 in 7,300 in Canada.

Child labor remains a reality today in many countries. The United Nations' (UN) International Labor Organization (ILO) estimates that there are at least 100 million child workers in the world (Hecht, 1996). In Africa, for example, the problem affects a minimum of 25% of all children between the ages of 10 and 14. In Senegal, the figure is as high as 40%. Child labor is a fact of life in Third-World countries. Children work to supplement the family income, and many rural families send children to work rather than to school. Child labor means work; it does not mean learning to read and write, playing, or resting when unwell.

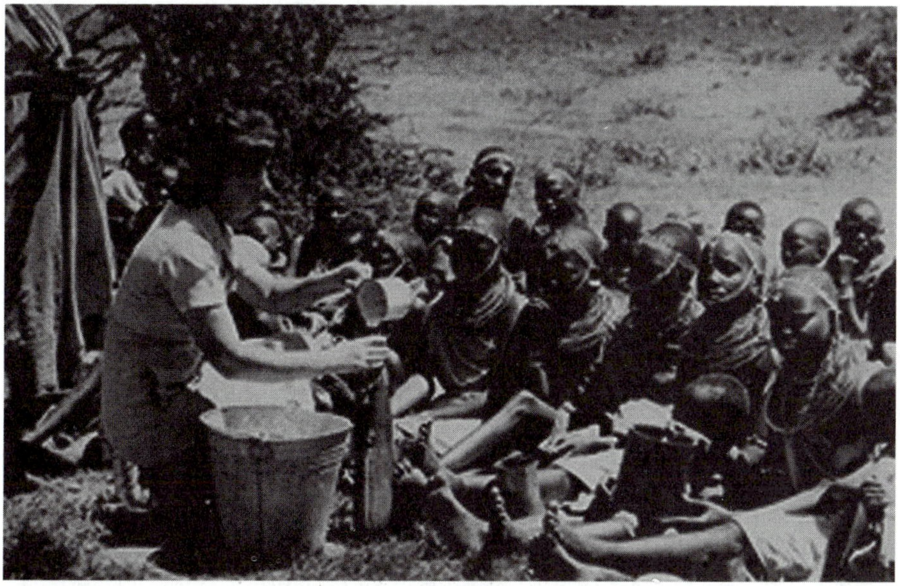

Poverty is prevalent in the Third World.

Child prostitution is a reality in Cambodia, India, China, Thailand, the Philippines, Taiwan, and other countries. Social workers and governments estimate that more than a million girls and boys, age 17 and younger, are engaged in prostitution (Kristof, 1996). Many enter the sex trade unwillingly, sold by parents to brothel owners, drugged, or kidnapped off the street. The fear of AIDS is one of several factors driving customers to younger girls and boys who are regarded as more likely to be disease free.

Education, particularly for girls, is by no means universal. Girls are far less likely than boys to attend primary school. Half of all girls in sub-Saharan Africa and 22% in North Africa, Asia, and the Middle East are not in school, compared with 14% of boys ("A World in Need," 1996). Girls are kept home to cook, clean, and mind younger children, or they work outside the home to bring in extra income.

The challenges in international human services continue to be great. The plights of refugees, those with AIDS, the homeless, drug users, and the displaced in the aftermath of natural disasters—in addition to the problems discussed here—are some of those challenges. Ishrat Husain, director of the Poverty and Social Policy Department at the World Bank in Washington, cites our improved understanding of poverty, the participation of the poor in the design and implementation of projects, and awareness of the damage done by discriminating against women and ethnic minorities as the keys to successful programs (Husain, 1996). He says:

> But all these strategies would serve no purpose if the poor cannot make a living. They can only do that if they have the health, strength, and

> education that will enable them to live and work productively. One of the most efficient ways to reduce poverty is to invest in the human capital of the poor. . . . No investment in education has a higher return than investment in educating girls. It has a powerful effect on almost every aspect of development. It lowers fertility rates, raises productivity, and helps the environment. Increasing female literacy in Africa could help lower infant mortality. (p. 19)

Influences in the United States

How does the international dimension of human services affect the United States? Although most of the information in this text concerns human services in this country, we must also be aware of the international dimension of human services. Immigrants to the United States increase our awareness of those nationalities that have become or are becoming part of our population. In the early history of the country, immigration was limited primarily to Europeans; 100 years ago, 90% of the immigrants to the United States came from European countries. By 1985, however, nearly one-half of all immigrants to this country were Asians. In addition to Chinese and Japanese, there are substantial numbers of Filipino, Korean, Vietnamese, and Indian immigrants. Today, people born in another country make up 9% of the American population, the highest figure since World War II. Latinos are the largest immigrant group, accounting for 46% of those born elsewhere (Grier, 1996).

We can continue to explore diversity in the United States by thinking about some population figures. America's population in the next century will experience profound shifts, making it more ethically diverse than ever before. By 2050, about half the population will be non-Latino whites, making the United States a "majority minority" nation (Friedman, 1996). This proportion is down from three-quarters today and is accounted for by high immigration rates and high birth rates among Latino women. The Latino and Asian portion of the population will grow fastest, while blacks will nearly double in number by 2050.

The population in the United States as a whole will grow from 262 million to 394 million, an increase of 50% (U.S. Census Bureau, 1996). This projection represents some of the slowest population growth in the country's history, but the Census Bureau notes that the United States is experiencing one of the most dramatic shifts in its racial and ethnic makeup since those brought on by the trade in slaves in the 17th and 18th centuries and the immigration from Eastern and Southern Europe in the late 19th and early 20th centuries.

Projections of population in the future are only that—projections. They are subject to change because of a number of factors. These include changes in legislation that regulates immigration and in fertility rates, and breakthroughs in medical care that impact life expectancy (Holmes, 1996). Nevertheless, the United States is the fastest growing country in the industrialized world today. After 2025, however, population growth will slow to an all-time low brought about by declining birth rates and increased deaths as the population ages. These changes will present new economic and social issues.

Today and in the foreseeable future, the United States must grapple with a number of issues related to diversity. Should changes in immigration laws reduce legal immigration rates? What efforts should be employed against illegal immigration? Do immigrants take jobs from unemployed citizens? Are immigrants entitled to public education and other benefits? Should English be the official language of the United States? What impact will these ethnic shifts have on Medicare and Social Security? While these questions are debated throughout the United States, we continue to be part of the global community and play a role in the international human services discussed earlier.

Managed Care

In the past decade, managed care has had a profound effect on the delivery of human services. Its influence is felt by both the client and the human service professional as they work together to plan and provide services. Today, managed care organizations administer over 70% of the group health insurance, and the movement of managed care into mental health care is also on the rise ("20 Hot Job Tracks," 1996). Let's look at managed care and how it has affected the delivery of health, mental health, and other services.

Managed care is a term used to describe a set of tools or methods designed to manage resources and deliver human services, especially in the areas of health care and mental health. It developed from the demand from the public for accountability of service delivery and from the rising costs in health and mental health care. Costs for health care are projected to use 15% of this country's financial resources by the year 2000, including expenditures by businesses of 60 cents on every dollar (Goodman, Brown, & Dietz, 1992). Costs in mental health services have also expanded, and in 1990, over $80 billion was spent treating mental health and substance abuse patients (Kessler, 1989). Prior to the use of managed care to allocate resources and services, most care was provided on a fee-for-service basis. In other words, a health or human service professional would provide a specific service and charge a standard rate. The payment for these services would come from the client, an insurance provider, or the agency or organization supporting the client care.

The Influence of Managed Care

A broad definition of managed care is that it involves "any patient care that is not determined solely by the provider" (Goodman, Brown, & Dietz, 1992, p. 5). In the case of human services, a provider is a professional who delivers services to a client or clients. Managed care influences the process of service delivery by *using external reviews, developing standards of good practice,* and *emphasizing a continuum of care.*

Managed care organizations provide several types of external reviews. One review authorizes the expense of needed services for a client. For the human service professional, this means that before a service can be provided and before the professional can be reimbursed or paid, the managed care organization reviews the requested service. According to Goodman, Brown, and Dietz (1992), those conducting this external review ask the following questions:

- What is the problem?
- What is the proposed treatment?
- Why is the proposed treatment recommended?
- What evidence supports the proposed treatment?

A guiding principle for managed care review is to approve the lowest level of care that will meet the client's needs. In other words, if hospitalization has been recommended, the managed care reviewer asks, "Could the client also be treated in the home?" If ten weeks of therapy is recommended, the question is, "Will four weeks be adequate?" If the client needs a vocational assessment, psychological assessment, physical assessment, and a social history, managed care reviewers may recommend conducting the physical and the psychological assessment first and then determining whether the others are needed.

Another component of the external review is related to the provision of good-quality services. The previously stated set of questions is asked *prior* to service provision; questions are also asked *after* service delivery. Goodman, Brown, and Dietz (1992, p. 21) listed the questions that guide the managed care organization as it determines whether good-quality care was provided to the client.

- Is the care appropriate (i.e., clinically necessary for the condition)?
- Is the provider competent to provide that care?
- Is the care effective?
- Is the care cost effective?
- Is the care accessible?
- Is the care safe?
- Is the patient satisfied?

Other considerations surround quality of care and many of those focus on fair treatment of the client, such as the ease with which the client can access the services, the meeting of client expectations, the attention to and fair disposition of client appeals and grievances, and client satisfaction (Schafer, 1996). Satisfaction within the service delivery system extends beyond the client to families of clients and to the human service professional.

Continuous review is another way managed care interfaces with service delivery. In continuous review, there is periodic dialogue between human service providers and the managed care personnel about the status of the client and the effectiveness of the services. The purpose of this review is to identify any problems with the assessment, the treatment plan, or its implementation. Another purpose of the review is to remind those providing services of the guideline that says to provide "the right services at the right time in the right amounts, no more, no less" (Schafer, 1996, p. 2). The following case illustrates what one client experienced:

Jimmy Jones, a 14-year-old, single, white male, has recently been truant from school and was caught fighting with other students. His difficult behavior began about the time his father, with whom he has a close relationship, was diagnosed with cancer. Jimmy's doctor recommended that he see a counselor who specializes in working with adolescents to help him cope with his father's illness. After an initial visit with the counselor, ten visits are authorized by the Jones's insurance company. Part of the authorization requires the counselor to file periodic progress reports. After the tenth visit, a review of the case will determine whether additional visits will be authorized.

Managed care also affects the way we think about and deliver services to specific client populations. Because managed care emphasizes appropriate services for clients and matching services to specific outcomes, both managed care personnel and human service professionals are working to develop *standards of best practice* for meeting specific client needs. In the past, human service professionals have had great difficulty stating clearly the appropriate services for addressing the needs of their clients—needs that stem from poverty, unemployment, illiteracy, juvenile delinquency, child abuse, and other difficulties. Further complicating the task of developing standards is the complexity and large number of problems that many clients face.

Examples of standards of best practice are provided by Barker (1996), referring to best practices in child welfare. For issues of access, he suggests that the current system is based on voluntary access, and that system does not always reach those who need care. The best practice would be good preventive and crisis services with access to all who are in need. The way managed care would be responsive to best practice would be to have a single point of entry to all who have needs and to provide services immediately after access. As you can see from this example, the standard of best practice is high, and in many cases, it is different from what is available for clients now.

Within the framework of standards of best practice and managed care, professionals are now being asked to specify their outcomes, relate those outcomes to services, and provide the services as efficiently and effectively as possible. Because resources are limited, managed care organizations suggest that only a few outcomes should be attempted and all services should be tied to outcomes. This limitation means that helpers may not be able to address all the needs of their clients. They must set and then focus on priorities. An example of the specific standard of practice is described in the following box, which describes a short-term, computer-based therapy, *Therapeutic Learning Program,* by explaining the focus of each session and the session's goals.

This therapy meets very specific needs and was developed to help "patients define a specific problem, propose an active solution and resolve their conflicts about taking action" (Gould, 1992, p. 351). The program focuses on three questions:

Therapeutic Learning Program (TLP) Session Goals

Session 1: Identifying stress-related problems, conflicts, and symptoms
- a. to identify sources of stress and ineffective responses
- b. to sort out stressful issues from developmental stress problems
- c. to prioritize one clearly stated stress problem that calls for some action

Session 2: Clarifying goals and focusing on action
- a. to identify the developmental goal that addresses the adaptational demand
- b. to clarify and define the action or behavior change that is necessary
- c. to build an action intention that represents the recovery of the underdeveloped function

Session 3: Thinking through the consequences of taking action
- a. to distinguish realistic dangers from exaggerated dangers
- b. to isolate and expose the fears as predictions confused with memories
- c. to reach a conscious cost-benefit positive decision about the intended action

Session 4: Uncovering hidden motives and fears of failure and success
- a. to clarify that certain strongly felt fears are not objective dangers
- b. to weaken the hold of irrational fears
- c. to learn to identify thinking errors as a useful concept
- d. to distinguish between healthy and unhealthy motives
- e. to demonstrate that fears of failure and success rarely point to real dangers

Session 5: Exploring anger and guilt as obstacles to action
- a. to clarify that certain strong anxiety feelings are not indicative of external dangers
- b. to demonstrate that angry feelings are controllable by rational considerations
- c. to demonstrate that the feeling of guilt is information that can be processed to clarify values
- d. to continue to confirm that the intended action is safe and doable

Session 6: Confronting issues of self-esteem
- a. to identify and acknowledge self-esteem sensitivities
- b. to begin to accept the universality and mystery of these sensitivities

(continued)

(continued)

c. to entertain the thought that this powerful inner voice represents a historical fiction
d. to understand that the self-esteem sensitivity is the biggest block to resolving the developmental conflict

Session 7: Examining old and detrimental patterns of behavior

a. to identify the deepest vulnerability that is being challenged by the action intention
b. to see how the self-doubt triggers the ineffective protective behavior
c. to examine and demonstrate how the self-doubt system feeds itself
d. to begin to challenge the automatic response

Session 8: Understanding the history of self-doubts

a. to expose the illusion of permanent damage
b. to see that responses to early events were limited and naturally protective
c. to see that these early protective behaviors were automatic responses to feeling inadequate
d. to view the self-doubt as an initial response to events by the immature mind

Session 9: Analyzing a current incident involving the self-doubt

a. to demonstrate and diminish self-fulfilling prophecies
b. to identify the erroneous thinking that currently feeds the powerful self-doubt
c. to understand that feeding the doubt by misinterpretation is a choice, not a necessity
d. to recognize that to continue to do this is to avoid growth

Session 10: Evaluating the changes experienced during the course

a. to see that fears are to be overcome and not submitted to
b. to see the action intention as part of ongoing recovery of function
c. to understand that recovery of function and individuation are necessary
d. to consolidate new views of reality

SOURCE: From "Adult Developmental Brief Computer-Assisted Therapy," by P. L. Gould, 1992, in J. L. Feldman and R. J. Fitzpatrick (Eds.), *Managed Mental Healthcare* (pp. 347–358). Washington, DC: American Psychiatric Press. Reprinted by permission.

- What is hurting you and how can you help yourself?
- Would the action you propose be a smart and safe one?
- What serious concerns do you have that keep you from acting?

At the conclusion of the ten sessions, clients are asked whether they can answer the three preceding questions. This is one example of focusing the service and then linking the service received to specific outcomes.

Another important concept for delivering human services within the managed care environment is *continuum of care.* During the assessment phase of the helping process, human service professionals and clients work together to identify the problems, assess their severity or seriousness, and decide on the type of treatment that is needed. Type of treatment includes a decision about the level or continuum of care. In the philosophy of managed care, an assessment should determine the intensity of care to be delivered to the client, and clients should not be given more treatment than they need. The level of care needed should also be continually reviewed, and client treatment should be moved along a continuum from more intense to less intense when appropriate. Of course, there are times when clients will require more elaborate interventions and will move from less intense to more intense care.

An abbreviated continuum of care for children and adolescents is presented in Table 3-2. Note in the left column that there is intensive treatment, inpatient/acute psychiatric care. This level of treatment is appropriate when children and youth need constant supervision, medical intervention, and therapy. Many times clients receive these services when there is a probable threat of violence to self or others. At the other end of the continuum is home-based therapy, which is appropriate when children and youth are in troubled situations that can be addressed with brief, short-term interventions.

As you can see, managed care is influencing the way human services are delivered by introducing or emphasizing such concepts as external review, standards of best practice, and continuum of care. These in turn affect the way human service professionals do their work.

Managed Care and the Human Service Professional

Managed care has affected the daily work of the human service professional, especially in providing direct service. This interaction has required a shift in the roles and responsibilities of the professional in five ways: an emphasis on case management responsibilities, increasing demands for documentation, growing use of gatekeepers, expansion of resolution-focused helping strategies, and continuing importance of confidentiality and providing high-quality services.

Today, more human service professionals than ever are using case management in providing services to their clients. With an emphasis on cost-effective service delivery, coordination of care through a case manager has emerged as a method to better ensure efficiency and high-quality service. The purpose of case management, discussed in Chapter 1, is to oversee the comprehensive care of a client. It can include assessment; planning, coordinating and monitoring of

TABLE 3-2 ✦ CONTINUUM OF CARE

Inpatient/acute psychiatric care	*Residential treatment*	*Partial hospitalization*	*Therapeutic respite care emergency shelter*	*Therapeutic foster care*	*Outpatient treatment*
• Suicidal attempts, threats, or ideation, with a plan and the likelihood of carrying out the threat, need for continued observation to prevent any at-risk behaviors. • Assaultive, aggressive, or self-destructive behavior, with the likelihood of harm to self or others. Need for continued observation to limit behavior and protect self or others. • Crisis stabilization with intensive individual, family, group therapy, and/or appropriate medication therapy.	• Client requires full 24-hour daily supervised care and treatment; not functioning adequately enough to benefit from treatment while living at home or alternative living situation. • Significant dysfunction in family or interpersonal relationships and/or in the school or community setting. • Not an imminent suicide risk, not physically abusive to self or others. • Not destructive toward other people or propriety. • Not a high-elopement risk (for unlocked programs).	• Client has symptoms and/or behavioral manifestations of such severity that there is a significant interference with social, family, and/or educational functions. • Client does not present significant danger to self or others, such as imminent suicidal risk, assaultive or homicidal behaviors, severe disorganization or disorientation, extreme impulsivity, severe uncontrolled substance abuse or acting-out behavior. • Client is not a high-elopement risk.	• Client required supervision and out-of-home placement due to an emergency situation or crisis in the family. • Client has a history of physical, emotional, and/or sexual abuse. • Client is experiencing mild or moderate emotional problems. • Client may be aggressive and oppositional but is able to respond to external control and structure of 24-hour program. • Client has not been successful with previous out-of-home placements.	• Client is in need of services more intensive than outpatient treatment, but less intensive than the level of care provided by partial hospitalization, or 24-hour residential or hospital treatment. • Client has a DSM Axis I diagnosis, with a history of neglect and abuse. • Client requires 24-hour supervision and support which the family is unable to provide. • Client presents mild to moderate risk of harm to self or others, with the need for observation and monitoring.	• Diagnostic evaluation establishes the presence of behavioral/emotional problems amenable to outpatient problem-focused psychotherapy. • Client's symptoms warrant a DMS Axis I diagnosis. • Client does not demonstrate problems of sufficient severity to warrant more intensive treatment. • Degree of danger to self or others is judged to be manageable. • Family is willing to participate in child's treatment plan.

SOURCE: From "The Management of Information," by B. Webb (1996), presentation conducted at the Managed Care Institute—Futurecare: Preparing for Managed Care and Children's Services, Nashville, Tennessee. Reprinted by permission.

treatment; and evaluation. The human service literature describes two types of case managers. One is a case manager in a human service organization who assumes many of the responsibilities described above, the other works for a managed care organization. The following examples illustrate their different responsibilities.

Chris Bachman, a rehabilitation counselor, has a caseload of 70 clients. Chris works with each client to develop a plan of services, some delivered by Chris himself, but most provided by professionals at other agencies. Chris monitors the delivery of services, authorizes payment on behalf of his agency, and evaluates with the client the services received. Tasha Jones is a case manager who works for Healthcare, Inc., a managed care organization that has clients in five counties. Her major responsibilities include external utilization review and resource allocation. Her contact with human service professionals like Chris Bachman is through applications, forms, or phone calls. She has never met a client or a human service professional in person.

As more services are regulated and directed by managed care organizations, the need for the services of both types of case managers will grow.

Another influence of managed care is the increased documentation associated with service delivery. The workload for many human service professionals has doubled as they use the managed care external review process. A request for services can include an initial assessment, a detailed description of the client's problem, a treatment plan, a periodic assessment of the implementation of the plan and status of outcomes, requests for reimbursement, and termination of clients. Often the documentation required for the managed care process is different from that required by the agency. Thus, unless the managed care organization has established the same information system as the organization, the professional may have two systems of documentation to maintain.

Another change that has emerged is an elaborate gatekeeping function for initial screening of clients. Gatekeeping in the managed care system, especially in the area of mental health, is a method used to control access to services. Often, to receive mental health services, clients must have a referral from a physician. The purpose of this physician referral is to decrease the utilization of mental health services, but the result has been to increase the client load of the physician who must sign the referrals (Schneider-Braus, 1992). Gatekeeping also occurs when a special service, not considered part of the "standard of good practice," is needed or recommended. The client is not free to take the initiative to seek that service but must have the permission of and referral from the primary caretaker—in most cases, the physician. The introduction of the gatekeeper to mental health services places hardships on both the client and the human service professional. Clients see this visit to the physician as a barrier to getting services, and they often encounter physicians who are not sympathetic to their nonmedical problems. Sometimes they must wait to see the physician, and this wait delays their receiving the mental health services they need. For human service professionals, the gatekeeper is another layer of bureaucracy between them and their clients. On a positive note, however, many of these professionals are working with the gatekeeper physicians to help them understand the mental health needs of their clients.

Another influence of managed care is the need to develop resolution-focused helping strategies that are limited in time and in scope. This brief counseling type of intervention focuses on reaching specific outcomes in a relatively short period of time. Because resolution-focused helping is becoming a viable way of providing treatment, this method of helping is described in detail later in the chapter.

Several legal and ethical issues, such as confidentiality, have emerged from the interface of managed care and human service delivery. Much of the information that is transferred to managed care organizations is sensitive and provided in confidence by the client. Human service professionals worry about who will see the information on clients that is transmitted to the managed care organization. They are also concerned about how the information will be used and how it will be stored. Most human service professionals understand well the importance of confidentiality of information, but they know little about the commitment to confidentiality of staff in managed care organizations.

Another concern that human service professionals have about the managed care system and its influence on service delivery is the impact on quality. One purpose of managed care is to contain costs, and professionals believe that this focus can lead managed care organizations to sacrifice quality in their services to clients. Those outside the managed care organization worry that these for-profit companies have financial gain as their primary goal. Human service professionals have expressed specific complaints about quality that include insufficient mental health treatment, insufficient reimbursement, rejection of justifications for services, and a resistance to approve treatment. They are concerned that specific populations, such as the elderly and the poor, receive less than acceptable care. They also have doubts about the professional qualifications of case managers in the managed care setting, especially when these professionals are conducting the external review and approving service delivery.

Many in the human service sector recognize the problems with managed care but also concede that it is now part of service delivery. If the problems are to be addressed to improve the quality of client care, human service professionals need to create a partnership with managed care organizations. The following strategies may help accomplish this goal:

- Human service organizations can hire consultants to help them work with managed care organizations.
- Human service professionals can contract directly with case management organizations to provide services.
- Human service professionals can work with managed care organizations to document client problems and possible options of treatment to help them define standards of best practice.

- Human service workers can learn more about the world of managed care, its language and business practices.

As discussed earlier, the broader use of resolution-focused helping has been a direct result of the growth of managed care. The following section explores this type of intervention and its use in the human services.

Resolution-Focused Helping

In response to declining resources and the pressure from managed care to provide more effective service delivery, a new framework for human service delivery has emerged. This method approaches the helping process from three perspectives: (1) making an immediate difference in the client's life, (2) targeting behaviors that need to be changed and facilitating those changes, and (3) helping clients make new choices about how to behave and think. Those who advocate the use of resolution-focused helping methods believe that professionals should use the best of what works to meet client needs more quickly. A key concept to remember is that help is delivered in a short period of time.

Resolution-focused helping has a long history in human services, especially in the area of crisis intervention. Several principles guide crisis intervention: clients receive help immediately after a crisis event; the help is time bound; a referral may be necessary if clients do not recover quickly or need long-term care. Today, with the advent of managed care, all areas of human service delivery are feeling pressure to adapt these principles to meet client needs as quickly as possible. Because every dollar must be well spent and must be linked to specific outcomes, human service professionals are beginning to use a resolution-focused model that defines a few specific problems, establishes outcomes, and develops and implements a short-term treatment plan. Many times this means only one session with the client, especially those who are mentally healthy. For others with more serious problems, such as chemical dependence, resolution-focused services may be extended to as many as 20 sessions.

One way to gain a better understanding of resolution-focused helping is to review the assumptions on which the method is based. According to Littrell (1996), these assumptions include the following:

- Clients are able to change quickly.
- To facilitate change, clients can use their own strengths and the supports that exist within their external environment.
- Clients want to solve their own problems and want some help when they cannot do this by themselves.

To achieve positive results in resolution-focused helping, the human service professional develops conditions that encourage clients to share their concerns and to take risks to promote change. These are conditions of trust, warmth, empathy, and genuineness that are discussed in Chapter 7. These are the same conditions used to establish relationships within the traditional helping model. Rapport and relationship with the client must be established very quickly and is critical to the success of the helping interaction, even if it is brief.

Action is central to resolution-focused helping. The resolution-focused helping model enables the client and the human service professional to target fairly quickly both the behavior and the thinking that are required for the client to change. The action within this model occurs as the professional actually has the client "do" something, and very often the client has a task or homework to complete. The task is very concrete and detail oriented, and it is always linked to the goals the client and human service professional have identified.

Using the resolution-focused model, the helper focuses on the strengths of the client and the positive interactions the client has with his or her own environment. One way to focus on strengths is to identify the behaviors and thinking that are working for the client at present. Describing the supportive aspects of the client's environment is also important. This information is used to determine how the change that is to be made can be supported by both the client and the environment.

The interaction between the client and the human service professional is time limited. Sometimes there is only one session from a duration of 10 minutes to an hour. Other resolution-focused helping includes 20 sessions, especially when the problems presented are more complex or require more detailed homework. There is little opportunity for interaction that does not focus on the purpose of the session and the way to reach the identified outcomes.

A five-stage process in resolution-focused helping assists clients in problem solving in a short period of time (Budman & Gurman, 1988; Littrell, 1996). In the first stage, developing a clear description of the problem, the client and the human service professional determine the nature of the problem, and the client is asked to state the problem in one sentence.

In the second stage, the helper and the client determine what has worked for the client in the past and what strengths the client and the client's environment have. This step allows the client to reflect on successes and brings a positive focus to the discussion. The client has the opportunity to assess how much he or she already knows about the problem and to generate possible solutions.

In the third stage, the human service professional and the client determine the goal and the outcomes directly related to it. For resolution-focused helping to be effective, the outcome must be within the client's control and must work for the client in the environment in which he or she lives and works. It is stated in positive, concrete, manageable terms.

As the client and the human service professional work through stage four, the client commits to the goal and the human service professional assigns tasks to help the client reach the goal. The helper also provides motivation and support to the client for actually changing behavior and thinking. The worker can do this by complimenting the client for working on change, by assigning tasks that help the client reach the goal, and by allowing him or her to practice the tasks before leaving the session.

The final stage is evaluation or actually matching the results of the work in phase four with the predetermined outcomes. During this time, the human service worker and the client review the goals and the previously defined outcomes and decide whether these outcomes have been reached.

Here's how Linda Raphael moves through the five stages as she deals with the problem of being taken advantage of by her boss:

Linda Raphael describes a situation that happened in her office earlier this morning. "I came to work on Monday morning and my boss told me we had this project to complete. She wants me to work all week, day and night, until the report is put in the mail. The problem is that I am a single parent and cannot stay during the evening to work. I also get paid for 40 hours a week and there is no overtime available. . . . This is not the first time that this has happened." She says the boss's behavior is representative of other times when she feels she has been taken advantage of and is angry for not standing up for herself.

Using resolution-focused counseling, how would Rosa Sims, a human service professional, work with Linda Raphael?

STAGE 1: DEVELOPING A CLEAR DESCRIPTION OF THE PROBLEM

Ms. Sims and Ms. Raphael together discuss the problem presented.

Ms. Raphael defines the problem in one sentence: "I do not stand up to my boss when she makes unreasonable demands."

STAGE 2: PAST SUCCESSES AND PRESENT STRENGTHS

Ms. Sims and Ms. Raphael discuss together past successes and present strengths of Ms. Raphael.

According to Ms. Raphael, past successes included confronting her ex-husband when he was abusing her daughter, taking flawed merchandise back to a store, and telling her best friend that she did not want to answer some of the friend's questions relating to Ms. Raphael's private life. She suggests that her strengths are her ability to get along with people, her willingness to work hard, and her commitment to doing things well. But she adds very quickly that she is really scared of her boss and that she cannot afford to lose her job. Ms. Raphael says she does not know very much about the project to be completed. There are really two problems: her boss's demands about the current project and the consistent demeaning way her boss treats her. She does know that this report is very important to her boss and that if the report is turned in on time and done well, her boss may be considered for a promotion.

Stage 3: Formulating Goals and Outcomes

Ms. Sims uses humor to help Ms. Raphael relax a bit and think about the goals she has for this problem. Ms. Raphael finally decides that right now she cannot focus on her long-term relationship with her boss, that she really wants to focus on how to help her boss complete the report and still have time in the evenings to be with her daughter. Her goal is to help her boss and still be able to care for her child.

Stage 4: Strategies for Goal Attainment

Ms. Sims suggests that Ms. Raphael can write out what she plans to say and then practice it right here and now. She lists several ideas that she wants to get across to her boss.

I need to talk with you and I need for you to listen to me.

I know this report is really important to you.

It is important to me, too, because I want it to be completed on time and to be a high-quality product.

I have to take care of my daughter at night, so I will not be able to work on the report in the evenings.

I can come to work one hour early and stay one hour late.

If you don't think we can complete the work in that time, maybe I can help you think about ways we can get some additional help for the office.

I have several ideas and would like to share them with you.

Ms. Sims and Ms. Raphael role-play this discussion. The first time, Ms. Raphael reverses her role and she is the boss while Ms. Sims assumes the role of Ms. Raphael. They practice and then switch roles.

Stage 5: Evaluation

There are two parts to the evaluation process. Ms. Sims asks Ms. Raphael to review her definition of the problem, her strengths, and the proposed solutions. Together they critique the plan and make changes. Ms. Sims also discusses ways Ms. Raphael can objectively critique her discussion with her boss after it has occurred. Ms. Raphael is encouraged to return for one more session if she needs more feedback and support.

Three applications seem to be appropriate for resolution-focused helping (Talmon, 1990). The first is in addressing a specific problem that can be easily identified. Clients can state clearly what the problem is, and the client and the human service professional immediately focus on the issue as defined by the client. The second application is with a mentally healthy client—that is, someone "who is experiencing normal emotional pain when facing a difficult developmental step (e.g., puberty or mid-life crisis), a significant life trauma/change, or a problematic interpersonal relationship. Without intervention, the individual will probably cope with the problem and tolerate the pain" (Schneider-Braus, 1992, p. 129). The third application is in using resolution-focused helping as a way to access the larger human service delivery system. This use is for clients who need to be referred to other sources, the worker helps the client determine the sources that are relevant.

Because resolution-focused helping is becoming a necessary tool for human services that are delivered within the managed care environment, its use is being expanded. It now appears in treatment for chemical dependence, in children and youth services, and in mental health services. The model is continuing to be developed to serve these populations, and future human service professionals will learn to use resolution-focused therapy as new applications develop.

The Impact of Technology

Recent advances in technology are beginning to change the delivery of human services, although not without cost. Many organizations are finding the initial investment in equipment, software, and training to be quite expensive. Even so, new technologies have been introduced into the human service delivery system in the areas of communication, information management, service delivery, and professional development. Many of these areas have experienced great changes; in others, change is predicted. Administrators of services, direct service providers, and clients are all "customers" of the new computer systems that have emerged during the technology revolution. We expect growth in the creative use of technology to continue occurring at a rapid pace through the beginning of the 21st century.

The primary goal for using technology in the human service delivery system is to provide services more effectively and efficiently. Human service professionals expect that using technology will help them provide better quality services in a more cost-effective manner. As these technologies become interwoven in our lives, they will also be used simply because they represent the standard way of doing business. Next, we examine several areas where computers and other new technologies have been integrated into human service practice and delivery.

Communication

Computer technologies and the advances in satellite communications have changed the ways many interactions occur in human service delivery settings. One innovation is electronic mail (e-mail) that is used for daily interactions with colleagues, whether they are in the same building or across the state, nation, or sometimes the globe. The advantage of e-mail is convenience. When a computer is linked to an e-mail service, users can write messages on the computer and send them immediately, any time of day or night. Recipients can open messages and read them at their convenience; often, they can do this at a different computer from their own—by signing on as a guest. Any message—incoming and outgoing—can also be printed if a paper copy of the message is desired.

Much of this communication focuses on understanding procedures to help clients, seeking services, acquiring information, and sharing ideas. One example is shown in Figure 3-2, which is a printed copy of an e-mail message from a supervisor to a child care worker with information about the new guidelines for foster care that have been implemented by the state.

From: Sunger

To: Sjonas

Subject: New Policy

Message: Thanks for letting me know about your confusion on the new policy. I will contact Donald and ask him to print you a copy from the new manual that we received last week. I am sorry that I am not there to explain this to you, but you can call me here and we can also talk when I return. This new policy refers only to children who have been in foster care for over five years and that may take care of your problem altogether since your child may not apply. But in case the child has been in our system for over five years, then here is the policy or at least my interpretation of it.

Figure 3-2 ✦ An example of e-mail communication

Human service professionals can use computer technologies in other ways to communicate. Distribution lists and LISTSERVs are used when individuals with a common interest wish to talk with one another and share ideas and concerns. One such LISTSERV is the International Counselor Network (ICN) (Granello, 1995). The members in this network are continually discussing issues such as ethics, treatment, managed care, and funding. When you belong to a LISTSERV such as the ICN, you can read all messages sent between the members, but you are not committed to responding in any way. You can also actively join the dialogue at any time by just writing a response to an issue being discussed or by raising a question. Each member receives your communication and is free to answer. The entire membership receives all the communications among members. Figure 3-3 shows an example of a message similar to those sent in the ICN. More than 850 counselors received the message (Marino, 1996).

Another way human service professionals in different locations can communicate with each other over great distances is by teleconferencing. Many large organizations find this technology a cost-effective way to conduct meetings and to talk with each other about service delivery, new programming for clients, and learning new knowledge and skills. Teleconferencing is used by many state agencies to stay in touch with their local branches.

Cellular phones and "beepers" are becoming increasingly popular communication tools for administrators and those providing direct services to clients. These devices allow professionals to be available at all times; they also provide many workers security when they are in dangerous or isolated situations.

Another method of expanding communication is through the worldwide web (WWW). Through individualized web pages, many individuals and organizations can provide information to those on-line. Public and private human

Date: Mon, 18 Sep 1995 20:02:57 -0500
Reply-To: XXXXXXXXXXXXXXXXXXXXXXXXXXXXXXX
Sender: "International Counselor Network (ICN)"
<ICN@UTKVM1.BITNET>
From: XXXXXXXXXXXXXXXXXXXXXXXXXXXXXXXXXXX
Organization: XXXXXXXXXXXXXXXXXXXXXXXXXXX
Subject: Sleepwalking
X-To: ICN <icn@utkvm1.utk.edu>
To: Multiple recipients of list ICN
<ICN@UTKVM1.BITNET>

Hello, I have two students ages 8 and 9 who have come to me and said they are concerned about their sleepwalking. I do not know anything about sleepwalking, so I am asking for your help. Any information about the causes or what contributes to it would be helpful. I would also like to know the counseling issues behind sleepwalking. Do you feel a school counselor should try to help the student or should they be referred to outside sources? I work in a school where most parents could not afford outside treatment. I will appreciate any information you might have.

Figure 3-3 ✦ Example of LISTSERV message

SOURCE: Reprinted from "Counselors in Cyberspace Debate Whether Client Discussions Are Ethical," by T. W. Marino, January, 1996, *Counseling Today,* p. 18. © ACA. Reprinted with permission. No further reproduction authorized without written permission of the American Counseling Association.

service agencies can use their web pages to advertise their services. As an example, the web page for the National Organization of Human Service Education (NOHSE) is found at http://www.nohse.com; it offers much information about the organization, including links to information about its role and mission, a listing of the board of directors, information about regional organizations, and membership.

Just as technology supports better communication, it also offers an improved way of managing information. There are many ways in which computers and their software help manage information within the human service delivery system.

Information Management

With computer technology, managers can coordinate information from a variety of sources and then organize the data to facilitate planning, decision making, and reporting. Information can also be managed to support evaluation and help tie service delivery to outcomes and cost. The information entered into a human service database can include a client's name and other relevant demographic data (age, gender, race, marital status), history of use of the human service delivery system, intake information and assessment results, problem identification, treatment plans, treatment records of services provided, and evaluation of those services according to outcomes reached and client satisfaction.

In addition, in this environment of managed care, the information system may also include service costs, payment, the cost of each service delivered, and a record of the interaction with the managed care organization. The interaction record may show the kinds of services authorized by frequency, duration, and definition of the provider of the services (Webb, 1996). Table 3-3 shows the types of information in an information management system that can be used for foster care (Webb, 1996).

Another example of an information system supporting the delivery of services is an information care network established in the Netherlands (Grebel, 1993). This system coordinates the care of people with mental disabilities who reside in institutional settings. It includes data for activity planning, electronic day journals of professionals, and evaluation of care planning. In addition, financial cost of care is part of the system. The care information system was written from the perspectives of the clients and the direct care workers. Training is a critical component in the use of this system, and standards were developed for the use of the system by human service workers. The human service professionals who use this information care system are medical and paramedical staff, social workers, nurses, and other helpers such as those who coordinate day activities and therapeutic recreation.

Another advantage of a management information system is its ability to transfer information electronically from organization to organization and from worker to worker. This feature benefits both human service professionals and clients in several ways. First, the client and the professional save the time and energy that would be required to generate the data for a second or a third time. If the data represent intake information or initial assessment information, the professional can review it with the client and request additional information to ensure accuracy. Second, work can begin with the client much earlier because, in some cases, much of the information gathering is complete. Access to broad information gives the human service professional a more comprehensive review of a client's experience within the service delivery system. Human service professionals are also able to provide better service because they can coordinate their care of the client with any other current services the client is receiving.

Just as technology is becoming an effective way to support human service work using management information systems, it is also being developed to provide services to clients.

Providing Services to Clients

The services available through new models of service delivery range from computer programs that assess client knowledge or skill and recommend a plan of action to actual counseling on-line in real time. The Missouri Automated Reinforcer Assessment (MARA) is a computer program that helps determine what reinforcers will work effectively with clients in programs that use behavior

TABLE 3-3 ✦ FOSTER CARE DATA ELEMENTS

Data elements	*Categories*
1. State	**General information 1–4**
2. Report period ending date	
3. Local agency FIPS code	
4. Record number	
5. Most recent periodic review date	**Child's demographic information 5–17**
6. Date of birth	
7. Sex	
8. Race	
9. Hispanic origin	
10. Child diagnosed with disabilities	
11. Mental retardation	
12. Visually or hearing impaired	
13. Physically disabled	
14. Emotionally disturbed	
15. Other diagnosed conditions	
16. Has child ever been adopted	
17. Age of child when adopted	
18. Date of first removal from home	**Removal/placement setting indicators 18–24**
19. Total number of removals	
20. Discharge date from last episode	
21. Date of latest removal	
22. Computer-generated date	
23. Placement date in current setting	
24. # of previous settings in episode	
25. Manner of removal for episode	**Circumstances associated with removal 25–40**
26. Physical abuse	
27. Sexual abuse	
28. Neglect	
29. Parent alcohol abuse	
30. Parent drug abuse	
31. Child alcohol abuse	
32. Child drug abuse	
33. Child disability	
34. Child's behavior problem	

(continued)

TABLE 3-3 ✦ *(continued)*

Data elements	*Categories*
35. Death of parent	
36. Incarceration of parent	
37. Caretaker inability to cope	
38. Abandonment	
39. Relinquishment	
40. Inadequate housing	
41. Current placement setting	**Current placement setting 41–42**
42. Out of state placement	
43. Most recent case plan goal	**Most recent case plan goal 43**
44. Caretaker family structure	**Principal caretaker information 44–46**
45. 1st principal caretaker birth year	
46. 2nd principal caretaker birth year	
47. Date of mother's TPR	**Parental rights termination 47–56**
48. Date of father's TPR	
49. Foster family structure	
50. 1st foster caretaker's year of birth	
51. 2nd foster caretaker's year of birth	
52. 1st foster caretaker's race	
53. 1st foster caretaker's Hispanic origin	
54. 2nd foster caretaker's race	
55. 2nd foster caretaker's Hispanic origin	
56. Date of discharge from foster care	
57. Computer generated date	**Discharge date 57–58**
58. Reasons for discharge	
59. Title IV-E (foster care)	**Sources of federal financial support/assistance for child 59–65**
60. Title IV-E (adoption assistance)	
61. Title IV-a (AFDC)	
62. Title IV-D (Child Support)	
63. Title XIX (Medicaid)	
64. SSI or other social security	
65. None of the above	

SOURCE: From "The Management of Information," by B. Barker (1996), presentation conducted at the Managed Care Institute—Futurecare: Preparing for Managed Care and Children's Services, Nashville, Tennessee. Reprinted by permission.

modification (Vatterott, Callier, & Hile, 1992). This information can be used with parents, child care workers, human service professionals, or others who are working with clients for whom behavior change is targeted. The program has been used successfully with various populations, such as individuals who are developmentally delayed, young children with behavior problems, or individuals who have suffered brain trauma (Vatterott, Callier, & Hile, 1992). This and other assessment programs are only one component of the assessment process and, as such, are interpreted as they relate to the other data gathered.

Many software programs and tools are available to teach clients specific knowledge or skills to enhance their daily living or increase their vocational potential. Many of the programs are designed for clients experiencing difficulties. One such program, BUSTED, was developed to reduce antisocial behavior of youth involved in the criminal justice system. The computer game SMACK was developed for at-risk teens to help them learn the consequences of bad decisions and drug use (Oalcley, 1994; Resnick, 1994). Some programs are proactive and promote good health and wellness. One of these is BARN, a health education game designed to teach adolescents about issues ranging from AIDS to sexual awareness and body awareness (Bosworth, 1994). HealthWorks is an AIDS education program for early adolescent middle schoolers (Cahill, 1994). Both SMACK and BARN are educational tools that can be used in the schools, in child and youth programs, and in family programs.

Technology has also influenced the delivery of counseling services. In many programs, the client uses an interactive computer program, followed by a discussion with a human service professional of his or her responses. One such interactive multimedia system, developed by the Beck Institute for Cognitive Therapy and Research, computerizes cognitive therapy and is used at the Norton Psychiatric Clinic in Louisville, Kentucky ("New Interactive Multimedia System," 1995). "The program instructs patients on how to recognize maladaptive thoughts and behavior thereby reinforcing the positive aspects of therapy, such as modifying 'automatic thoughts,' generating alternative thoughts and activity scheduling. Each time the patient uses the video, a printed progress report is generated to help therapists focus on key areas of concern" (p. 44).

Counseling services and other support services are also provided on-line. This allows human service professionals to be available by electronic mail and on the worldwide web to work with individuals who are experiencing specific difficulties. One example is a "chat group" for law enforcement officers and their families, inviting those with problems to share them electronically. A second example is a teleshopping and social services effort in the United Kingdom that makes shopping available for inner-city elderly and the disabled who cannot travel to major shopping areas. Clients can place orders by computer or by phone and can arrange a place to pick up their purchases or ask that they be delivered (Cahill, 1993).

Much assistive technology is available for clients with disabilities. Its purpose is to help individuals with handicaps to "increase, maintain, or improve

Assistive Technology Defined

- Defines assistive technology device to mean any item, piece of equipment, or product, whether acquired commercially off the shelf, modified, or customized, which is used to increase, maintain, or improve functional capabilities of individuals with disabilities (same definition as is used in PL 100-407, Technology-Related Assistance for Individuals with Disabilities Act [1988]).
- Defines assistive technology service to mean any service that directly assists an individual with a disability in the selection, acquisition, or use of an assistive technology device. Such term includes
  A. The evaluation of the needs of an individual with a disability, including a functional evaluation of the individual in the individual's customary environment
  B. Purchasing, leasing, or otherwise providing for the acquisition of assistive technology devices by individuals with disabilities
  C. Selecting, designing, fitting, customizing, adapting, applying, maintaining, repairing, or replacing of assistive technology devices
  D. Coordinating and using other therapies, interventions, or services with assistive technology devices, such as those associated with existing education and rehabilitation places and programs
  E. Training or technical assistance for an individual with disabilities, or, where appropriate, the family of an individual with disabilities
  F. Training or technical assistance for professionals (including individuals providing education and rehabilitation service), employers, or other individuals who provide services to, employ, or are otherwise substantially involved in the major life functions of individuals with disabilities.

SOURCE: From *Technology, Computers, and the Special Needs Learner,* by J. Ray and K. M. Warden, 1995, Albany, NY: Delmar, p. 4. Reprinted by permission.

their functional capacities" (Ray & Warden, 1995, p. 4). The next box offers a detailed description of assistive technology as defined and mandated by Public Law 101-476. These assistive devices are being developed or being upgraded continually and the list includes devices that support individuals in their learning and in their daily living.

Assistive technology addresses needs in the areas of vision, hearing, learning, speech and language, and mobility. One example of assistive technology is technology that supports the functioning of individuals with visual impairments. Many individuals cannot read regular print and need assistive devices to help them input data into the computer. One device is Braille-to-Print with six keys of the standard keyboard used to input braille with full access to the function keys. There is also special software such as BRLkeys for the IBM that makes this adaptation possible. Additional assistive technologies translate braille to print, braille, and to voice. Software allows the input to produce a printed copy and a braille copy.

There is a portable note-taking device. "The BrailleMate (TeleSensory) combines a portable note-taking device with braille keypad, voice output, and a single refreshable braille cell output. All of these devices have the capability of sorting information within the device itself or transferring the information to external disk drives, braille and print devices or other computers" (Ray & Warden, 1995, p. 114). These are only a few of the many assistive technologies available to facilitate the functioning of the visually impaired.

Technology not only facilitates the education and training of clients but is also used for the education and training of human service professionals who desire new knowledge, information, and skills to support their work with clients. Computers are also used in this area.

Professional Development

Professional development is an important aspect of lifelong learning, and technology has made it easier for human service professionals to take advantage of the latest information about populations being served as well as the knowledge and skills of emerging best practice. One way this information is available is by CD-ROM, compact disks filled with information and written texts. Most CD-ROMs of interest to the human service professional may be found in a local university or city library. One advantage of using these compact disks for research is the easy access to current information (Granello, 1995).

Another advancement in professional development is the availability of software that facilitates skill development. Programs are available to teach interviewing, problem solving, rehabilitation counseling skills, decision making, counseling, crisis counseling, organizational assessment, case management, and many other skills. Much of the software is interactive and uses simulation as the primary instructional tool. In teaching problem solving in case management, many programs use simulated cases of individuals with severe problems and difficulties. Students and practitioners are asked to identify and prioritize needs, and to choose alternatives and outcomes. Most programs provide the client's current status as well as other, more detailed information about client history (Gray, 1994).

In summary, the profession of human services is currently using technologies to improve the ways professionals communicate with each other, to expand the ways information is managed, to provide services to clients, and to engage in professional development. We predict that technology will continue to have an impact on the profession during the 21st century.

✧ Things to Remember

1. Human services are delivered to populations in a variety of settings, including industry, the military, schools, and other community-based settings, all of which increase the number of clients who can be reached.
2. Schools have become a site for service delivery as teachers and human service professionals share the same clients.
3. The trend toward providing more services in community-based settings and less in institutional ones is helping to serve clients in the least-restrictive environment.
4. Community-based services were first used with clients with mental illness who were deinstitutionalized; now, populations receiving community-based services include those in the criminal justice system, the developmentally disabled, and the elderly.
5. As technological advances draw the world closer together, we become more aware of the human service challenges in an international context that includes many individuals and families in war-torn areas, living in a disruptive and life-threatening environment.
6. In the international context, many individuals live in large cities in poor countries where they struggle to meet basic needs and have little access to housing, sanitation, and nutritious food.
7. The increased use of managed care organizations is dramatically changing the delivery of human services through the use of external reviews, the demand to develop standards of best practice, the need for better information management, and an emphasis on a continuum of care.
8. Managed care standards, developed for accountability in health and human services, can be summarized as "providing the right services at the right time in the right amounts, no more, no less" (Schafer, 1996, p. 2).
9. Resolution-focused intervention has emerged as a way to help clients change in a brief period of time.
10. Resolution-focused helping is represented by a five-stage process: developing a clear description of the problem; acknowledging the client's past successes and present strengths; formulating goals and outcomes; developing strategies for goal attainment; and evaluation.
11. Technology has begun to change the way human service professionals meet their responsibilities, particularly in the areas of communication, information management, service provision, and professional development.
12. Communication avenues used by human service professionals include electronic mail, LISTSERVs, the worldwide web, cellular phones, and teleconferencing.
13. Computer technology is available to help human service professionals manage information and use data to make decisions about planning programs, establishing costs, and reporting.

14. Technology is being effectively used to provide services to clients, including diagnosing and assessing, teaching new skills, and assisting those with disabilities or impairments.

Additional Readings: New Trends

Desjarlais, R., Eisenberg, L., Good, B., & Kleinman, A. (1995). *World mental health: Problems and priorities in low-income countries.* New York: Oxford University Press.

This report issues a call to action for individuals, communities, governments, and international agencies to take steps to stem the growing personal and social burdens due to mental illness and behavioral problems worldwide.

Leiderman, M., Guzetta, C., Struminger, L., & Monnickendaen, K. (Eds.). (1993). *Technology in people services: Research, theory, and applications.* New York: Haworth.

This book describes the many uses of technology in the human services. It discusses the future of technology and human services, ethical issues, and practical applications.

Mullahy, C. M. (1995). *The case manager's handbook.* Gaithersburg, MD: Aspen Publishers.

The author, believing that case management today is a rapidly growing service with a collaborative rather than competitive nature, has written a handbook that defines case management, examines the process, and presents practical procedural information.

Naisbitt, J., & Aburdene, P. (1990). *Megatrends 2000: Ten new directions for the 1990s.* New York: Avon Books.

This book identifies and describes the most important trends of the 1990s, the last decade before the millennium.

Chapter 4

Models of Human Service Delivery

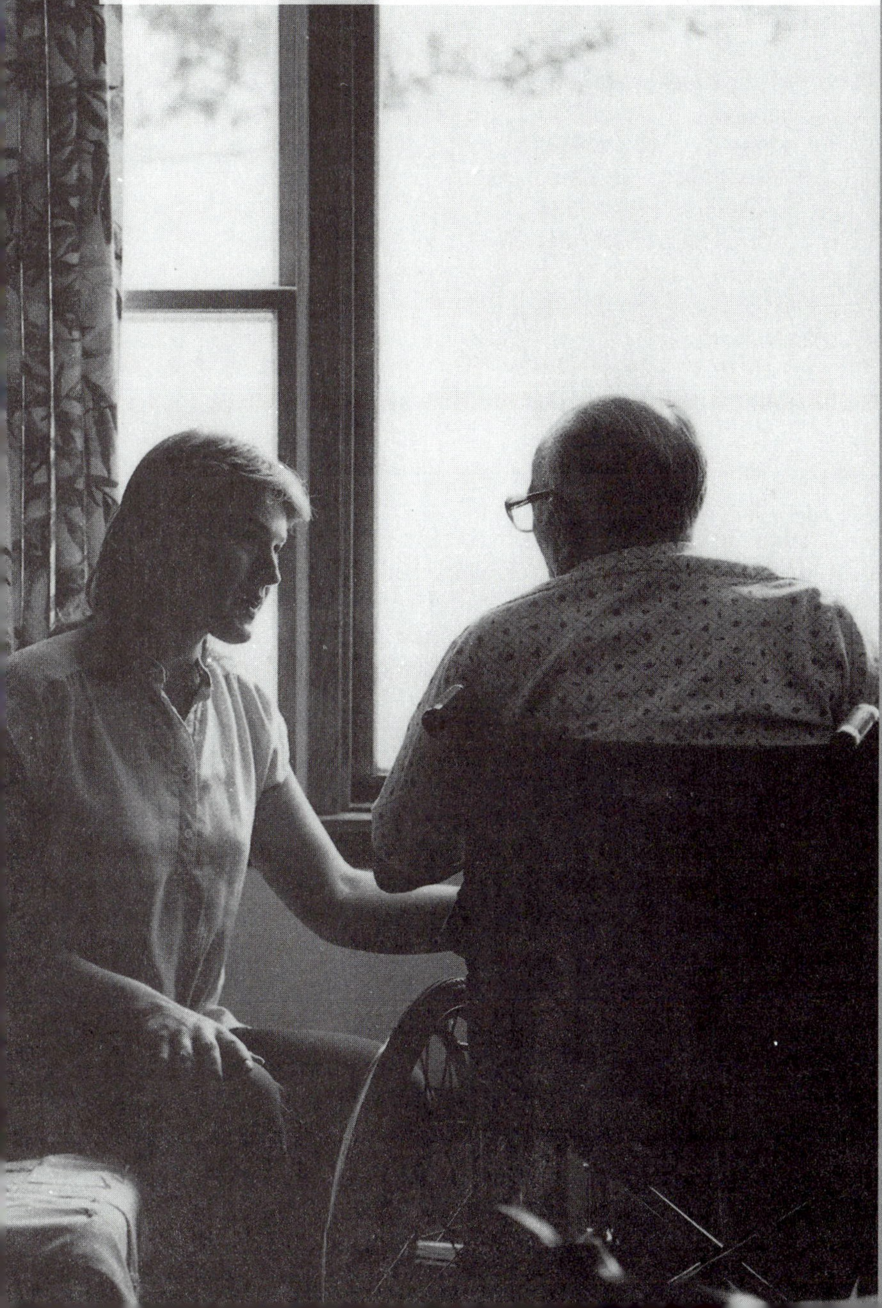

In developing a definition of human services, we have discussed its various characterizations, briefly traced the history of service provision, and explored 20th-century development, emphasizing human services today. Another approach to defining human services is to examine the way it benefits service recipients. This chapter describes three models that represent different orientations in service delivery: the medical model, the public health model, and the human service model.

All three models are used to deliver services today; some agencies may prefer one over the others, and one model may be more effective than the other two in some situations. Workers may be skilled in following one particular model, but you are likely to be working closely with practitioners who follow the other models. Therefore, you should know the characteristics of each model, its historical development, and how it is used. To help translate this information into human service practice, we examine a relevant social problem from the perspective of each model.

Introduction

Each of the three models of service delivery has certain philosophical assumptions that guide its practice. These assumptions reflect beliefs about the causes of problems, their treatment, and the role of the professional in the model. To illustrate, we can consider the nature of mental disorders from the perspective of each of the three models.

The medical model is based on an orientation developed by the medical profession; it assumes that mental disorders are diseases or illnesses that impair an individual's ability to function. The disease or illness, in this case the mental disorder, has an organic basis and responds to medical interventions such as medication, laboratory studies, and physical therapies. Often, the individual, called a *patient,* receives treatment from a physician in a hospital or medical clinic.

The public health model resembles the medical model in its diagnosis and treatment process, but the models differ in recipients of services and methodologies of treatment. Whereas the medical model emphasizes individuals, the public health model focuses on *groups* in the population, who may be identified by geography (community, country, region, or state), types of problems (abuse, poverty, specific illnesses), or specific characteristics such as age (children, the elderly). This model views mental disorders as the result of malfunctions or pressures created by the environment or by society. The mental disorder is evaluated for its impact not only on the individual but also on society at large. In addition to treating the individual, this model emphasizes preventing the problem through supporting activities such as use of films, speakers, school programs, and pamphlets, all aimed at educating the population about the problem.

The human service model is concerned with the interaction between the individual and the environment, it stresses the need for balance between the two. Although recognizing both the medical and the public health perspectives, this model focuses on the interpersonal and environmental conflicts that may result from the problem (in this case, a mental disorder). Perhaps the individual (called a *client* or *consumer)* has problems resulting from genetic predispositions, biochemical imbalances, faulty learning, lack of insight into behavior that may be inappropriate, a physical or mental disability, and/or influences from the social environment. Whatever the situation, the client is experiencing interpersonal and emotional difficulties that affect his or her behavior. Treatment in this model encompasses services to both the individual and the environment through work with the client as well as the people and the institutions with which the client is involved. Each model provides a different perspective on the same problem. We next look at the development of each one.

The Medical Model

Definition

The medical model sees the person coming for help as an individual whose problem is a disease or a sickness. The individual is "sick" or "ill," not healthy. Often called *patients,* these individuals depend on the physician or service provider to prescribe a treatment or cure for the "disease." This model can be summarized as a system that involves the following elements: symptom–diagnosis–treatment–cure (Reinhard, 1986).

The medical model, with a history that includes shamans, medicine men and women, and witch doctors, is perhaps the oldest of all treatment models. In fact, other models used it as they were developing. For example, Chapter 2 had a discussion of the beginning of the new profession of social work at the turn of the 20th century. Mary Richmond, author of *Social Diagnosis* (1917), used the medical model to describe social casework. Believing that the presenting problem was rooted in the individual, she suggested that pauperism was a disease. The friendly visitor, therefore, became a social physician whose duty was to heal the complex conditions of poverty (Zimbalist, 1977).

The corrections field also adopted the medical model during the 1930s, when its emphasis shifted from punishment to treatment. The change was based on the assumption that "criminal behavior is caused by biological or social conditions that require treatment" (Clear & Cole, 1990, p. 87). Theoretically, prisons were to become therapeutic communities, where inmates would be rehabilitated to reenter society. Unfortunately, budget constraints limited this change to one of name only; departments of prisons became "departments of corrections," but punishment continued to be the reality. Structurally, the system already included parole, probation, and the indeterminate sentence. All that remained to complete the incorporation of the medical model was the addition of a classification system to aid in diagnosis and treatment (Clear & Cole, 1990).

History

As mentioned in Chapter 2, institutions developed as a way to meet the needs of some segments of society. Asylums were established primarily to care for persons with mental illness, shifting care from the local community to rural institutions and replacing local financing with state funding. Responsibility for the care of persons with mental illness rested with the medical profession.

Psychiatry emerged as a discipline at the end of the 18th century when Philippe Pinel became head of the Hospice de Bicetre and later of Salpetriere (mental institutions in France). Some mental disorders had been recognized as such early on, but Pinel's removal of chains from patients and other humane acts emphasized the belief that pathological behavioral disorders had organic origins and that their treatment belonged to medicine. Accordingly, those

INTERNATIONAL FOCUS
Models of Service Design

Howard N. Higginbotham (1979) suggests three basic models of service design today: traditional psychiatry, the public health approach, and the village system.

The first model, traditional psychiatry, is similar to North American or European psychiatry, which has not been modified for use in non-Western settings. This model emphasizes residential facilities; the individuals who need these services must therefore leave their homes to get treatment. Unfortunately, long-term confinement often results. Treatment within such facilities varies from custodial management to programs of work "therapy," which may take the form of farming, sewing, or daily chores around the hospital. Programs of psychotropic medication and electroconvulsive shock (ECT) are often followed in the cases of new admissions and chronic patients. Less prevalent as a treatment modality is one-to-one psychotherapy.

The second model is a public health approach to services. In developing countries, this approach is characterized by its emphasis on primary prevention and the training of paraprofessionals. Consultation and educational activities are provided so as to maximize the utilization of resources. Maintaining the patient outside the hospital, by mobilizing and coordinating community resources, is also characteristic of this approach.

The third approach, the village system, developed as a response to frustrations in attempting to establish facilities based on Western models in areas such as Africa. In this system, patients live with relatives who reside near mental clinics. Treatment in the village system incorporates the use of native healers, therapeutic relationships, psychotropic drugs, and the natural therapeutic elements of the village, which include confession, dancing, and rituals.

SOURCE: Adapted by permission from "Culture and Mental Services," by Howard N. Higginbotham. In Anthony J. Marsella, Roland G. Tharp, and Thomas Ciborowski (Eds.), *Perspectives on Cross-Cultural Psychology*, pp. 205–236. Copyright © 1979 by Academic Press.

diagnosed as mentally ill were to be treated as patients by physicians in hospital settings, just like other patients with medical problems. Pinel, hoping to create a science of mental disease, is credited with introducing the medical model into psychiatry by stressing the clinical diagnosis and appropriate medical treatment.

Until the end of the 19th century, insanity was socially defined: "An insane was a person whose behavior for pathological reasons was so disturbed that he had to be segregated in special institutions" (Pichot, 1985, p. 10). With the emergence of psychiatry as a medical specialty, a body of knowledge was established to explain the nature and causes of insanity. The discovery and application of the most effective treatments became a priority. Insanity became medically defined, meaning that the institution of treatment had to be a hospital instead of a prison, and the care of the patient would be handled by a physician, not a warden.

Philippe Pinel

Philippe Pinel (1745–1826) is famous in the history of medicine and mental health. In revolutionary France, Pinel courageously campaigned to secure a new status for persons with mental illness as people suffering from disease rather than being possessed by demons or manifesting the consequences of sin. Pinel argued, practiced, and taught that such persons require medical care rather than persecution or punishment, and that they are entitled to be treated with respect as persons and citizens. This was a revolutionary idea.

Pinel was born into a modest family of surgeons in southwestern France. Initially trained as a cleric and destined for service in the church, he decided to study science in Toulouse. By 1773, he had acquired a doctorate of medicine, but he continued his studies for four more years in Montpellier under Barthez. Sickness and health became his lifelong concern, and he systematically applied himself to learning all he could about medicine from ancient as well as contemporary sources. He acquired the education of a classicist and a humanist in addition to his extensive knowledge of the practice of medicine in his day. He moved to Paris in 1778 and supported himself by translating scientific and medical works and teaching mathematics. Though extremely shy, he became a member of an important group of reformers and medical thinkers called the Ideologues. Benjamin Franklin tried to convince Pinel to go to America. However, Pinel was a patriot and wished to help modernize medicine in his own country. His interest in insanity derived from the suicide of a seriously depressed friend and patient in 1783.

In 1792, apparently because of his connections with the Ideologues, Pinel was appointed Physician of the Infirmaries to the Hospice de Bicetre, a huge Parisian custodial institution for indigent ailing men. In the same year, he wrote an essay on the subject of the clinical training of doctors. This essay remained unnoticed in the Archives of the National Academy of Medicine in Paris until 1935, when it was discovered by M. Gentry, curator of the academy. Translated and published in America in 1971, it gives a remarkable view of the attitudes, values, and practices of French medicine at the end of the 18th century.

Pinel's essay on the clinical training of doctors was written at the beginning of a period, 1794–1815, which medical historian E. H. Ackerknecht terms the "period of Pinel." During this time, Pinel managed two of the major hospitals in Paris and published three significant works: *Philosophical Nosography* (1798),

After the middle of the 19th century, use of the medical model to treat mental illness dominated. By the end of the century, however, the medical model was changing. A new school of thought rejected medical treatment and advocated psychotherapy for treatment of persons with mental illness. The new philosophy was based on the assumption that diseases of the soul were completely separate from diseases of the body. Psychiatry concerned itself with the medicine of the soul; psychosis was the disease of the soul, and neurosis was

Treatise on Insanity (1801), and *Clinical Medicine* (1802). The first book would serve for years as a text for the classification of diseases; the second would lay the foundation for modem psychiatry; and the third, published in three successively enlarged editions, would spread his methodology and fame among the next generation.

In 1794, Pinel transferred to the Hospice de la Salpetriere, an institution that housed nearly 7,000 destitute women. He administered, practiced, and taught in this hospital for 30 years, applying the principles that gave him the reputation as a founder of modern psychiatry.

In medical practice, Pinel practically invented the role of the full-time resident physician who teaches and trains students, interns, and fellow researchers in a hospital ward. Along with other reformers, he argued for national curricula, standards, and diplomas for medical education. Pinel insisted that such education should be conducted in French and based on clinical practice and observations. He viewed the natural sciences as "accessories" to the practice of medicine.

With regard to mental health, Pinel is often given credit for what he learned from the uneducated but experienced and successful Keeper of the Insane at Bicetre, J. P. Pussin (1746–1811): namely, that the mental patients could be managed without cages, chains, or cruelty. Pinel brought Pussin to Salpetriere in 1802 to aid him in caring for the many unruly patients. Pinel combined Pussin's practical management principles with his own medical knowledge to develop his famous "moral method" for treating mental illness. This method assumes that mental illness is due to some imbalance in the patient, which the physician can treat and rectify. The crux of this method is extensive observation and knowledge about the patient. This knowledge makes possible detailed therapy, which the physician must carefully supervise. Pinel's approach is a far cry from bleeding, beating, purging, and imprisonment, which had been the usual methods of treating the insane.

Pinel's methods and publications made him well known, and students flocked to him. Among them were the future leaders of French medicine. Pinel's concern for humane treatment of persons with mental illness was realized in France and made that country a world leader in the enlightened treatment of mental illness. When Dorothea Dix traveled in Europe in the late 1850s, extending her great American crusade to reform in the treatment of the insane, she had only small changes to recommend to the French, and to the Turks in Constantinople who had been trained by the French.

SOURCE: Used by permission of H. Phillips Hamlin (1985).

the disease of the nerves (Pichot, 1985). Sigmund Freud's work reflected this orientation.

Early in his career, Freud was a researcher and clinician in biology and neurology; he made outstanding contributions to both fields. He used the scientific method, insisting that medical problems of mental illness be studied in the rigorous laboratory setting.

Later, Freud rejected his earlier training and revolutionized the study and treatment of mental illness. He developed a method of therapy commonly known today as the *psychoanalytic method.* In this method, the client shares all thoughts with the therapist. The therapist interprets this material to explain to patients the nature of their repressions and the influence of these repressions on their present problems. Freud also developed a theory of neurosis and a theory of the normal mind, based on the assumption that mental disorders were psychologically based. Although Freud's impact was profound, psychoanalytic theory did not completely change the medical model or become the preferred method of treatment, for several reasons. First, its success was difficult to evaluate and to document. Second, it required too much time and expense to be a viable treatment for large numbers of people.

The treatment of persons with mental illness continued to develop in the 1940s; however, more psychiatrists and improved treatment were needed. A common treatment during this decade was electroconvulsive or electroshock therapy. This treatment involved administering an electric shock of 70–130 volts to the brain, leaving the patient unconsciousness and/or in convulsions. On regaining consciousness, the patient sometimes experienced confusion and memory loss, but problem behaviors diminished after several weeks of treatments. Electroshock therapy was effective with depressed individuals, but it was used less successfully to treat other mental disorders. Its abuse during the 1960s resulted in negative perceptions of this treatment method, and these perceptions contributed to the growing popularity of psychotropic medications.

Psychotropic drugs, which act on the brain, are now among the most widely used treatments for mental disorders. Because of the prevalence of these medications, *psychopharmacology,* the study of the effects of drugs on mental health, is an area of interest to human service workers. Ponterotto (1985) suggested that familiarity with this information will help human service workers communicate with medical personnel and better understand the uses and limitations of these medications as they relate to client behavior.

Psychotropic medications can be divided into four major classes: antipsychotic drugs, antidepressant drugs, antianxiety drugs, and lithium salts. *Antipsychotic drugs* are effective in managing psychotic disorders such as bipolar disorder (colloquially known as manic depression) and schizophrenia. Although these drugs do not cure psychosis, they help to control certain psychotic behaviors such as suspiciousness, hallucinations, and impulsiveness. Haldol (haloperidol), Thorazine (chlorpromazine), Clozaril (clozapine), and Mellaril (thioridazine) are well-known examples of antipsychotic medication.

Antidepressant drugs, the second class, relieve depression. There are two kinds of antidepressant drugs: the tricyclic antidepressants and the monoamine oxidase inhibitors. Human service workers will most likely come in contact with widely used tricyclic antidepressants such as Elavil (amitriptyline) or Tofranil (imipramine). However, Prozac (fluoxetine), Paxil (paroxetine), Luvor (fluvoxamine), and Zoloft (sertraline), antidepressants unrelated to tricyclic or monoamine oxidase inhibitors, have become increasingly popular in recent years because they have fewer side effects. These drugs are selective seratonin reuptake inhibitors.

TABLE 4-1 ✦ POSSIBLE SIDE EFFECTS OF PSYCHOTROPIC MEDICATIONS

Antipsychotic drugs	*Antidepressants*	*Antianxiety drugs*	*Mood stabilizers*
Feelings of heaviness	Dry mouth	Drug tolerance	Toxic warning signs
Sluggishness	Blurred vision	Stumbling gait	(nausea, tremors,
Weakness	Constipation	Slurred speech	muscle spasms)
Faintness	Urinary retention	Drowsiness	Thyroid disorders
Drowsiness	Lowered or raised	Conjunctivitis	Renal toxicity
Dizziness	blood pressure	Dry mouth	Nausea
Tremors	Agitation	Constipation	Vomiting
Seizures	Raised temperature	Urinary problems	Diarrhea
Tardive dyskinesia	Hallucinations		Sedation
Loss of muscle tone	Convulsions		Confusion

The most widely used psychotropic medications by far are the *antianxiety drugs, sedatives, and hypnotics.* Prescribed to relieve anxiety, fear, or tension, these medications may be classed as barbiturates, benzodiazepines, or antihistamines. Benzodiazepines such as Valium (diazepam), Xanax (alprazolam), Tranxene (clorazepate), and Librium (chlordiazepoxide) are especially popular, because they reduce anxiety without reducing overall performance.

The final class of psychotropic medication is *mood stabilizers.* They include lithium carbonate, calcium channel blockers (Calan, Isoptin), and anticonvulsants (Tegretol, Epitol). Used primarily in the treatment of bipolar disorder, these drugs are particularly effective in preventing the mania state, which is characterized by symptoms of extreme irritability, talkativeness, grandiose ideas, exaggerated self-esteem, and increased involvement in risky activities such as spending sprees or reckless driving.

Psychotropic medications have revolutionized mental health by facilitating deinstitutionalization, but the effects have not always been positive. For example, critics say that antianxiety drugs mask symptoms so that individuals avoid dealing with the real problem. Individuals who take major tranquilizers over a long period of time may suffer dangerous side effects. Tardive dyskinesia, a neurological disorder characterized by abnormal, involuntary mouth or tongue movements, is one such side effect. Table 4-1 lists other common side effects of the four major categories.

Today, those delivering services in the medical model face a number of challenges. One is that the symptom–diagnosis–treatment–cure process more realistically leads to cure *or* control. Particularly with psychiatric illnesses, controlling the illness and making the patient functional are the guides for treatment. Complicating this issue are the numerous new drugs that appear with frequency. There are now many drugs that do not fit neatly into the four categories of psychotropic drugs just described. For example, the new seratonin drugs (Prozac, Paxil, and Zoloft), which don't fit one category, are broadly prescribed today to treat bulimia, obsessive-compulsive disorders, and anxiety disorders.

A second challenge is determining who controls medical services. Is it the physician, the patient, insurers or managed care organizations, employers, and/or the government? To varying degrees, all seem to have a role. For example, the intrusions of government become greater each year. Although it is sometimes difficult medically to separate the organic and psychiatric states, it has happened at some state government levels; that is, diagnosis and reimbursement guidelines have differentiated physical and mental conditions. A second example is the impact of managed care discussed in Chapter 3. Typically, in a managed system, physicians receive a fixed amount per patient to take care of medical problems. A small part of the capitation fee is for behavioral health care. Once again, physicians are faced with an arbitrary separation between physical and psychiatric conditions. They also grapple daily with wanting to do the right thing but at the same time contain costs. Achieving this balance is difficult when physicians attend to the "whole" patient, which includes a consideration of the patient's environment and social circumstances.

The past 30 years have demystified psychiatric illness and its acceptance is widespread. The future may include new perspectives. One may be an awareness that we treat mild disease too aggressively. A second perspective is that in some cases it is society that is malfunctional, not the individual—that is, society places people in situations that are not normal but expects them not to behave abnormally. For example, think about the malfunctional mother who has a full-time job as well as responsibility for the home and the children. The problem may not be that she is malfunctional but that society's expectations are unrealistic.

Case Studies

One obvious example of the medical model's application to human service problems is its use in treating mental illness. Two illustrative case studies follow. The case of Robert Smith describes the mental illness and treatment of a man in the late 1870s. This narrative not only illustrates the orientation of the medical model but also expresses the attitudes of that time toward mental illness. The case of Ralph Jones represents the use of the medical model 100 years later, in the 1970s. The use of the medical model in the second case is especially reflected in the prescription of medication and other physical treatments for Ralph's illness. In both cases, note that the clients are considered ill and that their treatment reflects this diagnosis.

ROBERT SMITH

Robert Smith was the fourth of six children and the third son. His family, third-generation immigrants from England, lived in Philadelphia. Robert was quiet and withdrawn as a child, and while he did the work the family found for him, he was never very energetic in seeking it out.

Used by permission of H. Phillips Hamlin (1985).

The Smith family was relatively poor. Their fortunes improved somewhat during the Civil War, when they were able to find employment in the war-related metal industry, but after the war they descended again into poverty.

In his late 20s, Robert began to have episodes of "mania," as a doctor later called it. While still usually quiet and withdrawn, Robert would become violent and aggressive if crossed by members of his family or neighbors or if frustrated by events. These episodes of mania cost him his job, and soon the family was having to watch him all the time. During an episode, he would sometimes attack anyone who tried to communicate with him; when the episode passed, he would again become withdrawn and listless.

When Robert's aggressiveness began to be expressed toward the neighbors as well as toward family members, the family began to seek help for him. They took him to physicians, who examined him but did not know what to do for him.

By the time he was 32, Robert Smith's behavior had become so distressing that his family was desperate. He had been arrested more than once for destroying property in the neighborhood and threatening neighbors. His family had only barely kept him out of prison. His father took him to the county commission, which, after hearing the testimony of the family and the local sheriff, agreed to send him to the Blockley Almshouse in the fall of 1875. Blockley Almshouse was a huge collection of buildings maintained by the city of Philadelphia for its insane poor. When it was time for Robert to go there, the combined efforts of several family members and neighbors were necessary to overcome his resistance and subdue him.

At first, Robert was kept in the general hospital to recover from the injuries he had received in resisting the move to Blockley. Then he was transferred to a crowded asylum building, where he was nominally under the care of Dr. Isaac Ray, whom he actually never saw except from a distance.

Robert had to sleep in a night bed put on the floor in a corridor. When his violent episodes occurred, he was put in a straight waistcoat, which reduced his ability to attack other patients or attendants. The ward was generally noisy and turbulent. There was little chance for a good night's sleep, nor was there anything much for the patients to do during the day except to excite each other, creating almost continual disturbances.

After a year in Blockley, and weeks in a straitjacket, Robert became less violent and more depressed. Cold-water treatments seemed to reduce his violent episodes while he was in Blockley. His family noticed that he had lost weight and became worried about his physical health. They found the hospital dreary and depressing, but they were reluctant to have Robert discharged because they were afraid of what he would do outside. They were torn by their desire to get help for him and their concern that conditions at Blockley were unhealthy.

In the fall of 1876, the Smiths decided to move to Albany, New York. Because Robert seemed more manageable, if not better, they decided to take him with them. He made the journey all right, but the new environment seemed to bring on upsetting manic episodes such as he had had in Philadelphia. Within months, the family was again trying to decide what to do with him.

The business they had joined, begun by Mr. Smith's oldest brother, was modestly successful, so the family's financial resources were improved. When Robert's condition worsened, his family took him to a well-known local physician. After futile attempts to treat Robert, the doctor suggested that they take him to the Lunatic Asylum for the State of New York at Utica. The physician assured them that this asylum was a reputable one, much better than Blockley, and he signed a Certificate of Insanity, which helped them get Robert's admission to the asylum approved by a justice of the court.

In the early summer of 1877, Robert was taken to Utica by his father, uncle, and two older brothers. They traveled by boat, a short distance up the Hudson River, and then west on the Mohawk, a journey of some 150 miles.

The Smiths were impressed and encouraged by the asylum at Utica. They were shown the ward where Robert would stay; it was large, cheerful, and well furnished with large windows. None of the other patients were in straitjackets, and the Smiths were told that Dr. Gray, the superintendent, did not believe in mechanical restraints. Rather, he believed in an organized regimen of treatment that involved engaging the patients' minds and bodies in healthy activities, such as walking, bowling, gardening, and the mechanical arts.

Robert improved somewhat at Utica. The frequency and intensity of his manic episodes decreased, and within a year he was able to go home on a parole of about six months. However, he was never able to remain outside the asylum longer than that because his mania would return and intensify. He spent most of his remaining life in the asylum at Utica and died in 1890 from pneumonia, which he caught after a bout with influenza (Hamlin, 1985).

Ralph Jones

Ralph Jones has had a hard life. The third youngest of seven children, he apparently witnessed the suicide of his natural mother when he was 6. His natural father was either unable or unwilling to keep the family together, and all the children were sent to foster homes and orphanages.

Ralph was adopted at age 10 by a minister and . . . a psychiatric social worker. He had a hard time getting along with them. He began dealing and using drugs when he was about 13 years old, abusing pot, phencyclidine (PCP), acid, and alcohol. He may have become an alcoholic by the age of 16. Ralph says that his adoptive parents were kind to him, but he just could not seem to do what they wanted, and after a while relations between them became very strained. At 16, Ralph was brought to the local youth program at the mental hospital because of his drug problems and violent acting out.

He did not complete high school but managed to get a GED while studying mechanics at a local vocational school at the truant home. Ralph served 18 months in the Army. He was discharged with partial disability, caused by an injury to his left leg which he incurred playing football.

Ralph tends to be violent and lacks self-control when he has been drinking. Because of this behavior, he has lost many different jobs. Once, while drunk, he robbed and assaulted an elderly man in Florida—a crime for which he spent one year in jail. Also, he has been in several accidents, suffering injuries to his head and his back. He complains frequently of back pains.

Within the last five months, Ralph has been in jail twice and also in the state mental hospital. He was jailed on charges of driving while intoxicated. While there, he committed acts that were taken to be suicidal gestures. The first time, he cut his wrists superficially, and the second time, he slashed his throat with a razor blade.

Both times, Ralph was brought straight from the jail to the mental hospital. The second incident occurred only three days before his jail term was to be completed.

A case review was undertaken after three weeks at the mental hospital. Admission notes were reviewed: Ralph was unclean, nonverbal, depressed, and lacking in judgment. He claimed to be suffering from alcohol withdrawal at the time of admission. The doctor who admitted him said that Ralph looked "psychotic" at the time.

A number of features of Ralph's situation came out during the case review. During his previous stay at the mental hospital, he had received shock treatments and was heavily sedated most of the time. He was given Thorazine, a tranquilizer used to control psychotic behaviors and calm patients down, and another drug to counter the side effects of Thorazine. The two psychiatrists he saw noted that he was uncooperative and lacked understanding of his suicidal, violent, alcoholic, abusive behavior.

Today his situation remains complex. First, Ralph admits to several suicide attempts or gestures, dating back to when he was 18, but he is not willing to talk about them other than to say that he is depressed all the time. Second, he has a fiancee, whom he plans to marry within a year. She visits him regularly, dominates communication between him and the staff when she is around, and believes that he would be better off discharged. Also, she reports that he is well behaved, even gregarious, around her family. Ralph has virtually no other social contacts. She has been encouraging him to go to AA meetings and accompanies him when he does attend. In a conversation with a social worker, Ralph said he was afraid that she would press charges for a beating he gave her eight months ago.

Third, Ralph's contacts with his siblings and adoptive family have been minimal. He says he would like to live with his adoptive family, but they absolutely refuse to have anything to do with him. He has had no contact with any of his siblings in over two years. Fourth, Ralph apparently does well at skilled manual work and is only about one term short of completing training as a mechanic at a vocational school. When asked about his plans for the future, he says that he wishes to complete his schooling, get a job, and then get married. Fifth, he was married in his late teens and fathered two children (ages 7 and 8 now) before getting divorced at age 22. However, it is unknown where this family is and what connection, if any, he has with them.

Last, it seems clear that Ralph is a depressed, angry person who can be dangerous to himself and others. His antisocial tendencies seem to have been established early in his life, and they are exacerbated by his alcohol problem. It is not at all clear that he has even begun to work through what was perhaps the central trauma of his childhood, his mother's suicide. The treatment team, composed of nurses, physicians, social workers, psychologists, and others, is not sure whether Ralph should be discharged so that he can pursue the goals he articulates. The team is not convinced that he can handle life outside the hospital. The alcohol problem remains and seems to precipitate actions dangerous to Ralph and others. Yet he does have goals, and apparently his fiancee is supportive. If he were to establish a relationship with someone at a mental health center to secure help for him at his lowest points, and if he were to attend AA meetings and stop abusing alcohol, some members of the treatment team feel that he might be able to get his life together (Hamlin, 1985).

These case studies describe two treatments of mental illness. As you answer the following questions, you will come to understand better the characteristics of the medical model.

What problems did Robert Smith face? Ralph Jones?
What treatments did Robert receive? Ralph?
Why are these treatments classified as part of the medical model?

The Public Health Model

Definition

Public health is a concept that is sometimes difficult to define. One challenge in defining it is its multidisciplinary nature, which leads to difficulty in understanding it as a whole and defining its operations. We can approach its definition in three ways. One is to define public health by examining its historical development, achievements, and health successes. The next section will provide a brief review of this perspective. A second approach is to examine its goal, which is to provide the opportunities and conditions for health as a basic human right. The goal is reflected in its mission: to fulfill society's interest in assuring conditions in which people can be healthy (Committee Study of the Future of Public Health, 1988). Because the concept of health has changed during the 1800s and 1900s, a third approach to defining public health reflects its dynamism and adaptability. For example, until the past few decades, health has meant the absence of disease and disability. Today, health has a more positive meaning—the capacity to live fully, which entails maintaining the physical, mental, and social reserves for coping with life's circumstances in a way that brings satisfaction (Afifi & Breslow, 1994).

The public health model bridges the medical and human service models but is more obviously linked with the medical model. Diagnosis and treatment of individuals using medicine and surgery are the core of clinical medicine. Physicians have delineated parts of the body (anatomy), how they function (physiology), their disorders (pathology), and the agents of disease (etiology). Their goal is to combat disease by repairing the breakdown of the "machinery" (Afifi & Breslow, 1994). Those physicians who are cognizant of social, environmental, and biological factors and see disease as it affects populations have moved toward the public health model.

Public health is sometimes not separable from human welfare, either. Improving public health means improving education, nutrition, safe food and water supplies, immunization, and maternal and child health. It is particularly difficult to dissociate ill health from poverty.

In conclusion, a number of characteristics of the public health model distinguish it from the other two service delivery models. The public health model, like the medical model, is concerned with individuals who have problems, but it extends the concept of heath care beyond the traditional medical model (Pinkstaff, 1985). In the belief that individuals' problems may be linked to other social problems, the public health model serves larger populations rather than just individuals. Societal control is a prime concern of the public health model, as it attempts to solve many of society's social problems. This model is unique in that it approaches social conditions or problems in two ways. Data are collected from the public at large as well as from examination of the individuals who have the problem in question (Pattison, 1984).

The public health model applies a multicausal approach to studying the causes or origins of problems and emphasizes prevention. The preventive component also distinguishes this model from the medical model. The general aims of the American public health service system include not only a more equal distribution of health care services to all segments of the population (including the elderly, persons with disabilities, and the impoverished) but also identification of social, nondisease problems and methods of attacking their causes and contributing factors. The objective of the public health model is to improve the present and future quality of life and to alleviate health problems that have consequences for society in general.

History

Communicable diseases, poor sanitation, and lack of medical knowledge have been community health problems since ancient times. During the colonial period in North America, smallpox, yellow fever, and cholera were major health problems. Laws such as the Massachusetts Poor Law of 1692 gave local authorities the power to remove and isolate the afflicted. By the end of the 18th century, establishment of the first dispensaries and the first local boards of health had laid the foundations for voluntary organizations and public health agencies.

In the early 1800s, people migrated from the country to urban areas around burgeoning industrial plants. Severe disease outbreaks resulted from the poor

The Public Health Service

The Public Health Service has a distinguished history that dates back to the late 1700s, when many merchant seamen arrived ill and unattached in American port cities that had little capacity to care for them. In 1798, adopting the British tradition of caring for sick mariners at public expense, Congress enacted a measure, which President John Adams signed into law, that provided for "the temporary relief and maintenance of sick or disabled seamen." The first hospital dedicated to the care of merchant sailors was a building purchased near Norfolk, Virginia, in 1801. The first public hospital actually built with tax revenues, however, was in Boston.

Since that time, almost 200 years ago, the Public Health Service has grown to prominence as a federal enterprise dedicated to promoting and protecting the public's health, with a mandate that often embroils its agencies in controversy. The eight agencies of the Public Health Service are the Agency for Health Care Policy and Research, the Agency for Toxic Substances and Disease Registry, the Centers for Disease Control and Prevention (CDC), the Food and Drug Administration (FDA), the Health Resources and Services Administration, the Indian Health Service, the National Institute of Health (NIH), and the Substance Abuse and Mental Health Services Administration.

SOURCE: From "Health Policy Report: Politics and Public Health," by John K. Iglehart, 1996, *Health Policy Report, 334*, p. 203.

nutrition, overcrowding, filth, and excessive work requirements of the inhabitants living in these slums. In 1842, Edwin Chadwick, an English social reformer, wrote a grim account of the conditions in England's slums, a document that profoundly affected the development of public health and led to the enactment of the English Public Health Act of 1848. On this side of the Atlantic, Lemuel Shattuck, a Boston city councilman, prepared a report financed by the Massachusetts legislature that presented the first plan for an integrated health program in the United States. The 1842 Chadwick Report in England and the 1850 Shattuck Report in the United States precipitated both a sanitary awakening and social reform that constituted public health at that time (Afifi & Breslow, 1994).

The social philosophies of the early 19th century impacted public health as they reflected two beliefs about disease. The first was that disease was providential. Like poverty and natural disasters such as floods, disease occurred as a result of God's wrath toward an individual. Therefore, the obvious solution to the problem was improved behavior. The second belief linked disease to the disorderly and filthy cities with their unpaved streets, poor drainage, untethered animals, and outside privies. Intuitively, people realized the impact of environmental factors on disease. Many believed that the solution was to eliminate dirt and filth to create a healthier environment.

A report by Lemuel Shattuck in 1850 declared the need for improved sanitation and disease control in Massachusetts and recommended establishment of state and local boards of health, collection of vital statistics, institution of sanitation programs, and prevention of disease (Shirreffs, 1982). Although widely ignored at the time, Shattuck's report has come to be considered the most farsighted and influential document in the history of the public health system (Committee Study of the Future of Public Health, 1988). By 1868, Massachusetts had established the first state public health department in the country.

A second important event was the organization in 1861 of the United States Sanitary Commission, the first major public health group in America. It is significant to the public health movement because its efforts were primarily preventive; it alerted the public to the benefits of preventive sanitary measures. Appalled by the poor conditions in army camps and hospitals, a group led by Dr. Henry Bellows, Louisa Schuyler, and Dr. Elisha Harris organized this voluntary citizen effort. A central focus of the commission was to unite all voluntary groups to aid governmental agencies in meeting the physical and spiritual needs of men in uniform. Initially, their efforts were directed toward teaching proper personal hygiene and inspecting and supervising living arrangements in camps and field hospitals. Their later efforts included recruiting nurses, distributing supplies, and assisting in communication between soldiers and their families.

Prevention emerged as a major component of the public health movement when Dr. Louis Pasteur and Robert Koch demonstrated that germs—not God or dirt—cause disease. The "golden age of public health" (1890–1910) included the discovery of causes for typhoid, tuberculosis, and cholera. Personal cleanliness, inoculations, serums, and hygienic laws became the basis of reform, and preventive medicine developed beyond research and lab diagnosis. Preventive medicine included a social focus, with well-organized public health education programs (Trattner, 1994). Today, the Public Health Service is part of the Department of Health and Human Services (see Figure 4-1). It focuses on interventions aimed at disease prevention and health promotion that shape a community's overall profile.

Industrialization and its spread around the world during the 19th and 20th centuries stimulated the problems of communicable disease; these were followed by the difficulties that accompanied epidemics of chronic disease—coronary heart disease, cancer, diabetes, and chronic obstructive lung disease. Public health responded to the first set of problems and has made strides toward controlling the second. A third group that has emerged in the past two decades consists of HIV/AIDS, domestic and street violence, and substance abuse.

Many changes have occurred in public health over the years. In 1789, the Reverend Edward Wigglesworth assessed the health of Americans and produced the first American mortality tables. By 1900, influenza, pneumonia, tuberculosis, and gastrointestinal infections were the main cases of death in the United States. Average life expectancy at birth was 47 years. This statistic has seen a phenomenal rise, with life expectancy at birth extending to 68 years by 1950, a

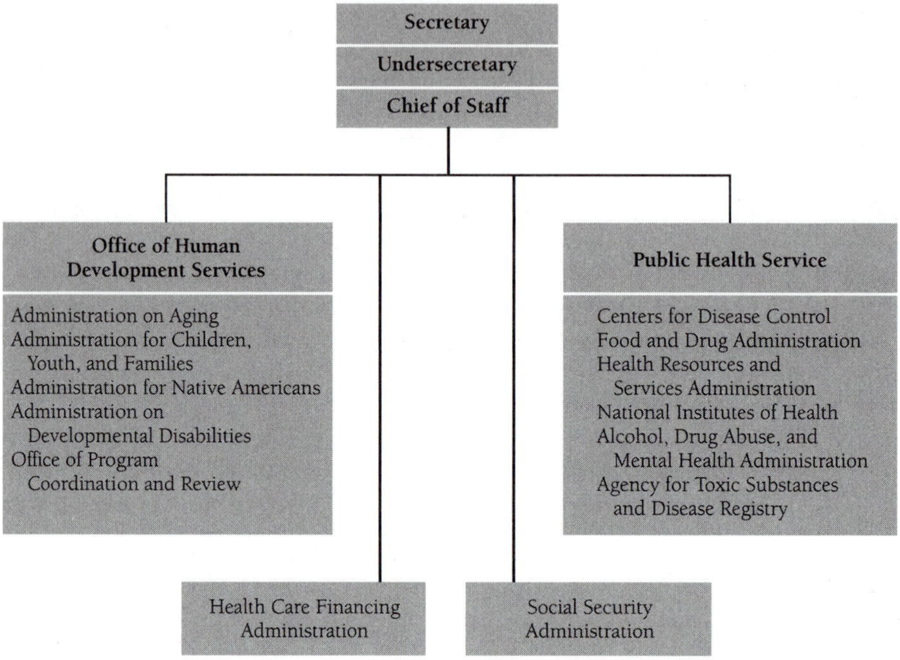

Figure 4-1 ✦ Organization of the U.S. Department of Health and Human Services

SOURCE: From "The Future of Public Health," by Committee Study of the Future of Public Health Institute of Medicine, 1988, Washington, DC: National Academy Press.

change attributable to improvements in diet and sanitation and the development of antibiotics and vaccines. By the 1990s, life expectancy has grown to 75 years. Leading causes of death are heart disease and cancer. The leading health problems are chronic diseases (*Healthy People 2000,* 1995).

Healthy People 2000 is a national effort to provide a vision for improving the health of all Americans. Led by the Public Health Service, this effort began in 1979 with the publication of *Healthy People: The Surgeon General's Report on Promotion and Disease Prevention.* The initial objectives for 1990 were established in 1980 with the publication of *Promoting Health/Preventing Disease: Objectives for the Nation.* These objectives were expanded for the year 2000 to include topics such as HIV infection and cancer. Participants in defining and pursuing a prevention agenda for the nation come from every level of government, from professional groups, and from American communities. Their primary task has been to set objectives for the year 2000. The midcourse review and 1995 revisions charted progress and assessed the challenges that remain.

A major challenge is to shift the national emphasis to prevention. Here are some of the successes. Since the 1970s, stroke death rates have declined by 58% and coronary heart disease death rates by 49%. Tobacco use among adults declined from 34% to 25% between 1974 and 1993. A 32% decline in the death rate from car crashes is attributed to the increased use of safety restraints. Unfortunately, cases of AIDS, tuberculosis, asthma, and birth defects have increased.

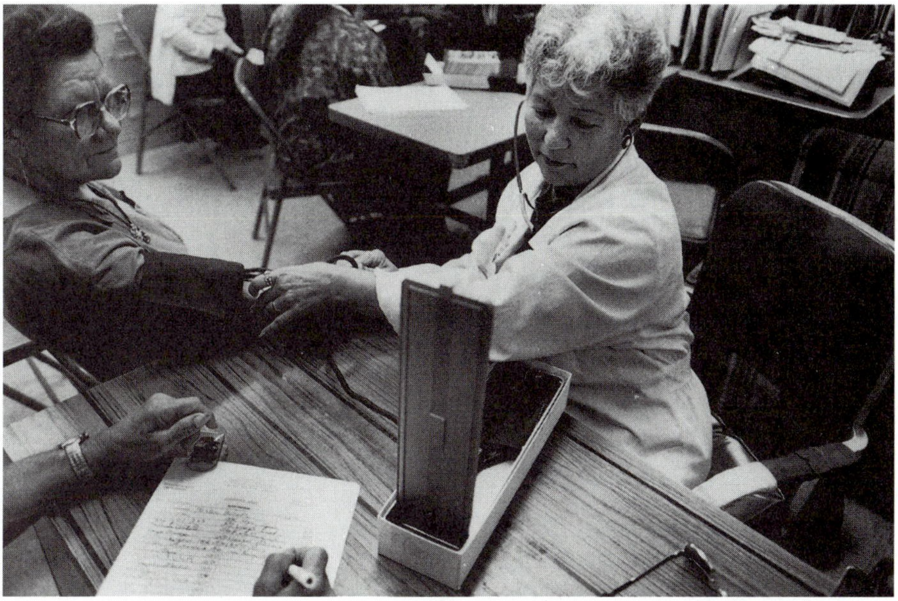

Medical screenings are part of the preventive focus of the public health model.

A 1974 assessment by the Centers for Disease Control and Prevention estimated that nearly 47% of premature deaths among Americans could have been avoided by changes in individual behaviors (for example, quitting smoking and beginning to exercise regularly) and another 17% by reducing risks, such as by wearing seat belts and by changing to a healthier diet. Improvements in access to medical care have prevented an estimated 11% of premature deaths among Americans. Consider that in the United States in 1990, the most prominent causes of mortality, to which more than half of all premature deaths were attributed, were these:

- Tobacco use (400,000)
- Poor diet and lack of physical activity (300,000)
- Alcohol abuse (100,000)
- Infectious agents (90,000)
- Toxic agents (60,000)
- Firearms (in homicides, suicides, and unintentional deaths) (35,000)
- Unprotected sexual intercourse (30,000)
- Motor vehicle injuries (25,000)

(McGinnis & Foege, 1993).

Case Studies

The following case study illustrates the historical problems that are the primary focus of the public health model. It tells of Sean O'Reilly, and the setting is the

1850s in New York City. The study illustrates the living conditions that called attention to public health concerns in America. Especially in larger cities, the problems of immigrants living in poverty greatly challenged public health professionals. The second and third cases illustrate two public health efforts today.

SEAN O'REILLY

Sean O'Reilly, age 25, was the first member of his family to emigrate from Ireland to America. He joined the great numbers of Irish who came to America in the wake of the potato blight that devastated Ireland in the middle of the 1840s. His journey, in a wooden sailing vessel from Liverpool, took 40 days. The voyage was very difficult. Like most poor immigrants, he traveled in steerage, a lower deck below the water line, reserved for third-class passengers. The space was four to six feet high and lined with two berths of wooden bunks. The floor was crowded with baggage, water, and cord wood. The only fresh air for the steerage area came from the hole in the deck for the hatchway.

After the six-week crossing, Sean emerged from steerage pale, weak, and 20 pounds lighter than when he started. He had not succumbed to cholera or dysentery, as had several other passengers. The starvation, filth, and crowded conditions he had encountered during the passage to America were just a continuation of the hardships he had experienced in Ireland, which had driven him to emigrate.

The ship docked in New York. Even though Sean did not feel well, he was not eligible for medical treatment from the Marine hospital on Staten Island, as he did not have a communicable disease. Nor did he have enough money to enter Bellevue, the city hospital. He ignored the "runners" who accosted him on board, trying to get him to travel to other cities for a "small" fee. He left the ship and joined hundreds of other new arrivals, mostly Irish like himself, in search of a place to live and a job.

Although Sean had been a farmer in Ireland, he felt that the land had somehow rejected him. He wanted to stay with other Irishmen, near the sea, so he decided to remain in New York City. Sean found work before he found lodging. The first night, he slept in an alley, and the next day he joined a construction gang, moving earth to build roads in the city. The men he met at work suggested that he live with them in a tenement building housing other newly arrived Irish immigrants. His first Saturday night in America, he was invited to and attended a "kitchen racquet" (get-acquainted party) organized by the family who lived downstairs.

Housing was the most difficult problem Sean faced; laborers' jobs, the sort of work he could do, were plentiful but irregular. Slum lords, taking advantage of immigrants in dire need of housing, crowded families into small, filthy, dimly lit, poorly ventilated tenements situated on narrow, unpaved streets with inadequate drainage. Partly because there was no integrated health program or municipal board of health, the city was disorderly, dirty, and disease-ridden.

From the time he landed, Sean became part of the considerable Irish community in New York. He shared two rooms with a family of six. His living conditions never significantly improved. He held several jobs, constructing roads, buildings, and sewage ditches. The jobs involved long hours, hazardous working conditions, low wages, and frequent short periods of unemployment.

Any money he made beyond bare living expenses went to the church and to his small account in the Emigrant Industrial Savings Bank of New York. This account enabled him to bring his family to America through the system known as "one bringing another," in which each immigrant worked and saved for a prepaid ticket for the next member of his family to come to America. By the late 1850s, most of Sean's family had joined him in New York.

A CHLAMYDIA SCREENING PROGRAM IN THE PACIFIC NORTHWEST

In 1988 in the Pacific Northwest, a public health family planning program began screening for chlamydia. In a grassroots program designed to detect chlamydia among asymptomatic women, more than 100,000 women who attended 150 family planning clinics in Alaska, Idaho, Oregon, and Washington were tested for the disease as part of their routine gynecological health care. Through early detection and treatment, the rate of chlamydia infection among these clinic patients dropped by 58% from 1988 to 1992. This decrease occurred among women of all social, economic, and age groups (CDC, Region X Chlamydia Project Report). The screening program reduced the incidence of chlamydia infection, PID, and infertility.

The screening program includes a health services quality assurance component. Participating public health staff evaluate available tests for chlamydia, and through centralization of testing and bulk purchasing arrangements, have reduced costs of high-performance test kits by more than 50%. A regional advisory committee of family planning and STD [sexually transmitted disease] leaders oversees the program's activities. These collaborative efforts have led to consistency in screening, which will result in quality care for all participating women.

The Pacific Northwest story illustrates how current and especially innovative public health programs can prevent and control STDs. The Preventive Health Amendments of 1992 authorized implementation of the Pacific Northwest model for infertility prevention in other regions of the country.

SOURCE: From *For a Healthy Nation: Returns on Investment in Public Health,* by U.S. Department of Health and Human Services, Public Health Service, p. 29, Washington: DC: Author.

CALIFORNIA'S TOBACCO CONTROL PROGRAM

California took an aggressive step in 1988 when it passed the Tobacco Tax and Health Protection Act, aimed at decreasing tobacco use among California residents. This act increased the excise tax on cigarettes by $.25 a pack, *and earmarked 20% of these funds for use in antismoking activities. Local health departments are the lead agencies for regional tobacco-control education programs funded by the act, and they have worked with more than 300 community-based organizations to implement tobacco-control interventions. The resulting coalitions have fought tobacco industry sponsorship of sporting and other events designed to attract large numbers of youth and minority populations. Local health departments are also responsible for promoting tobacco-free work sites and public places in their communities.*

Another activity funded by this public health initiative is a statewide media campaign that strips the glamour from using tobacco through a combination of dark humor aimed at the tobacco industry and more traditional health messages. An innovative, competitive grants program for projects that target high-risk populations was also established. Funded projects include the Asian American Health Forum, which formed an ethnic network and created a multiple-language telephone hotline; Project Trust in San Diego, which targeted 400 stores for merchant education and reduced the number that were selling cigarettes to minors from 73% to 30%; and Fantasy Theatre in Sacramento, whose anti-tobacco plays were seen by nearly 12,000 children.

The program has resulted in numerous successes:

- *Smoking prevalence in California decreased by 28% between 1988 and 1993. An estimated 173,000 people credit their decision to quit smoking to the media campaign.*
- *The largest declines occurred among minority populations, which were targeted by the competitive grant program.*
- *In response to actions by local health departments, the proportion of smoke-free workplaces almost doubled between 1990 and 1993, with exposure of nonsmokers to environmental tobacco smoke decreased by 23%.*
- *The increase in smoking seen among adolescents in the period 1988–1990 has been halted.*

California has set several goals related to smoking, including banning free distribution of tobacco products and tobacco sales from vending machines and establishing tobacco-prevention policies in all public schools. By 1999 the state hopes to reduce the smoking prevalence in California by 75%.

SOURCE: From *For a Healthy Nation: Returns on Investment in Public Health,* by U.S. Department of Health and Human Services, Public Health Service, p. 16, Washington, DC: Author.

The following questions will help you clarify the role of public health today:

How do the public health problems in the last two case studies compare with those Sean O'Reilly encountered?

How do these three case studies illustrate what you have read about the history of the public health model?
How do the solutions in public health in the 1850s differ from those in the 1990s?

The Human Service Model

Definition

A primary focus of the human service model is to provide services that help individuals solve their problems. As Table 4-2 shows, this model differs considerably from the medical model and the public health model. According to the human service model, problems are an expected, even necessary part of everyday life. They occur because human existence is a complex process, involving interaction with other individuals, groups, institutions, and the environment. The human service model considers the problem of the client within the context of the environment. If a client must be temporarily removed from the environment to provide effective treatment, treatment within the context of the environment will continue once the client reenters that environment.

Individuals are one of the *client* groups of the human service system. Clients can include smaller groups, such as families; larger geographic populations, such as neighborhoods or communities; and populations having problems in common, such as the homeless and substance abusers.

The primary method of treatment is problem solving, a process focused on the here and now. Problem-solving models range from three phases to six phases. Generally, the flow of all these models begins with problem identification and advances to decision making and implementation (McClam & Woodside, 1994). It is important, however, to remember that these three phases are not truly discrete units of activity. During problem solving the boundaries between the various phases and activities are blurred. For example, "problem definition and goal setting are directly related, and the generation of alternatives can occur early in the goal-setting process" (McClam & Woodside, 1994, p. 12). Another example is evaluation, which is not always distinct from implementation and, in fact, occurs throughout the process.

The first phase, problem identification, is particularly critical to the entire process because identification of the problem directs the phases that follow. This phase also includes preparing to solve the problem, a step that often occurs before the client enters the process. Decision making follows problem identification and includes setting goals, generating alternatives, and making a decision. After a decision is made, the third phase, problem resolution, begins. Activities in this stage are planning, implementing, and evaluating the solution.

The problem-solving approach is used in this model for a number of reasons. First, the process provides a systematic way of thinking about very complex situations. Problem identification suggests ways to describe situations in clear, understandable terms, encouraging the client and the worker to

TABLE 4-2 ✦ AN OVERVIEW OF THREE MODELS OF SERVICE DELIVERY

	View of the problem	*Who is the client?*	*Who is the worker?*	*Where treatment occurs*	*Method of treatment*	*Goal of treatment*
Medical	Individual has a physiologically based illness or disease	Individual who receives services is called *patient*	Trained professional in health sciences (doctor, nurse, dentist, psychiatrist)	Office Institution	Diagnosis Treatment Behavioral prescription Medication Psychoanalysis	Return individual to prior state
Public health	Individual, groups, and society have disease or illness. Environmental and social pressures also contribute to problem	Individuals and special populations or geographic areas (community, neighborhood, state, nation)	Public health training combines medical knowledge with community action skills	Office Community	Medical diagnosis Prescription Education Mobilization of resources Advocacy for special populations	Prevention Social action
Human service	"Problems in living" Problems may be internal, environmental, and/or intrapersonal	Individuals, families, special populations, and environment can be clients	Volunteer Paraprofessional Entry-level human worker who works with abuse, rehabilitation, education, etc. Professionals (rehabilitation or mental health counselor, social worker, psychologist)	Offices/agencies/ institutions serving individuals, families, children Community	Problem-solving process	Enhance client's well-being, quality of life Teach client problem-solving skills Prevention

prioritize the problems that need to be addressed and discouraging impulsive, reactive behaviors. Second, the effectiveness of the process can be assessed at each stage. If the worker or the client discovers new information or if the problem or the environment changes, the process can be revised. Third, clients can learn this problem-solving process and use it themselves when they no longer require services. Clients have the opportunity to improve their own problem-solving skills by working with a human service worker to solve problems and by rehearsing the behaviors under the worker's direction. Fourth, the outcomes of the process support the philosophy of human services by fostering clients' self-esteem and sense of personal responsibility as they work successfully through the process. In addition, the results of the process improve the quality of life for the client. Fifth, the approach is a tool for identifying other problems that may occur and determining strategies to prevent future problems.

Philosophy

In its broadest sense, the philosophy of human services was solidified during the 1940s. It included the following beliefs:

- People had the right to expect their society, through its technology and other resources, to prevent their deprivation and provide for their basic human needs.
- The society, through its government, had the irrevocable responsibility for providing people with adequate human services.
- Meeting people's needs comprehensively and effectively required an understanding of the "whole person" and his [or her] relationship to [the] environment.
- Meeting the "whole person's" needs meant that the resources of many disciplines should be cooperatively mobilized for him [or her]. (Eriksen, 1981, p. 53)

Other factors contributed to the development of a human service model. One factor was the community mental health center movement, which grew out of the public health model (Rapoport, 1962). This movement broadened the definitions of care, services, recipients, and goals of intervention (English, Kritzler, & Scherl, 1984). A second contributing factor was the medical field's recognition of the goals of the human service field. The medical profession began stressing patients' responsibility for diet, exercise, recreation, and rest. A third contributing factor was the support of President Jimmy Carter, as expressed in his message introducing proposed legislation to improve the provisions of mental health services and to promote mental health (1979, p. 2):

> Substantial numbers of Americans do not have access to mental health care of high quality and at reasonable cost. For many, this is because of where they live; for others, it is because of who they are—their race, age, or sex; for still others, it is because of their particular disability or economic circumstance.

This reflected the human service philosophy of the 1940s, with its emphasis on both the responsibilities of society and the importance of working with the whole person.

Most texts agree that a model of human service delivery should include the following characteristics or themes (Eriksen, 1981; Harris & Maloney, 1996; Mandell & Schram, 1995; Mehr, 1995; Schmolling, Youkeles, & Burger, 1997):

1. The *generic focus* is critical in both human service training and human service delivery. This focus allows for the application of basic helping skills to serving different populations as well as other models to provide services to clients most effectively.
2. Services should be accessible, comprehensive, and coordinated. Prevention, restitution, and rehabilitation are equally important parts of an *integrated* service system.
3. The *problem-solving approach* emphasizes the here and now. Included in this approach are helping the client solve the problem and teaching the client problem-solving skills.
4. Taking into consideration the impact of social institutions, social systems, and social problems, the model works with the person and the environment. Treating *the* whole person is best accomplished when the worker recognizes the client's needs in relation to others and to the environment.
5. Human services is *accountable to the consumer.* Clients are active participants in the human service model, making decisions, taking action, and accepting responsibility for themselves.

Case Study

The following case study illustrates several concepts you have read about in this chapter. There are four possible clients in this case study who are experiencing problems and who have different perspectives on the problems. This situation also illustrates the individual as client as well as the family as client. Let us focus first on the human service model of service delivery.

Consider yourself the human service professional who has received this case. As you are reading it, think about the following:

Describe how Susan, Ted, Justin, and Matthew have solved problems in the past.

How do you think each person in the case study will define the problems?

As you consider problem solving as a systematic way of thinking, how would you as a human service professional approach the problem Susan faces?

How will the themes and characteristics of human services guide your work with this case?

Susan and Ted met in college, where she was studying to be a teacher and he was studying to be an engineer. Ted was from an upper-middle-class family;

Susan, from a religious, working-class family. Even while they were dating, Ted was a heavy "social drinker," but Susan ignored his drinking. She wanted to marry a man with a college education and have a large family. She came from a small, close-knit family and had only one sister. She remembered her family as having few luxuries while she was growing up but much love and nurturance. Ted's family was also small, but not close. Ted had no contact with his family, even though they lived in the same town as the university.

During Ted's and Susan's sophomore year, Susan's grades began to fall. She was on a partial scholarship and was in danger of losing it. She dropped out of school and moved out of the dorm into an apartment with Ted. Then Susan became pregnant. Ted dropped out of school and got a job as a draftsperson for a small local firm. They married.

Leaving behind a happy, carefree life without responsibility, they now faced an uncertain future. Susan tried to be the "perfect wife" her mother had been. Ted began drinking heavily. He lost several jobs during Susan's pregnancy and often took his anger out on her by hitting her and keeping her constantly tense and fearful. He turned to drugs, and the relationship deteriorated further. After losing several more jobs, Ted had to take a menial, low-paying job just to make ends meet, and his resentment increased. He spent more time away from home, leaving Susan without money for food or transportation. She was alone and depressed but did not confide in her family, because she did not want to upset them.

Often Ted was away for days. As Susan's pregnancy progressed, he became more violent. Once, he beat her so badly that he cracked two of her ribs and broke her nose. He also attempted to strangle her. She told no one and lied to her doctor and friends about the injuries. Ted "came to his senses" and tried to make amends. But he began drinking heavily once again and in a fit of rage kicked her in the stomach, bringing on labor. Susan delivered a son in the sixth month of her pregnancy. Justin weighed 3 pounds, 2 ounces, and had difficulty breathing. He was placed in an intensive-care nursery for six weeks before his parents could take him home. Justin continued to be sickly, suffering from chronic ear infections and colic. Ted had trouble adjusting to his new son, so Susan took care of him alone.

Justin had many health problems and was constantly under the care of physicians. He was often hospitalized with pneumonia and severe dehydration. When Justin was 14 months old, Ted deserted them. Susan had no money and no car. She turned to her parents for a small loan and got a job in a department store making minimum wage. She had to work, but it angered her to leave Justin with a baby-sitter. Being a single parent was difficult. By the time she paid the rent, the bills, and the baby-sitter, there was no money left. She was desperately unhappy but determined to make the best of things.

Several months later, Ted returned. He had a new job making good money and was ready to "work things out." He continued to drink, and he still beat her, but she now wanted him at any cost. He soon learned this. One year later, Susan had another son, Matthew. At this point, Ted and Susan bought a house in a small town near the university and proceeded to raise their family. For Ted, this consisted of nightly bouts with the bottle in front of a television set and of forcing himself sexually on Susan. The years passed, and Susan continued to put up with his drinking and rapes. Eventually, Ted's drinking became uncontrollable, and he started abusing the children. One night he came home late, pulled a gun, and shot at Susan. A neighbor called the police; he was handcuffed and arrested. Ted's father, who had previously been completely out of the picture, now came to Ted's aid by paying his bail. This became a regular routine. Each time Ted was out of jail, he would return home to drink and terrorize Susan and the children. After six months, Susan told Ted she wanted a divorce. He became enraged and threatened her. She persisted and engaged a lawyer. Her intention was to return to the university to finish her education and continue with her plans to be a teacher. She had less than two years to go and was confident that with child support, income from a job, and financial aid, this plan was feasible. Until the divorce, Ted refused to leave the house. The boys suffered terribly, seeing their mother beaten and their father handcuffed and taken to jail in a police car.

Currently, the youngest child, Matthew, now 14, works part-time while attending high school as a sophomore. He is doing poorly in school but is managing to pass his courses. He likes his job and the money he makes. He is able to help pay for some of the things the family needs. He no longer has plans for college and, indeed, intends to continue working at the pizza restaurant if and when he graduates from high school. Although Matthew's grades have recently dropped from A's to C's and D's, Justin's grades have suffered the most. He is now failing all his classes and has developed severe behavioral and emotional problems. He skips school, refuses to do his homework or schoolwork, and "hangs out with the wrong crowd." He takes drugs at home as well as at school and sells drugs to his classmates. Justin is extremely depressed and hostile. He carries a knife to school and threatens classmates with it. During one incident, when the victim's parents pressed charges, Justin was suspended from school and referred to the juvenile correctional department. He was placed in a program for adolescents dependent on alcohol or drugs. School officials realize that Justin "has problems" but have offered Susan no guidance or support, taking action only when Justin's behavior is life threatening.

Justin received correctional treatment in a private residential hospital. One condition of Justin's admission into the private hospital was coverage under his father's insurance plan. As Justin started to improve slightly, Susan discovered that the boys were not, and never had been, covered by their father's insurance. She did not tell the hospital personnel for fear that Justin would be dropped from the program. She felt that the program was his only hope. She has now received bills totaling more than $8,000 that she is expected to pay. She knows she will soon have to admit to the hospital that she cannot pay.

Susan is in trouble financially. She receives free medical aid from the university student clinic but has to find the money for her children's medical care. Last Christmas, a church she joined took up a collection for her and the *children and bought them $200 worth of groceries. She requested one month of subsidized utilities from the local utilities company but is eligible for this assistance only one time. She is concerned that she will not be able to afford utilities this month. Ted pays child support only sporadically, and he moves from town to town. Susan never knows where she can find him in case of an emergency and is not certain he would even help. Ted continues to have visitation rights, because he "sometimes" pays child support. She is furious about this privilege but keeps thinking he will eventually take more responsibility for his children. Constantly depressed because of this situation, Susan also fears that bill collectors will start to hound her and that, if an emergency occurs, she will not be able to handle it. She does not know what to do.*

As you think about these clients' needs from the human service perspective, you quickly realize that $200 for groceries and one month of subsidized utilities solve only immediate problems. The larger problems that Susan, Ted, Justin, and Matthew face are much more complex and will require comprehensive, coordinated service delivery.

You have learned in this chapter that human service professionals use three primary models of service delivery. In taking charge of this case, you will function within the context of the human service model. To promote the well-being of the whole person and to provide the comprehensive services necessary to that end, you may rely on professionals whose service delivery is guided by the public health model or by the medical model. To minimize duplication of services and to promote coordinated service delivery, you need to maintain active links with other professionals who may work with the same clients you do.

Now that you are familiar with the history of Susan, Ted, Matthew, and Justin, review the problem-solving process. Select one of the individuals in the case study as your client and ask yourself the following questions:

What is the mind-set of this client now?
What problems and subproblems does the client face?
What alternatives are possible to solve these problems?
How would you as the helping professional use the human service model in this case?
How might professionals from the public health model or the medical model facilitate the delivery of services your client needs?

Using models is a helpful way of identifying the different approaches to clients' problems. The distinctions among the models are not arbitrary, for each has a separate history and has developed in response to different social needs. From the human service perspective, however, each model has a part in the problem-solving process. The worker is responsible for blending the models and the treatments they represent in response to clients' needs. Indeed, one of the strengths of human services is the focus on clients' needs and the flexibility to use approaches from various models to meet those needs.

✧ Things to Remember

1. Three different models represent orientations in service delivery: the medical model, the public health model, and the human service model.
2. Underlying each of the three models is a set of philosophical assumptions that guide the delivery of services and shape beliefs about the causes of problems, their treatment, and the role of the professional in the model.
3. The medical model views the person coming for help as a *patient* whose problem is diagnosed as a disease or sickness and treated by a physician or service provider who prescribes a treatment or cure for the "disease."
4. At the turn of the century, Mary Richmond, author of *Social Diagnosis,* used the medical model to describe social casework.
5. Until the end of the 19th century, insanity was socially defined, but when psychiatry emerged as a medical specialty, insanity became a medical label.
6. Psychotropic drugs are now among the most widely used treatments for mental disorders. Psychopharmacology, the study of the effects of drugs on mental health, is an area of interest to human service professionals.
7. The public health model, like the medical model, is focused on individuals as well as larger populations; it attempts to solve many of society's social problems.
8. Communicable diseases, poor sanitation, and lack of medical knowledge have been primary community health problems since ancient times. Laws such as the Massachusetts Poor Law of 1692 in North America and the Public Health Act of 1848 in Britain initiated efforts to improve public health conditions.
9. The United States Sanitary Commission was the first major public health group in the United States. Its efforts were primarily preventive, alerting the public to the benefits of preventive sanitary measures.
10. A primary focus of the human service model is to provide services that help individuals solve their problems, including a consideration of client problems within the context of their environments.
11. Individuals are among the clients of the human service system, as are small groups, larger geographic populations, populations defined by lifestyle, and populations that have problems in common.
12. The primary method of treatment is problem solving, a process focused on the here and now and encompassing three phases: problem identification, decision making, and problem resolution.

13. The human service philosophy emphasizes both the responsibilities of society and the importance of working with the whole person.

14. Themes characteristic of human service delivery are *its generic focus; its accessible, integrated services; the problem-solving approach; treating the whole person; and accountability to the consumer.*

15. Using models is a helpful way to identify the different approaches to clients' problems.

Additional Readings: Focus on Mental Illness

Gibbons, K. (1995). *Sights unseen.* New York: Putnam.

The subject of this novel is a manic-depressive mother and the havoc she wreaks on her family.

Isaac, R. J., & Armat, V. C. (1990). *Madness in the streets: How psychiatry and the law abandoned the mentally ill.* New York: Free Press.

The authors believe that public interest lawyers, influenced by false and destructive antipsychiatric doctrines, have corrupted the law and have made it impossible to provide patients with the treatments they require but lack the insight to accept.

Slater, L. (1996). *Welcome to my country.* New York: Random House.

This book is a chronicle of the author's early days as a therapist in Boston when she ran a group therapy session for men and dealt with clients with a range of disorders, including schizophrenia, depression, and personality disorder.

Styron, W. (1990). *Darkness visible: A memoir of madness.* New York: Random House.

The author's account of his own bout with debilitating depression, which began in 1985 and soon made him unable to function.

Winerip, M. (1994). *9 Highland Road.* New York: Pantheon Books.

This book was written after the author had spent two years following the daily lives of the residents and their 24-hour-a-day counselors in this group home. Winerip spent time talking to them; eating with them; following them into and out of psychiatric hospital wards, day programs, schools and jobs; reading their records; visiting their families; and talking to their social workers and psychiatrists.

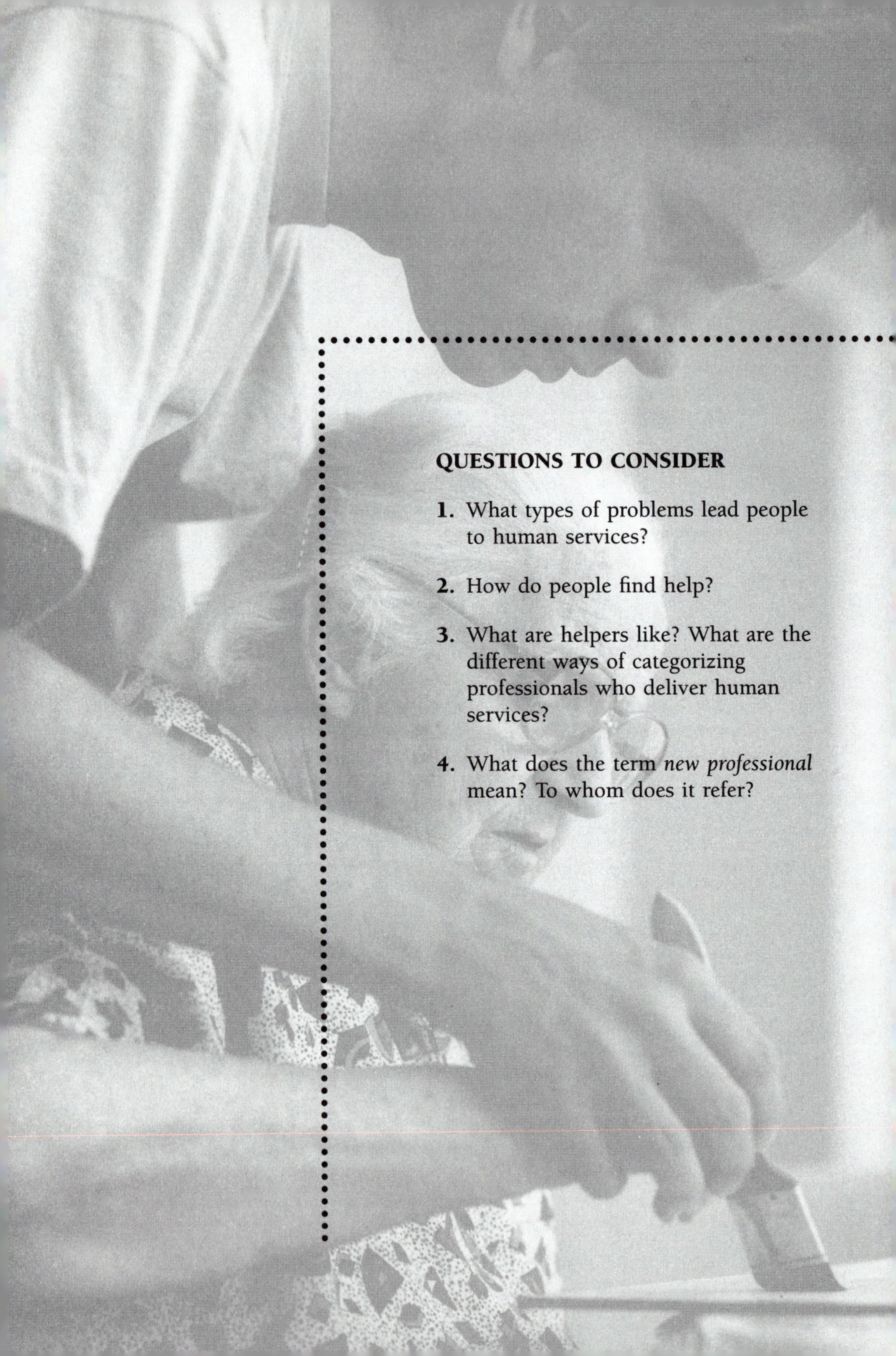

QUESTIONS TO CONSIDER

1. What types of problems lead people to human services?
2. How do people find help?
3. What are helpers like? What are the different ways of categorizing professionals who deliver human services?
4. What does the term *new professional* mean? To whom does it refer?

PART TWO

Clients and Helpers in Human Services

Part Two focuses on the people who are involved in the practice of human services, either as recipients or as service providers. Chapter 5 introduces the client or consumer—who may be an individual, a group, or a population—and gives examples of these different types. The chapter examines how they get help, barriers they encounter, and their perspective on help.

Chapter 6 shifts to the human service professional, the provider of human services, with an examination of helpers' motivations, values, and characteristics. It also provides an overview of the categories of human service professionals and insights about them. The chapter concludes with a description of the beginning professional in the field.

The primary purpose of Part Two is to further refine the definition of human services by considering the individuals who are involved in service delivery. As you read the two chapters in this part, think about the questions on page 138.

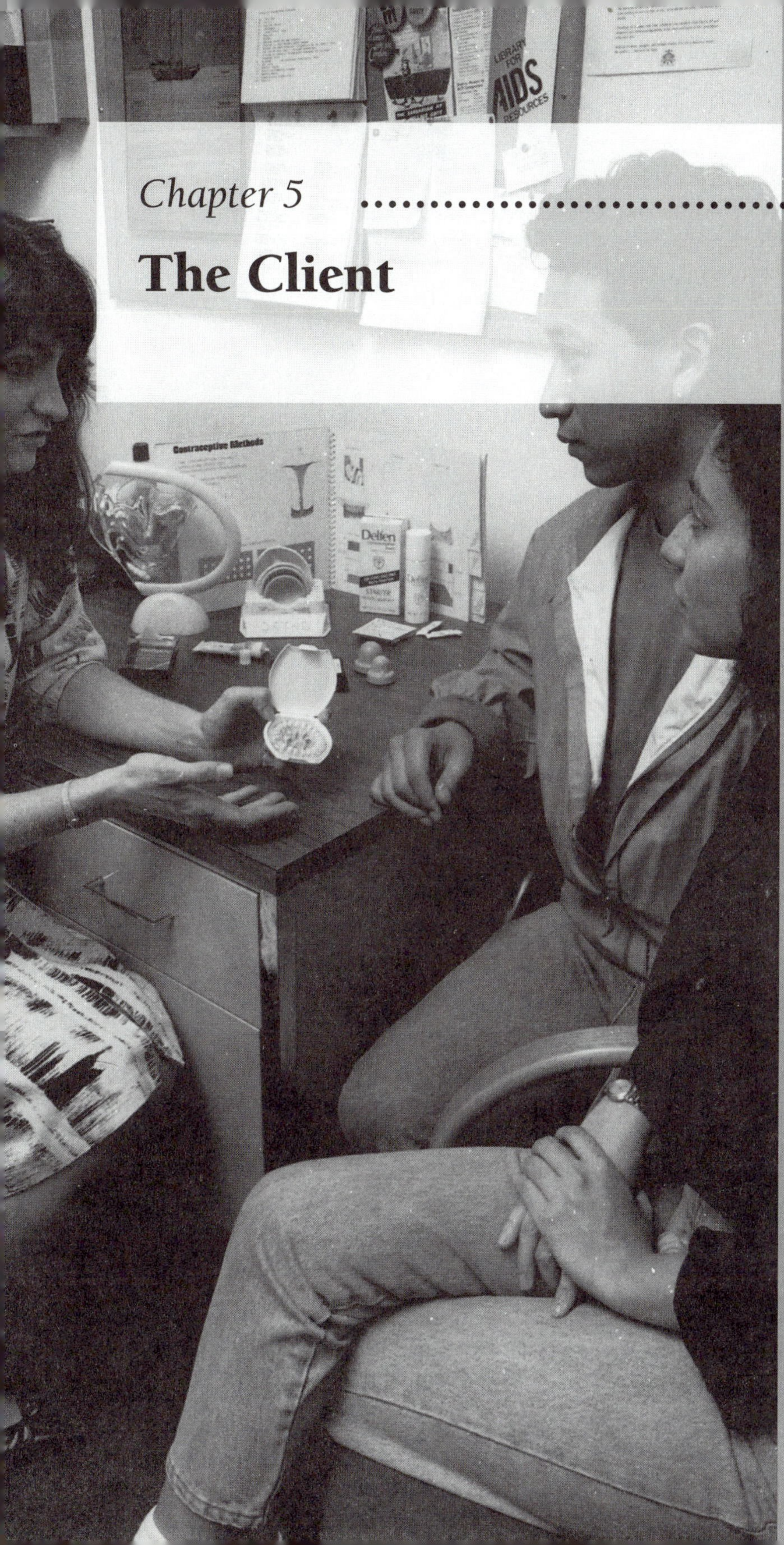

Chapter 5

The Client

The purpose of this chapter is to explore the client in the human service system. Understanding the client is critical to any study of human services. Indeed, the client is the reason there are helpers and a helping process. Part One has already established that some people, in some circumstances, need assistance from others to survive and to develop the ability to help themselves.

In an effort to define the term *client* comprehensively, this chapter introduces several ways of thinking about the user of human services. One way of viewing the client is to study the meaning of the phrase "working with the whole person." This is a guiding principle in human services because it focuses on the many components that define an individual and the areas of support a helper must consider when providing assistance.

Describing the problems that clients experience is also an important consideration in defining the client. And problems can be considered in various ways. Several possible theories can be used to define the problems and difficulties that confront individuals. A developmental theory approaches problems from the life span perspective and defines problems in terms of life crises or tasks that occur during a lifetime. The situational perspective describes problems that occur from accidents and other traumatic points in time. Meeting human needs, both physical and psychological, is another approach taken to explain the problems that individuals encounter. Finally, one theory posits that social change has a primary effect on the problems individuals experience. Each of these perspectives is defined and its impact on the delivery of human services is described in this chapter.

The term *client* has many meanings. In some cases, clients are individuals; in others, the client may be a small group, such as a family, or even a larger population, such as the residents of a geographic area. Descriptions of these different types of clients illustrate more clearly the range of meaning encompassed in this term.

Finally, in defining the client, we explore the experience of getting help from the client's perspective. Sometimes it is difficult for human service professionals who themselves have never been clients to understand thoroughly what it is like to ask for and receive services. We discuss the many ways of getting help, the barriers to be surmounted, clients' expectations, and their evaluation of services.

The Whole Person

Clients enter the human service delivery system as individuals with multifaceted perspectives that include psychological, biological, social, financial, educational, vocational, and spiritual components. All these perspectives are integrated within the individual to form the "whole person" that the human service professional encounters. During the helping process, the professional is continually aware that the client does not simply represent "a housing issue," "a food stamp dilemma," or "a child care consideration." Problems for clients are rarely single issues, and the human service professional should approach each client with the expectation of more than one problem. In fact, one problem can cause, influence, or at the very least, be related to other difficulties.

The case of Rufus is a good example of how problems in one area influence problems in other areas. The following is from the official record.

> "The client, a 38-year-old white male, was involved in a motor vehicle accident while riding his motorcycle. He sustained severe head injury, multiple orthopedic fractures, and cardiac arrest at the scene of the

> accident . . . evaluated the client in an acute rehabilitation facility 18 months after injury. The client had completed the acute rehabilitation phase of recovery, but because of funding issues, discharge had been delayed. The client was nonverbal . . . although he had some automatic activity of daily living, ambulation and communication functioning. The client needed 24-hour supervision for activity and safety. He was newly married, and his wife worked full time. (McBride, 1992, p. 72)

Rufus was involved in a motorcycle accident and the initial concerns for him were physical. He sustained multiple injuries and experienced cardiac arrest on site, so attention to his physical well-being was of primary importance. Once his physical condition stabilized, human service professionals involved with planning and providing his care, using the "whole person" perspective, established the following treatment plan that addressed other issues:

> *Current treatment plan.* Client receives 0.5 hour of occupational therapy 1 day a week. Client receives physical therapy for 2 hours per day, 5 days per week or as tolerated. Client has not been able to be tested by speech therapist nor does he respond to attempted intervention.
>
> *Immobility.* Client is at risk for complications due to immobility. . . .
>
> *Nutrition.* Client's usual weight is approximately 190 lbs. Client has a very poor appetite . . . current weight is approximately 170 lbs.
>
> *Verbal communication.* According to therapists and physician, client appears to withdraw from social stimulation . . . been observed to read a newspaper . . . consistently not engaged in eye contact or verbalized with therapists. . . .
>
> *Bladder and bowel impairment.* Client is incontinent of urine . . . and of bowels.
>
> *Self-care deficit.* Client is able to assist in bathing and dressing activities . . . he has not demonstrated any consistency in follow-through in step-by-step procedures. . . .
>
> *Psychological assessment.* Client has been consistently followed by a psychiatrist while in the acute rehabilitation facility. Multiple medical regimens have been utilized. . . .
>
> *Potential injury.* Client is at risk for potential injury . . . appears to need 24-hour supervision and care. . . .
>
> *Family/parenting.* Client was newly married prior to injury . . . on home visits . . . major problems included mobility . . . and client's behavior. (McBride, 1992, p. 73)

This treatment plan illustrates the multiproblem client receiving services in the human service delivery system. Note that, in this case, severe physical problems affect other areas, such as psychological functioning, relationships with family, vocational limitations, and financial difficulties. Although the financial and vocational are not addressed specifically in the treatment plan, advocates for the client are currently trying to find financial resources for him as he does not have long-term care benefits or home care benefits. Vocational needs are addressed by recognizing that the client will not be able to work and will need 24-hour supervision or care.

As a human service professional working with clients, the critical point to remember is that the client is an individual made up of psychological, social, economic, educational, vocational, and spiritual dimensions and possibly will have needs in many of those areas. Even if a client appears only to be looking for housing, the helper realizes that the client may possibly have other difficulties, such as unemployment, illiteracy, or a lack of child care. If single problems are solved with little attention to the other difficulties the client is experiencing, that person may not be able to become self-sufficient.

A majority of clients enter the human service delivery system because they are experiencing problems. There are many ways those problems can be defined.

Perceptions of Client Problems

Problems are a normal part of life. This concept is central to understanding who a client is and what problems the client encounters. As you recall from Chapter 1, the "problems in living" approach, which is basic to our definition of human services, has been a major factor in shaping the human service model (described in Chapter 4).

Defining Problems

Several definitions of *problem* are useful in discussing problems in living. For example, Epstein (1981) defined a problem as "a situation that is causing trouble, discomfort, difficulty" (p. 170). *Webster's Third New International Dictionary* (1986) expands that definition to include "an unsettled matter demanding solution or decision and requiring considerable thought or skill for its proper solution or decision" (p. 1807). These definitions suggest that problems in living can have two components: a description of the problem and a course of action leading to its resolution. First, the problem is described as a situation, event, or condition that is troublesome for the client. It can be as simple as a pregnant 20-year-old married woman's request for information about prenatal care programs or as complex as an unmarried, pregnant 15-year-old's need for counseling. The second component occurs in several stages: the problem is identified and discussed, solutions are formulated and implemented, and the results are evaluated.

One complicating factor in identifying and resolving problems is the difficulty of predicting what the client will experience as a problem. Factors such as the cultural values of the society and the developmental needs of the individual influence how problems are defined. For example, an increasingly common problem in this society is care of the elderly. The extended family that once cared for elderly relatives has been replaced by the smaller nuclear family, a unit whose living space and lifestyle are sometimes not suitable for the care of others. American society also tends to view the elderly as people who have already made their contributions and have retired from productive activity. In some cultures, the elderly continue to work; in others, the elderly have a high status though they have stopped working. Pinpointing a problem is also hard in this example because of the difficulty of predicting when elderly individuals will need care and what care they will require. Some people live in nursing homes at 65, unable to manage independent lives; others are living alone with minimal support at the age of 90.

How clients view their own situations and what they perceive to be problems are important factors in problem identification. Epstein (1981) suggested that client problems have two components. First, the person lacks the resources to solve the problem, and second, the person lacks skills to do so. Given Epstein's definition, the client and the helper may disagree about the client's situation. For example, the helper may believe the client lacks resources or skills, while the client may perceive no problem at all. In the client's environment, unemployment, poor school attendance, and illiteracy may be normal conditions among neighbors and family members. The client experiences these conditions as a way of life, not as situations that must be corrected or problems that need to be solved. The helper, on the other hand, may view these conditions as problems that should be faced and resolved.

Even if clients recognize the existence of problems, there is no guarantee that they will seek assistance. If they do ask themselves whether help will alleviate the problems they have, they may conclude that it will not. They may see the condition as something to be endured, or they may feel that having the difficulty is preferable to seeking assistance.

Categories of Problems

Despite the difficulties of problem identification, problems are still a useful way to address the identity and needs of the client. It is because individuals have unmet needs that they come in contact with the human service delivery system. The system uses a variety of conceptual frameworks to aid in identifying problems. This section introduces models to address three types of problems: developmental and situational problems, hierarchical needs, and needs created by social change.

A DEVELOPMENTAL PERSPECTIVE

According to developmental theorists, individuals engage in certain tasks or activities at different points in their lives. Describing the developmental process, Sheehy (1995) said, "We continue to develop by stages and to confront predictable crises, or passages, between each stage" (p. xi). Of the same process Levinson (1978) wrote: "An incomplete, highly dependent child grows in complex biological, psychological, and social ways to become, in greater or lesser degree, an independent responsible adult" (p. 1). The change of dependent children into independent adults was studied by Erik H. Erikson, a psychoanalyst and expert in adult development, whose major contribution to the understanding of human development was his description of the "eight stages of man" (Erikson, 1963). These stages, summarized in the list that follows, reflect the tasks through which individuals work during the different stages.

Basic trust versus basic mistrust. Infants learn to trust in an environment that consistently provides for their needs—that is, one in which the caretaker is sensitive to the needs of the infant. A person who does not experience this warmth and caring in infancy will have difficulty trusting others in later years.

Autonomy versus shame and doubt. In this stage, the toddler wishes to "let go" and try new things but does not know the alternatives and consequences of such actions. The child at this stage needs both urging to try new things and gentle protection from the consequences of his or her lack of experience. A toddler who does not experience such support may later be reluctant to try new things and may doubt his or her abilities.

Initiative versus guilt. The child who moves beyond the stage of autonomy is able to define a task and work to complete it. *Initiative* means cooperative effort, enthusiasm for new things, and acceptance of responsibility. When a person experiences success at this stage, he or she will generally become an adult who is willing to accept moral responsibility and takes pleasure in developing his or her abilities. A child who does not develop the ability to take initiative becomes an adult who is unable to take risks and meet new challenges.

Industry versus inferiority. In this period of growth, the child begins to experience life as a worker and provider. Receiving instruction and evaluation (in the culture, in school), the child learns to enjoy work and develops good work skills, such as the ability to concentrate and to manipulate the tools of the society. If the child does not develop a sense of being capable, he or she may later have a fear of inadequacy, resulting in poor performance, low expectations, or both.

Identity versus role confusion. In this stage, the adolescent begins to combine the identity formed in the previous stages with the work he or she must accomplish in the future. The stage is complicated by physical growth and sexual maturation. The adolescent rebels against those who previously provided support and relies on peers and heroes and heroines for guidance and care. During this stage, the individual struggles to make sense of an adult world in terms of childhood experiences.

Intimacy versus isolation. The young adult, having formed an identity during the previous stage, desires to establish intimate relationships that may include the components of mutual love, sexual intimacy, and parenting. An inability to establish intimacy with others may result in isolation.

Generativity versus stagnation. The adult assumes the responsibility for "parenting" the next generation, guided by the children's needs, as described for the previous stages. This parenting responsibility is required of all adults, not just those who are biological parents. During this stage, acceptance of this role helps the adult avoid stagnation and loss of purpose.

Ego integrity versus despair. The ego integrity that is possible at this stage represents the culmination of the successful development of identity through the previous seven stages. The older adult understands and accepts life as it has been experienced, assumes responsibility for that life, and accepts death as the final part of the life cycle.

Developmental theorists view life as a *process* from birth until death, from the beginning to the end. Although everyone goes through the same developmental stages, individuals experience these stages in different ways. Development may be affected by the social context in which the individual lives—the home, family, community, culture, country, and sociopolitical climate. The individual's characteristics, including his or her traits, wishes, values, and childhood experiences, may also influence the way he or she experiences each stage. Determining the stage on which the individual is working is sometimes difficult. Moving from task to task and from developmental stage to developmental stage are not activities as discrete as having a birthday or completing a list of jobs or chores. Sometimes an individual is deeply focused on the tasks of a certain developmental stage, but there are also times of transition between stages, when the tasks are being completed and the individual is only beginning to formulate the questions that will signal the next stage (Levinson, 1978).

An individual is deeply focused on a specific developmental stage at a time of intense questioning and exploring. A developmental stage begins when the tasks of that stage are of primary importance, and the stage ends when the individual's focus has changed (Levinson, 1978). For example, a toddler who has learned to walk may want to explore every nook and cranny at one instant but be paralyzed by a new environment a moment later. When the child's focus changes from the independence of walking to the independence of exploring new environments, his or her developmental tasks have changed.

There is a dimension of quality to the completion of developmental tasks: Even if a task is finished, it is not necessarily finished well. As mentioned earlier, developmental tasks are addressed within the individual's social context, and that context may not support individual development. In addition, how the individual has completed previous developmental tasks affects his or her work on the next stage. An individual may not reach the next stage with the necessary skills or confidence to continue developing.

Sheehy (1995) suggested that, in Western culture, the "normal activities and tasks for each stage are changing." Citing examples of 9-year-old girls developing breasts, 9-year-old boys carrying guns to school, 40-year-old women having their first children, and 50-year-old men being forced into retirement, she sees a life cycle that has changed. Puberty is earlier, adolescence is extended into the 20s, middle age extends well into the 50s, and the activities of the elderly are broadening. According to a recent population study, there has been a ten-year shift in the life stages. When developmental theories are used to identify problems that individuals experience, an important point to remember is that these traditional stages are changing. Even the concept of "elderly" or "being old" is shifting as we see increasing longevity.

One way to understand the concept of defining problems by theories of development is to study specific examples, such as the relationship of middle-aged mothers and adolescent daughters, which follows. It illustrates the developmental tasks of individuals in the *identity* (adolescent daughter) and the *generativity* (middle-aged mother) stages. Bassoff (1987) explained the problems that may arise when individuals work on particular tasks in their developmental stage and described how additional problems can develop when individuals in a family are focused on the tasks of different stages.

According to Bassoff (1987), adolescent development is a difficult period for young people, who are involved in a struggle for identity. Family harmony and individual well-being are threatened during this adolescent rebellion. Mother-daughter relationships are particularly vulnerable, because the daughter rejects not only adults in general but in particular the one adult with whom she has greatest similarity—her mother. The daughter's developmental tasks in the *identity* stage focus on separation from parents, which involves a growing independence. The adolescent daughter rejects her previous world of family and forms her own world with personally chosen friends of both sexes.

During this time, the middle-age mother is involved in developmental tasks of her own, as she reassesses her purpose in life. She is facing the end of her power as the "giver"—relinquishing her role as a primary caregiver in the family. (This assessment applies both to women who remained home to raise their children and to those who held outside jobs and pursued careers while raising their children.) The mother must change roles and develop new ways of relating to her family and friends. Time that had been devoted to caregiving tasks is now freed up, and she may begin to use that time for her own personal growth and development. Also in this stage, the mother begins to understand that life is not perfect and tries to view relationships and situations more realistically.

An ideal situation exists when the daughter and the mother can grow together. During this time, each may be involved in developmental tasks that can complement the other's. When the tasks are in step, the mother allows the daughter to separate, for two reasons. The mother understands that the daughter's separation is a necessary (albeit difficult) growth process for the daughter. Also, the mother does not feel personally hurt when the daughter rejects her, because the mother is attempting to reduce her role as caregiver and to relinquish the power as "giver" that she has held over others. The mother uses her daughter's questioning as an occasion to reevaluate her own life plans and purposes. The daughter is allowed to rebel and to reject the family and the tradition it represents without losing the basic support of the family. At the same time, the daughter is given more control and autonomy; as she separates, she also assumes more responsibility for her actions (Bassoff, 1987).

Unfortunately, most individuals do not operate in the world of the ideal. Problems arise when, as in this example, individuals are engaged in difficult developmental tasks. If the mother is feeling insecure about losing her primary role as a caregiver, she may continue to smother the daughter and resist any independent actions the daughter takes. When the daughter rebels, the mother, who views herself primarily as a caregiver, feels personally rejected by the daughter. The daughter may intensify her rebellion by running away, acting out in school, and verbally and physically abusing the mother. The daughter may also refuse to assume any responsibility for her behavior. Pressure from the mother-daughter conflict not only can ruin that relationship but can also threaten the stability of relationships with other family members.

The problem just described is just one example of the problems in living that arise as individuals work on developmental tasks. Using the developmental model to view problems may be helpful to the human service worker, because it provides the worker with a basic understanding of the process of growth and change that individuals normally experience. Workers can use the stages to help describe problems in terms of current tasks that require the client's focus, as well as to determine whether the previous developmental tasks have been adequately completed.

Human service professionals can also use developmental models to provide a framework for identifying problems not regarded as normal. For example, certain problems associated with mental illness (such as hallucinations and delusions) and with criminal behavior (such as aggressive, violent behavior) are labeled deviant. In any attempt to account for this deviance, the developmental model is a starting point for identifying whether a problem can be categorized as a problem in living or as a departure from the expected. With clients who have very serious problems not classified as problems in living, it may be necessary to use more than one problem identification model.

A SITUATIONAL PERSPECTIVE

Another way of viewing problems in living is from the situational perspective. Problems resulting from accidents, violent crimes, natural disasters, and major changes in life—such as a move, job change, or divorce—are all defined as situational problems. The characteristics of these problems are very different from those of the developmental problems discussed in the preceding section. First, these problems usually occur because the individual is in a particular place at a particular time. It is difficult for individuals to "be in the world" without experiencing some situational problems. Such problems can occur even if the individual has not done anything to contribute to or cause them. In such cases, individual responsibility begins once the situation has occurred and is identified as a problem situation. Linking situational problems with a specific event may be difficult because the event might be only a marker of a more complex situation. For example, with divorce or a geographic move, there are obviously contributing factors that precede the event. However, the problem may still be characterized as situational because of the existence of the marker, a clear problem on which the client and the human service professional can focus.

Another characteristic of situational problems is that they can lead to short-term and/or long-term difficulties. Most such problems require, at a

Andy and Bob's Story

Wrightstown had long been known as a tough, blue-collar suburb. Residents rarely ventured downtown, with its open-air drug markets and drive-by shootings. Still "men were men," and their reputations depended on toughness, sexual and beer-drinking prowess, and family honor. Big Sunday afternoon beer parties were a local ritual, and everyone knew that some of the biggest and wildest happened at Andy's house.

In a tough town, Andy's friend Bob was one of the toughest. Like his father before him, Bob had begun drinking heavily as a teenager and had accumulated records of school fights and simple assaults. He nearly always won the fights, but had recently lost his job for missing work—he had been in jail after a bar brawl that got out of hand.

Late one Sunday afternoon, on a run to replenish the beer supply, Andy ran into his out-of-luck friend and invited him back to join the party. Once there, Bob quickly drank up a six-pack and began making passes at Andy's sister, Charlene. Charlene had never liked Bob. The more she resisted his advances, the more aggressive he became, until she slapped him hard across the mouth. Bob stepped back and tripped over a coffee table. As he picked himself up, half the crowd was laughing at him. The other half was yelling at Charlene to "make it up to him like a good girl," but Andy saw his sister's honor at stake.

Andy came at Bob. The two fought in the living room until Andy's older brother told them to "take it outside" after they broke the coffee table. As the crowd moved out to the porch to watch and cheer, Bob yanked a tire iron out of his trunk and used it to knock Andy to the ground, unconscious. The crowd fell silent only after Bob jumped into his car, ran over Andy twice, and roared away. After what seemed like forever, an ambulance responded and took Andy to the hospital emergency room, where he died four hours later of massive internal injuries.

SOURCE: From "Understanding and Preventing Violence," by J. A. Roth, 1994, *Public Welfare*, 52(4), pp. 33–43.

minimum, immediate action. The complexity and quantity of assistance required depend on the severity of the problem and the state of the client when the situation occurs. Situational problems may require additional help after the short-term assistance has been provided. Yet another characteristic is that individuals experiencing situational problems are often viewed as victims, persons who suffer injury from their own fault or that of others. One of the first responsibilities of the helper is to move the client from the role of victim to the status of taking responsibility for personal actions and thoughts.

Violent crime is a situational problem experienced by Americans every year. According to research by Roth (1994), the United States has the highest per capita murder rate of any industrialized country, and—in 1990—23,438 people were murdered. In addition, approximately 2.9 million individuals were victims of nonfatal crimes, such as rapes, personal robberies, and aggravated assaults. Over 3.1 million simple assaults were reported—defined as such because they do not involve a weapon or an injured victim. These statistics account for the violent crimes that were reported, but do not include the unreported violence that occurs behind the doors of homes, workplaces, and institutions.

According to Berglas (1985), the emotional sufferings of victims of violent crimes are the most serious result of violence. One explanation for this finding is the damage that occurs after the crime to previously psychologically healthy individuals. After the crime, even healthy individuals are likely to experience depression, anger, shame, and anxiety. They begin to question their previous sense of social order and to redefine their ideas of fairness and justice. Women in particular experience a sharp increase in physical and psychological stress after such victimization. In a study of the effects of crime on women, Berglas found that rape is a particularly traumatic event, as 80% of the rape victims surveyed reported they either had a nervous breakdown or thought seriously of suicide or actually attempted suicide.

For some groups, violence is a more realistic danger than for others. The probability of being a murder victim is most serious for teenagers and young adults and nonwhite males, especially black males. Murders of black males have, in most cases, exceeded those of whites during the 1900s. The black-white difference appears to relate primarily to conditions in low-income neighborhoods, and homicide is documented as the leading cause of death for black males between the ages of 15 and 24. Roth (1994) estimated that a black male has a 1 in 21 lifetime chance of being killed, probably by one of his contemporaries.

Another situation that creates problems is unemployment. Corporate downsizing, closing of mills and factories, and the high rate of small-business failures are factors that have made unemployment a situational crisis for many individuals. One example is Don Harris of Joliet, Illinois.

> As the morning sun glints off the windshield of his rusty brown van, Don Harris crosses the hump of the steel drawbridge on the Des Plaines River into Joliet, Illinois, with a load of magazines he delivers for $72 each week. The job helps Mr. Harris soothe a stung pride. After 26 years with one company, he recently lost a $29,000 position as a grocery-store manager and had to resort to food stamps. (Tyson, 1995, p. 10)

These new unemployed are finding it difficult to secure jobs comparable to the ones they lost. Many are now working in retail outlets and shopping malls. Their jobs are part-time or temporary, pay less than their previous jobs, have fewer benefits, and often provide less job satisfaction (Tyson, 1995). Overall, the affected individuals feel ashamed and unappreciated. The situation also creates economic difficulty that the whole family faces as the chief breadwinner's ability to provide the basics such as food, clothing, and shelter is threatened.

Another example of a situational problem is divorce, a serious dislocation experienced by many individuals in this society. As mentioned in Chapter 2, futurists predict that the trend will continue for one out of every two marriages to end in divorce. Divorce is complicated when the divorcing couple has children. The actual situation of divorce causes many short-term problems, such as emotional trauma resulting in anger, confusion, and guilt; financial disability; redefinition of the parent-child relationship; and the need to determine parental visitation with children. Long-term problems may involve continued parental disagreements, remarriage and adjustments to stepfamilies, and geographic relocation. Children and parents may need assistance during this time.

MEETING HUMAN NEEDS

Another way of defining human problems is to identify basic human needs and ask, "Which of these are being met and which of these are not being met?" Abraham Maslow developed a hierarchy of needs that is helpful in the problem identification process. Maslow's hierarchy begins with the most basic of physical human needs and ends with the need of individuals to become self-actualized, to strive to develop their understanding of themselves and their environment (see Figure 5-1).

According to Maslow, these needs exist in a hierarchy, which means that individuals cannot address higher-order needs until their most basic needs have been met. If an individual is hungry, or cold, or scared, or in a life-threatening situation, he or she will have difficulty concentrating on love and belonging needs. Likewise, people who get little acceptance or respect from others will have difficulty involving themselves in activities that will lead to self-actualization. Brammer (1995) suggested that the needs can be divided into two categories: "D" needs (*deficiency* needs) and "B" needs (*being* needs). "D" needs comprise the first four levels, wherein an individual seeks to achieve calm and satisfaction. After these "D" needs are met, the individual seeks to achieve the "B" needs and concentrates on developing the self.

The importance of meeting basic needs is a primary consideration in the case of child abuse and neglect. According to the National Committee to Prevent Child Abuse, reported abuse has tripled since 1976, and in 1994 abuse affected 3 million children (Gardner, 1996). When children are abused and neglected, many of their basic needs are threatened, including their physical, safety, social, and self-esteem needs. Even though experts agree on the needs that are not being met, they have not always agreed on the way to restore children to a supportive environment.

During the 1960s and 1970s, the emphasis was on removing the child from the home and placing the child in foster care. During the 1980s, the approach was to leave children in the home and provide services to parents that helped them better meet their children's needs. Today, there is continuing debate about whether foster care or family reunification is the best approach to use the meet the children's basic needs.

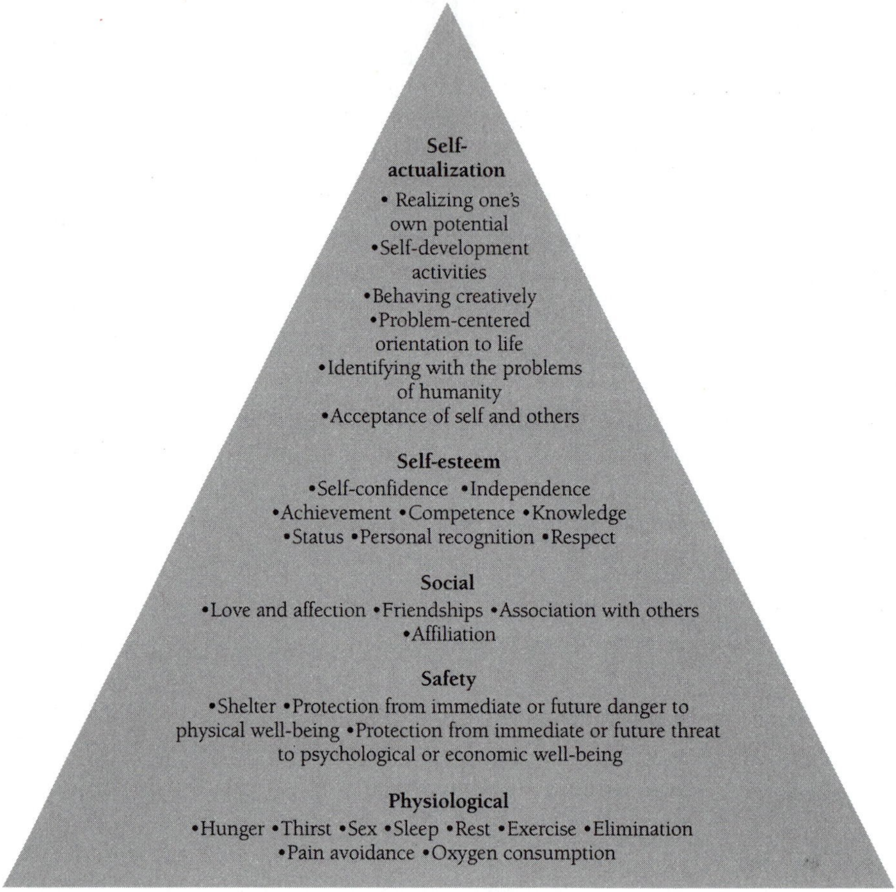

Figure 5-1 ✦ Maslow's hierarchy of needs

SOURCE: Adapted from *Fundamentals of Psychology,* by A. Haber and R. P. Runyon, p. 304. Copyright © 1983 by McGraw-Hill Publishing. Adapted by permission.

SOCIAL CHANGE AND ITS EFFECTS

Axelson (1985) suggested another view of the problems of human existence. Human beings experience problems not just because of their needs as individuals but also as a result of rapid social changes, the breakdown of many traditional forms of society, and conflicts between old and new values. In this century, many changes have occurred rapidly in society—sometimes explosively. Rapid social change leaves individuals in unfamiliar situations. Often, people do not have the skills, self-confidence, and support from others to adjust to changing demands. You can imagine the alienation and isolation experienced by people who retain the "old" way or who are no longer part of the mainstream of society as a result of changing urban areas and population shifts to suburbia. The homeless constitute one such group. Today that definition has expanded to include children, individuals with a dual diagnosis of mental illness and substance abuse, and those who live in the rural areas.

Homeless people have a variety of needs. This group can serve to illustrate the developmental and situational perspectives, as well as the approaches of Maslow and Axelson. Most people know there are homeless individuals, either from seeing coverage of their situation in the media or actually seeing homeless people in their community. In the discussion that follows, you will see that the homeless have multiple needs. Very basic survival needs come first; without a home, existence becomes a struggle to secure food, shelter, rest, and safety. However, homeless people also need recognition and acceptance by the community.

Few people choose to be homeless, yet many individuals find themselves in this situation as the result of rapid social change, unemployment, fire and flood disasters, or eviction. The homeless population includes single men and women and poor elderly who have lost their marginal housing, ex-offenders, single-parent households, runaway youths, "throwaway" youths (abandoned by their families or victims of family abuse), young people who have moved out of foster care, women escaping from domestic violence, undocumented and legal immigrants, Native Americans leaving the reservation after federal cutbacks and unemployment, alcoholics and drug abusers, ex-psychiatric patients, and the so-called "new poor" who are victims of unemployment and changes in the job market (Rivlin, 1986, p. 4).

Accurate statistics describing the homeless have been difficult to obtain; the very nature of the problem makes counting difficult. According to the 1990 census, 200,000 individuals fit into this category (Pendleton, 1992), and other experts speculate that more than 1 million people are homeless. According to a survey issued by the U.S. Conference of Mayors (1995), homelessness is on the increase, and 28 American cities saw a request for emergency shelter rise 13% from 1993 to 1994. The increase in requests for nonemergency shelter was 21%. According to this survey, individuals remain homeless for an average of nine months, and that length of time is increasing (U.S. Conference of Mayors, 1995).

There are several reasons for the increase in the homeless population. One is that the technological society in which we live has eliminated many unskilled and semiskilled jobs; downsizing and closing of factories has been the direct cause of job loss. In fact, employment-related problems such as unemployment and low wages represent the primary reason that individuals are homeless. A second reason is urban renewal or gentrification, which many municipal governments promote as a way to revitalize the downtown areas of cities. This movement has brought a decrease in low-cost housing, displacing individuals without providing any alternative affordable homes. Even in Atlanta, Georgia, in preparation for the 1996 Olympics, a new ordinance was passed prohibiting living on the streets, and there was stricter enforcement of the antiloitering and panhandling ordinances (Smothers, 1996). The changing structure of the American family has also contributed to the growth of this population. Because the nuclear family is more isolated than in previous generations, such events as divorce and the death of a spouse have forced individuals (and in some cases, whole families) to adapt to a lower level of survival (Fischer et al., 1986).

INTERNATIONAL FOCUS
Third-World Poverty

The following case study illustrates the effects of poverty on the physical and mental development of some citizens of the world. As you read about Fatima, Jaime, and Francisco, consider the following questions:

1. Which of Maslow's needs have been met? Which have not been met?
2. What are the consequences of these unmet needs?
3. How do the unmet needs influence Francisco's ability to develop according to Erickson's model?

HOW PEOPLE UNDERDEVELOP
Francisco's mother, Fatima, is small for her age. She is visibly weak, distant, yet easily irritated by the children. Years of pregnancy and menstruation, along with an iron-poor diet of maize, have made her chronically anaemic. Her husband Jaime is a landless laborer, with a low, erratic income barely enough to keep them all alive and clothed. No one eats enough, and when there's not enough to go round Fatima goes without, even when she's pregnant. And that is frequently, as the couple uses no form of contraception. They have had ten children, six of whom survived to adulthood.

Fatima went through several periods of undernourishment while Francisco was in her womb. There were times when Jaime could not get regular work and everyone went hungry. Fatima also had several attacks of stress and anxiety when Jaime beat her. Francisco probably suffered his first bout of growth retardation, both mental and physical, before he even saw the light of day.

He was born underweight, and his brain was already smaller than normal size. For the first few months he was breast-fed and suffered few infections, as he was partly protected by the antibodies in his mother's milk. Then he was weaned onto thin gruels and soups, taken off the breast and put onto tinned evaporated milk, thinned down with polluted water from the well. His diet, in itself, was inadequate. Then he started to get more and more infections, fever, bronchitis, measles and

Finally, deinstitutionalization, which many blame for most of the homeless population, in fact accounts for only 20% or 30% of this group (Kondrates, 1991; Nooe, 1996; Rivlin, 1986). The plight of people who are homeless for one or more of these reasons continues to be a problem as the number of public support programs decreases. As this group becomes more visible and society better understands their situation, perhaps more assistance will become available to help them reenter the mainstream of life. Today, almost one-half of all psychiatric patients are substance abusers and are categorized as dually diagnosed individuals who are difficult to serve. They have greater risk than any regular bouts of gastroenteritis. With well-fed children these pass within a few days; but in his case they went on for weeks and sometimes a month or more. In these periods he could tolerate no milk and few solids, and so was given weak broths, tea or sugar water. By now he was 25 percent underweight. Because of poor nutrition, he was even more susceptible to infection, and each time he was ill, he lost appetite, and ate even less. Then he got bronchitis which developed into pneumonia. But Fatima borrowed money off a relative, went to town and got antibiotics for him.

So he survived. But malnutrition made him withdrawn and apathetic. His mother got no reward from playing with him, so he received little of the stimulation his brain needed to develop property. As he grew older, infections grew less frequent, but by the time he went to school, aged eight, he was already a year behind normal physical development and two years behind mentally. The school, in any case, was a poor one, with only three classes, no equipment, and a poorly qualified teacher. As Francisco was continually worried about whether and what he was going to eat that day, he was distracted, unable to concentrate, and seemed to show little interest in schoolwork. The teacher confirmed that he was a slow learner, and could not seem to get the hang of math or reading and writing. As the family was poor, they did not want to keep him on at school. He was doing so badly anyway that there seemed no point. He did a year, then was away for three years helping an uncle who had a farm, then did another year, then left for good, barely able to read or write more than a few letters. He soon forgot what little he had learned. So, like his father, he began tramping round the local ranches asking for work. Without any educational qualifications or skills, that was all he could ever hope for. And because so many were in the same boat, pay was low. When he was twenty-two he married a local girl, Graciela, aged only fifteen. She too had been undernourished and was illiterate. She soon became pregnant and had to feed another organism inside her before she herself had fully developed. Graciela had heard about family planning from a friend, but Francisco would not let her use it and anyway she was not sure she wanted to. So, by the age of only twenty-five, Graciela already had five children and had lost two. The children had every prospect of growing up much as Franciso and Graciela did, overpopulating, underfed, in poor health and illiterate.

SOURCE: Excerpt from *Inside the Third World: The Anatomy of Poverty,* by P. Harrison.

other single group for rehospitalization, violence, suicide, poor self-care, and homelessness (Blankertz & Cnaan, 1995). The homeless individuals who are dually diagnosed also have high rates of interaction with the criminal justice system and have few family relationships they can use for support. Because of their history of medical noncompliance, they are never stable enough to receive services for any substantial length of time and they usually enter the human service delivery system only in a crisis (Blankertz & Cnaan, 1995).

INTERNATIONAL FOCUS
Children as Major Victims of Wars

A report issued by UNICEF in 1996 says that children are now the major victims of war. According to the report, during the last ten years, over 2 million children have been killed in wars that have devastated civilian populations. The report also stated that from 4 to 5 million children have been disabled, 12 million are homeless, and over a million have lost or become separated from their parents. In addition, over 10 million of these children are suffering psychological effects resulting in trauma caused by their war experiences. The report proposes that an antiwar agenda be adopted that targets improving and protecting the lives of young children (Crossette, 1995).

Some of the recommendations are these:

- Raise the age of military involvement from 15 to 18 years of age
- Draft a child impact statement each time economic sanctions are considered internationally
- Outlaw land mines, which maim or kill children
- Prosecute those who commit war crimes against children
- Allow children to reside in "zones of peace" where they can receive food and medicine during wartime
- Impose limited cease fires to protect and serve children's needs
- When war is over, provide rehabilitative services to children

A poignant story of one young Vietnam girl's experience illustrates the pain that children experience (Sciolino, 1996). Documented on film by American

One way to understand exactly who the homeless population are is to examine the ways they have been categorized. One method of categorization is to examine the personal attributes and life histories of individuals who are homeless (Fischer et al., 1986; Kiesler, 1991). In the early 1990s, this type of assessment identified four subgroups: the chronically mentally ill (including the dually diagnosed), street people, skid row alcoholics, and the situationally homeless (such as the unemployed or the evicted). By the mid-1990s, there had been a rise in the number of children and youth in the homeless population (McChesney, 1995; Nooe, 1996).

Families with young children are the fastest growing group of homeless. Many of these children enter the system with a single parent, usually the mother, but there is a growing number of two-parent families who are also homeless (McChesney, 1995; Nord & Luloff, 1995). Although some are without family and friends, many have relatives or other social ties, but they believe those in their support network would not "take them in" for more than a day or two.

journalist Nick Ut, 9-year-old Phan Thi Kim Phuc was running into the camera; she was naked and her arms were waving, she was caught by the lens screaming in agony with napalm burns over her body. In June 1972, there was fighting between the North and South Vietnamese troops in the Central Highlands of the South. The order was made to drop napalm bombs and they fell near a pagoda where Phan Thi Kim Phuc and her family were hiding. Two of her brothers were killed and she and another brother survived but were badly burned. The photographer took her to the hospital where she spent the next 14 months in rehabilitation. She had numerous grafts in an attempt to rebuild her body. During that time she was in intense pain and the medical staff said that she fainted and lost consciousness whenever her wounds were touched or washed. The world lost sight of her until a Dutch film crew found her in 1984. Later she moved to Cuba and tried to study, but she had to quit after she developed severe asthma attacks and diabetes that impaired her sight. In Cuba, she married a fellow Vietnamese man and traveled to Moscow for the honeymoon. When the plane landed in Newfoundland for refueling, they did not reboard. She sought her freedom in Canada, where she and her husband for a time were on welfare. Today he holds two jobs. She recently returned to the United States in an effort to forgive those who injured her and others in her country (Sciolino, 1996).

Today, she is still not free of reminders of the war. She has constant problems with asthma, diabetes, and migraine headaches. She also does not have sweat or oil glands and is in constant pain. "When the weather changes, the pain comes—like I am cut, cut . . . I try to keep down my pain, thinking, thinking to control my pain. I ask my husband, Tell me stories, funny stories, or ask me something, so I have to answer him. And that is the way I can live day by day. And I never think something sad" (Sciolino, 1996, p. A8). But she says that she is blessed, for she is a wife and a mother of a son, 3-year-old Thomas. She says that in her house she is always smiling.

Urban schools are struggling to provide educational opportunities for homeless children. The schools are faced with a challenge to educate during a time when children do not have a stable home and do not know where they will be living from day to day. There is also a growing number of teens who are homeless and not living with a parent or older adult.

Many refer to children in homeless situations as victims for they have "high rates of developmental lag, academic failure, shyness, dependent behavior, aggression, short attention span, withdrawal, depression, and anxiety" (Nord & Luloff, 1995, p. 462). The following story illustrates one teen's experience. Elizabeth became homeless when her parents threw her out of the house with only the clothes on her back:

> From April to October, Elizabeth lived in eight different places. She has lived in houses and trailers, with friends and alone. She lived in a friend's trailer by herself during the summer. He used the trailer every

Abraham Maslow

Abraham Maslow was born in Brooklyn, New York, on April 1, 1908. He was to become part of a wave of psychologists who challenged conventional psychology's most basic concepts. From his study of "self-actualized" people, Maslow theorized that all people have common psychological needs and that these needs are the foundation of human values. Lowry's (1973) biography of Maslow provides an interesting account of his professional development. Maslow first attended City College of New York in 1927 and became fascinated by anthropology—an interest he would retain throughout his life. In 1928, he transferred to the University of Wisconsin, where he became a devoted disciple of Margaret Mead, Branislaw Malinowski, and Ruth Benedict, who became close personal friends. While at Wisconsin, he lectured on various aspects of what would later become the psychology of culture and personality. In 1937, Maslow accepted a teaching position at Brooklyn College, where he worked with some of the greatest names in the fields of anthropology and psychology: Alfred Adler, Karen Horney, Margaret Mead, and Ruth Benedict.

His interests now turned from experimental psychology to the newer fields of social psychology, abnormal psychology, and human personality and motivation. He refined his theories on dominance into theories on self-esteem. He had found his true direction. In 1954, his first book, *Motivation and Personality,* was published; in it, he emphasized human freedom and human beings' potential for self-actualization. According to Maslow, self-actualized people are those who utilize their human capabilities to the fullest extent. However, this higher need cannot be achieved unless lower needs have been met. Maslow felt that therapy should be directed toward helping people understand their psychological needs and fulfilling them in constructive ways.

Maslow himself was no stranger to insecurity and low self-esteem. As a child, he had felt unloved and unlovable, because of his physical appearance and his father's scorn for it. Nevertheless, Maslow felt that people were basically good.

Maslow continued to write books as well as many articles for scientific journals and magazines. In 1967 and 1968, he served as president of the American Psychological Association. Maslow's ideas were to have a great impact on the newly emerging field of humanistic psychology, as well as on the literature of education, child rearing, and criminology. He died in 1970 in Menlo Park, California, where he was resident scholar of the W. P. Laughlin Charitable Foundation.

SOURCE: Adapted from A. H. *Maslow: An Intellectual Portrait,* by R. J. Lowry. Copyright © 1973 by Wadsworth Publishing Co., Inc. Reprinted by permission of Brooks/Cole Publishing Co.

> weekend, so she would have to move out during the weekends. Elizabeth lived with some friends for a couple of weeks, then would have to find a new place. She lived with one boyfriend and his parents for over a month. Currently, she lives with a boyfriend and his two siblings; she has lived there for 2 weeks. "I'm very embarrassed about my situation and I always try to hide it from the other kids. It's really not my fault, but I feel guilty," she says. "I don't have hardly any clothes so I don't feel I look as good as the other girls at school. If some of the people I lived with hadn't given me a few clothes I wouldn't have anything to wear." (Nord & Luloff, 1995, p. 469)

Homelessness, once thought of as an urban problem, has now become a serious problem for those in the rural areas. The rural homeless population has a higher percentage of homeless females and families than are found in the urban areas. Although few studies have been conducted about the individuals and families who are part of this growing segment of the homeless population, three factors have been isolated for female, single-parent, homeless women: residential mobility, residential insecurity, and residential inadequacy (Nord & Luloff, 1995). More information is needed to determine whether the rural homeless experience is different from the urban one.

A second way to categorize this population is based on the amount of time individuals are homeless, the alternative shelter available to them, and the nature of their social contacts (Rivlin, 1986; U.S. Conference of Mayors, 1995). Chronically homeless people with marginal social contact make up one group, which is associated with alcohol and drug abuse. This group may have some support from individuals with similar problems. The second category includes those who are homeless periodically. This means their homelessness is of limited duration and fairly predictable. A person who leaves home when the pressures become too great for him or her would be in this category. Usually, such a person has alternative shelter. The third category includes those who are temporarily homeless, usually as the result of a crisis such as a fire. They are homeless for a limited time only, and their roots are damaged but not destroyed. Finally, the fourth group comprises those who suffer total homelessness. For the most part, their situation results from the sudden and complete loss of their homes through disasters, which may be economic or interpersonal. These individuals have no support left. This is a fast growing group.

To improve your understanding of how human service workers understand this complex client group—the homeless—think of some of the homeless people in your community. As this group becomes more numerous and more visible, you may see them sleeping beside buildings or rummaging through garbage cans. Think of an individual you have seen, and describe his or her physical appearance. How old do you think he or she is? How do you imagine this person spends an average day? Where in your community do these people stay at night? How might this individual fit into the categories of the homeless described above? Identify five problems that your homeless individual has. Which problems are represented in Maslow's hierarchy? Which problems are associated with rapid social change?

Examples of Client Groups

This chapter has presented approaches to identifying problems through understanding human needs. This section examines examples of client groups with whom you may work in the field of human services. Before we discuss these clients, however, a brief review of the human service philosophy is useful.

Human services is concerned with the whole person. This means assessing the environment and the client so that he or she can be provided with comprehensive, coordinated services. Included in the provision of services is a focus on prevention by teaching the client to develop problem-solving skills as well as helping the client address present problems.

In many cases, the client will be an individual, but a broader definition of *client* is considered here as we examine some groups as clients. Such groups may be families, neighborhoods, problem populations, or even large geographic populations.

As you read the following examples of clients from the perspectives of individuals, groups, and populations, remember that knowledge builds compassion, and that what you learn about a particular client may transfer to other settings, situations, and clients. Ask yourself the following questions as you read each example:

1. Who is the client or client group?
2. How does this client group differ from other client groups? What similarities are there among these groups?
3. What is the stereotype of this group? What information contradicts these stereotypes?
4. What problems do the client groups face? Which models for defining problems may be helpful with this client group?
5. How are the perspectives of Erikson, Maslow, and Axelson represented in the problems of each group?

The Individual

The *African American male* is at risk for several reasons, including unemployment (20–30%), poor education, inadequate health care facilities, and discriminatory judicial processes and incarceration practices. Although some areas have improved, such as increased job programs and a greater number of African American judges, politicians, and businessmen, little attention has been directed at the African American male as an individual at risk. Life expectancy, health, and education have been identified as immediate areas of concern for the African American male (Hacker, 1995; Joint Center for Political and Economic Studies, 1994; Parham & McDavis, 1987).

African American males have a shorter life expectancy than white men or white or African American women. One reason for this is a higher homicide rate; 42% of all homicide victims are African American. As stated earlier, a black male's chance of being killed, probably by one of his contemporaries, is estimated at 1 in 21 (Roth, 1994). The problem is more acute among African American youths, who are 50% more likely to die before the age of 20 than are young whites. Homicides, drug abuse, suicide, and accidents all contribute to this statistic. The physical health of the African American male is endangered by a higher rate of cancer than for any other group in the United States. However, physical health is not the only concern; alcohol abuse and suicide are both significant mental health problems in the African American community. In fact, there is evidence of an increasing suicide rate among African Americans, which poses a serious concern (Blake & Darling, 1994).

Education in the United States is a primary socializing agent. However, the school system negatively affects the achievement and self-concept of many African Americans (Hacker, 1995; Parham & McDavis, 1987; Wilson & Lemann, 1991). Consequently, African American males are among the groups lowest in college matriculation and attendance. The implications of limited educational preparation for the African American male pervade all areas of life—reducing job possibilities, eliminating opportunities for vocational and social advancement, and determining future options for housing and children's education (Mortenson, 1996).

The *Vietnam veteran* is another client who is at risk in this society. United States involvement in the Vietnam War lasted approximately 13 years (1960–1973), and that war was especially stressful for several reasons. More than 50,000 Americans were killed, and far more were seriously wounded. The very nature of the combat contributed to the brutality of the war; sudden, unexpected guerrilla attacks made up much of the fighting. The war was controversial, so there was a lack of support within the United States for those fighting it. For the individuals who served in Vietnam, returning home to hear criticism and attacks from the public was often confusing and sometimes demoralizing. Because of air travel, their adjustment to civilian life was abrupt; soldiers were asked to make the transition from a jungle existence, fighting guerrillas, to their homes and families in little more than one day. Some estimates say that 850,000 of the 3,400,000 Americans who served in Southeast Asia during this time were affected by the stress of this experience and received either no treatment or inappropriate treatment (Department of Veteran Affairs, 1996; Hayman, Sommers-Flanagan, & Parsons, 1987).

Vietnam veterans may suffer severe psychological reactions, with symptoms that include depression, amnesia, fear of losing control, flashbacks, and sleep disturbance. Not surprisingly, some have turned to alcohol or drugs for relief, complicating their problems. The fourth edition of the *Diagnostic and Statistical Manual of Mental Disorders* (DSM-IV) (American Psychiatric Association, 1994) includes war trauma among the catastrophic traumas that trigger posttraumatic stress reactions. Such reactions are characterized as an anxiety disorder.

Today there are 189 centers for military veterans—at least one in each of the 50 states. They were established in 1979 to facilitate the adjustment of veterans by providing counseling services. In addition to this service, many medical centers run by the Department of Veterans Affairs have established

Department of Veterans Affairs: Readjustment Counseling Service

The Vet Center Program was established by Congress in 1979 out of recognition that a significant number of Vietnam era veterans were still experiencing readjustment problems. Vet Centers are community based and part of the Department of Veterans Affairs. In April 1991, in response to the Persian Gulf War, Congress extended the eligibility to veterans who served during other periods of armed hostilities after the Vietnam era. Those other periods of armed hostilities are identified as Lebanon, Grenada, Panama, the Persian Gulf, and Somalia. The goal of the Vet Center Program is to provide a broad range of counseling, outreach, and referral services to eligible veterans in order to help them make a satisfying post-war readjustment to civilian life. You are not forgotten.

In addition, Public Law 103-452 authorizes sexual trauma counseling for veterans who have experienced acts of sexual violence or harassment while on active duty.

ELIGIBILITY FOR SERVICES

All veterans who served during the Vietnam era (August 5, 1964 to May 7, 1975) or participated in the listed areas of armed hostilities since the Vietnam era are eligible for Vet Center services.

Eligible Areas of Armed Hostilities

Lebanon: August 25, 1982, to February 26, 1984
Grenada: October 23, 1983, to November 21, 1983
Panama: December 20, 1989, to January 31, 1990
Persian Gulf: August 2, 1990, to date of presidential proclamation ending Operation Desert Storm
Somalia: September 17, 1992, to date of presidential proclamation ending Operation Restore Hope

The Women Veterans Health Program Act of 1992 authorizes counseling for women veterans who have experienced acts of sexual violence or harassment

outpatient services for veterans. In another recognition of veterans' problems, President Clinton has announced new benefits for Vietnam veterans for illnesses and disabilities related to exposure to Agent Orange. Veterans with prostate cancer, subacute peripheral neuropathy, and seven other Agent Orange–related illnesses are entitled to these disability payments (Department of Veterans Affairs, 1996).

Another individual at risk who has received much recent attention in the media is the *anorexic or bulimic female*. Anorexia nervosa is self-imposed while on active duty. In addition, the Womens Health Extension Act of 1994 authorizes sexual trauma counseling for all veterans who experienced acts of sexual violence or harassment while serving in the military.

OBJECTIVES

To promote clinically sound services to veterans and their families. In order to meet the goal of the program, the Vet Centers have the following objectives:

- Outreach to locate eligible veterans to engage them in programs that meet their readjustment needs.
- Provide counseling and other services to eligible veterans and their families.
- Refer veterans to appropriate community agencies and service providers.
- Serve as a liaison between veterans and other VA facilities.
- Provide follow-up to ensure that eligible veterans receive adequate service.
- Offer community education to inform the public of the needs of veterans who served in combat or other situations of armed hostilities and the services of the Vet Center.

SERVICES PROVIDED

- Individual Counseling
- Group Counseling
- Sexual Trauma Counseling
- Marital/Family Counseling
- Alcohol/Drug Counseling
- Spouse/Significant Other Group
- Benefits Assistance and Referral
- Job Referral
- Employment Counseling & Guidance
- Community Education
- Liaison with VA Facilities
- Referral to Community Agencies
- Information regarding local & national veterans organizations & projects.

SOURCE: From "VA Fact Sheet," by the Department of Veterans Affairs, 1996, Washington, DC: Office of Public Affairs News Service, p. 1.

starvation, and bulimia is cyclic binging and purging of food (Frey, 1984; Martz, Handley, & Eisler, 1995). These "sister disorders" are fostered by our society's emphasis on thinness, beauty, and success; they result from an interaction of psychological, physiological, developmental, and cultural forces (Lenihan & Sanders, 1984; Shisslak, Crago, & Estes, 1995; Vandereycken, 1993).

One of the first signs of the presence of an eating disorder is a change in the person's personality. In some cases, developmental transitions such as leaving home or entering college may act as catalysts for one of these disorders to appear; frequently, the individual's family is also dysfunctional in some way (Brisman, 1996; Lenihan & Sanders, 1984). Some of the characteristics identified in clients with eating disorders are hyperactivity; limited range of affective responses; negativism; defiance; and the absence of pleasure, humor, or smiling. Periods of depression, mood fluctuation, and low self-esteem may also occur (Bruch, 1983; van Strien, 1996). Those most likely to develop eating disorders are students engaged in activities such as cheerleading, wrestling, track, and the performing arts (Frey, 1984). There are various treatments for eating disorders, including behavior modification, family therapy, hypnosis, and individual therapy. In addition to counseling, the professional involved with clients who have eating disorders coordinates treatment and collaborates with others as necessary.

Groups as Clients

Clients are often groups, such as the family, rather than individuals. This section describes some of the family problems in which human service intervention is appropriate.

The family is "a system with specific properties unto itself, and one that has developed rules, roles, and ways to communicate, negotiate, and problem solve so that its members can function effectively in the environmental context they share" (Baruth & Huber, 1984, p. 244). Composed of subsystems such as a marriage, which itself comprises two individual subsystems, the family is a hierarchical system. Its organizational structure may best be described as one of "wholeness," where the behavior of individual family members can be understood only within the context of the group.

The family as client comes to the attention of human service agencies for a variety of reasons. Divorce, abandonment, unemployment, unruly or delinquent children, adoption, and violence are some of the problems families may experience. The one we explore here is family violence, which occurs in all types of social groups. It is not determined by geography, economics, or age, and many families face such problems as child abuse, spouse abuse, and abuse of the elderly.

The literature on family violence recognizes each type of family violence as a serious problem. The 1960s focused on child abuse, and the 1970s concentrated on exposure of wife beating. Abuse of the elderly was the most publicized concern of the 1980s. Each type of abuse presents an example of the family as the client; the family *system* is dysfunctional in some way.

As many as 2 million children per year are physically battered by their parents. There appears to be a self-perpetuating cycle of abuse. Compared with individuals raised in nonviolent homes, victims of child abuse are 1,000 times more likely as grown-ups to use violence against a child or spouse (Gelles, 1981; Smith, 1996; Whipple & Wilson, 1996). The problem of *child abuse* is surrounded by many myths. For example, many people believe that child abuse occurs only in lower socioeconomic strata. Serving to perpetuate this myth is the stereotype of families at lower socioeconomic levels as uneducated, transient, and prone to violence. In contrast, families at middle and high socioeconomic levels are viewed as educated, resourceful, and able to control impulsive or violent behavior. In fact, child abuse occurs at all socioeconomic levels and among all races, nationalities, and religious groups.

In *spouse abuse,* the problem most often studied in the 1970s, the wife is usually the victim, although husbands can be victims also. Women usually receive the worst of the violence because they are smaller, less likely to be trained in the use of weapons, and sometimes more vulnerable due to pregnancy. Today the leading cause of injury and death to women is violence by intimate partners. This issue has become transnational in focus and is of concern to human service professionals and governments alike (Mills, 1996).

The highest rates of marital violence are among the following groups: urban families, minority racial groups, individuals with no religious affiliation, people with some high school education, low-income families, blue-collar workers, and families in which the husband is unemployed. One possible conclusion is that greater stress produces greater family violence. (Bennett, 1995; Gelles, 1981; Weaver, 1994).

The latest form of abuse to receive national attention is *parent abuse* or *elder abuse and neglect.* In some abusive families, children learn that hitting is an accepted part of family relations, and striking out at parents seems appropriate behavior to them. Most commonly, however, the elderly are the victims. In particular, elderly parents who reside with or are dependent on their adult children are targets. Those who are more likely to abuse the elder populations have difficulty with the law, have been hospitalized for psychiatric illness, or have difficulties with substance abuse (Conlin, 1995).

How prevalent is abuse of the elderly? To answer this question, we must consider three problems identified by Myers and Shelton (1987). One problem is defining abuse. What behaviors are abusive, and how can these be documented? A second problem is identifying those who are abused and those who are at risk. Finally, what interventions are appropriate and effective?

The categories of abuse are physical violence, negligence, psychological abuse, violation of rights, and neglect (Conlin, 1995). Hazzard (1995) estimated that 2% of the population over the age of 65 may be victims—more than a million individuals per year. Although elderly abuse occurs at a lower frequency and rate than child abuse, it is also less likely to be reported; one in three child abuse cases is reported compared with one in six cases of elder abuse.

Victims usually have physical or mental weaknesses, are widowed, are of advanced age, have had previous abusive relationships, or have a limited financial status. They are also over 75 years of age, female, white, middle class, and generally dependent on the caretaker adult son or daughter. Many are suffering from dementia (Cooney & Howard, 1995). The abuser is typically a middle-aged daughter who is the primary caretaker.

Several factors contribute to elder abuse. One of these is sociocultural factors. In American society, the prevalent attitude toward old age and the process of growing old is negative. Our mobile society is not really suited for care of the elderly in the home; the family is often unable to handle the financial difficulties or dependencies involved. Situational factors may include the increased stress of caring for children as well as older adults. Caretakers whose children have left home and who are looking forward to freedom may resent having to care for an elderly relative, resulting in "benign neglect" (Campbell, Harris, & Lee, 1995; Henton, Cate, & Emery, 1984; Sijuwada, 1995).

As more is learned about the abuse of the elderly, similarities between the battered child and the battered parent become apparent (Conlin, 1995; Steinmetz, 1982). Both victims are in dependent positions and assumed to be living in a loving, caring family situation. In many cases, the elderly recognize their dependence on the abusing caretaker and refuse to report the abuse. According to Steinmetz (1982), their reasons may include "fear of retaliation, lack of alternative shelter, fear of the unknown, and the shame and stigma of having to admit that they reared such a child" (p. 259). At the same time, however, both a dependent child and an elderly parent can be a source of emotional, physical, and financial stress to the caretaker. The elderly (like the abused child) may thus be in a double bind: the abuser is providing financial and other resources for the victim's survival.

In conclusion, family violence occurs in dysfunctional family systems. The most important step in coping with this problem is protecting the victim. The second step is preventing the violence by providing assistance to the abusers.

Populations as Clients

Three groups can provide examples to help us explore populations as clients: the new poor (or the "working poor"), single-parent families, and the underclass. All three of these populations experience multiple problems that are difficult to address.

THE NEW POOR (OR THE "WORKING POOR")

Individuals among the new poor are at the poverty line or slightly above. This is not a homogeneous group, but its members do have two things in common: They are poor, and they work (Chilman, 1995; Joe, 1984; Jones & Wattenberg, 1991). Such people can be found in cities, suburbs, and the country. They are African American, white, and Latino. Educationally, this group ranges from college graduates to people with only an elementary school education. The number of children who live in poverty, and whose parents work, has risen from 3.4 million in the mid-1970s to 5.6 million in 1994, an increase of 65% (Holmes, 1996).

Although economically vulnerable, the new poor are not eligible for Medicaid or welfare and are not perceived as truly needy. Carolyn Chute, author of *The Beans of Egypt, Maine,* a novel about the working poor, stated in an interview about her book: "Either people blame all the country's ills on them or they don't see them. Give the poor a little dignity. Anybody who works for a minimum wage is quite helpless. People say everybody has choices. But some have more choices than others. We are not all born equal" (Stevens, 1985, p. 7).

At the federal level there have been programs such as the "earned income tax credit of 1993, the small rise in the minimum wage, the increased public funding of child-care facilities . . . expansion of low-cost health-care resources and increased funding of the food stamp program" to aid the working poor (Chilman, 1995, p. 516). What is unclear at present is how the new political philosophy of reducing aid will affect this population.

SINGLE-PARENT FAMILIES

The program most people have generally thought of when they used the word *welfare* was Aid to Families with Dependent Children (AFDC). It was the principal program that gave money to people who are neither sick nor disabled; they qualified solely because they had children they could not support. The new welfare bill limits the time recipients may receive welfare. The challenges to this reform are to provide clients with education, job skills, quality day care, and ultimately a job so they can become self-sufficient.

The growing number of single-parent families headed by women is called the *feminization of poverty,* a condition suggested by Ken Auletta (1982) to be the greatest change in American poverty. Many families headed by women are impoverished, and the issue is not one of sexism but of economics. This term has expanded beyond the concept of mother-only families and has now begun to focus on men who do not provide support for their former wives and children. Foster (1995) suggested that five myths surround these single-parent families: children in single-parent families always have deficits; single parents cannot be both parent (nurturers) and breadwinner; single parents themselves are sometimes psychologically traumatized; children in single-parent families are expected to do poorly in school and to suffer emotionally and behaviorally; being a single parent means that life is horrible. Although in many cases single mothers are successfully raising their children, at times, the difficulties of single parenting and poverty are overwhelming. According to a report issued by the National Center for Children in Poverty (1994), poverty rates for children under 6 have risen dramatically in the past two decades and today there are over 6 million of these children. By the year 2000, some projections are that mothers and children will make up almost 100% of the families living in poverty (Sallee, 1986). In addition, the new welfare reform bill is predicted to leave a large number of children in poverty.

THE UNDERCLASS

A term popularized by Ken Auletta's 1982 book of the same name, *underclass* refers to a group of people known by a variety of names: the dependent poor, the acute poor, the bottom of the barrel, the disadvantaged. The term *underclass* is also used by the National Urban League and other civil rights leaders to describe the people left behind in urban areas as upwardly mobile African Americans move to better neighborhoods. Such people have been described as stripped down and socially disabled (Figueira-McDonough, 1995).

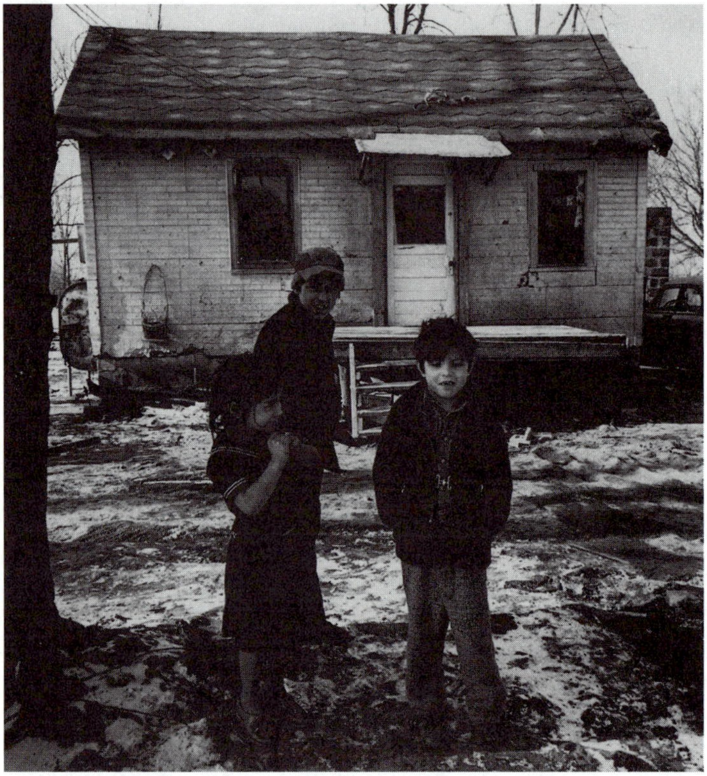

People living in poverty face many difficult problems.

There is vagueness about the identity of the underclass (Swisher, 1991). Some definitions include the working poor and single-parent families as part of this segment of society. There is no agreement on the size, definition, or causes of the underclass, nor is there any consensus as to whether its members' behavior is adaptive or cultural or whether its existence is society's fault or the fault of individuals. What is known is that it is an urban, poor, multiracial population estimated at 2.5 million (Gelman, 1988; Massey, 1994).

The underclass appears to be defined more by behaviors than by poverty. Although most members of this group are poor, they need not be so; street criminals, for example, are part of this population but they are by no means poor. The behavioral deficiencies observed in the underclass seem to be a more consistent measure of membership. The underclass typically operates outside the generally accepted boundaries of society, exhibiting deviant or antisocial behavior. Poor work habits, hostility, passivity, drug or alcohol addiction, and low self-confidence are common. It is also defined by social disorganization including unemployment, lack of family support, and living in rented housing. Dropping out of school is also considered a defining behavior (Figueira-McDonough, 1995).

In defining this group as clients of the human service system, a helpful start is to examine the categories of the underclass suggested by Auletta (1982). The passive poor, long-term welfare recipients make up the first category. Street criminals make up the second category; such individuals are usually high school dropouts and drug addicts. A third group, hustlers, earn a living in the underground economy and may even be prosperous. They rarely commit violent crimes. The last category includes the homeless, released mental patients, drifters, and drunks.

What are the consequences of the underclass? As a group, it is outside the mainstream of the economy and the labor force. For the individual members of the group, a lifetime of deprivation leads to dysfunctions such as low self-esteem, an inability to defer gratification, and avoidance of responsibility (Figueira-McDonough, 1995; Fordham, 1993; Sherraden, 1984). One approach to assisting this group is by reestablishing or redeveloping the inner cities, thus bringing people, businesses, and institutions to the underclass. This concern has yet to be addressed in American society.

This population is an important client group for the human service professional; although some statistics suggest that poverty has declined, the underclass has grown. It represents a minority of the poor, but it threatens to become a permanent class of individuals who require human services. The underclass may be very difficult to assist; the poor in the United States today are unlike the immigrant poor of the 19th and early 20th centuries, discussed in Chapter 2. The present group has little strong family support, little motivation to succeed, and little desire to become part of the mainstream. Assisting this group as a whole with one solution or program may also be difficult because the problems and the populations are so diverse.

Getting Help

Having discussed *what* problems clients face and *who* the clients are, we now address the question of *how* clients get help. The answer is not simply that clients experience problems and then find the appropriate human service agency because people do not always use the services they need. Gross and McMullen (1982), in describing the help-seeking process, raised the following questions: "Why don't people use available services? Why don't they ask for what they need if it is not available?" A discussion of the conditions under which clients enter the human service system, the barriers clients experience as they enter the system, and clients' perspectives on human services immediately before and after receiving assistance will provide answers to these questions.

Ways of Getting Help

As stated earlier, people do not experience problems and automatically go directly to the appropriate human service agency. Individuals can become involved with the human service delivery system in several ways, including self-referral and referral by other professionals. Clients can also be forced to receive services or can receive services inadvertently as members of a larger population.

REFERRAL

Referral, a common method of getting help, includes self-referral and referral by others. According to Boy and Pine (1968), "a counseling relationship that has been initiated by the client is built on a firmer footing than one into which he has been forced" (p. 144). Individuals may voluntarily seek assistance from human service agencies because they are desperate and confused. They have experienced a traumatic event or are in a situation so intolerable that they can no longer ignore it. Self-referral typically occurs when a client has tried every way she or he knows to cope, to no avail, and has no other ideas about how to address the problem. Some potential clients have heard about services from their friends and neighbors or through TV, radio, or billboard advertising and know exactly what their problem is and where to go. Others in desperate condition stop at the first agency available, regardless of its function, hoping that someone will be able to refer them to the right service.

Another type of referral is from another professional to a human service agency. Ministers, physicians, mental health workers, and other helping professionals often see an individual who needs assistance for problems beyond their expertise. The referring professional first assesses the client's complex situation and then refers him or her to one or more additional human service agencies. For such a referral to be successful, the referring professional must help the potential client clarify his or her problems and begin to provide some alternative solutions. (Referral may be one of those solutions.) This action may preempt the next professional's work, but it assures the client that the referring professional is not just "passing the buck." The referring professional should also provide the potential client with as much information as possible about the agency to which the referral has been made. If the client is somewhat reluctant to go to another professional for help, more assistance from the referring professional will increase the probability that the referral will be successful.

INVOLUNTARY PLACEMENT IN THE SYSTEM

Another way of getting into the human service system is to be placed in the system by others. *Involuntary* clients—referred by schools, prisons, courts, marriage counselors, protective services, and the juvenile justice system—are potentially difficult to work with because they have not chosen to receive services. The service to which they are referred usually offers only part of the treatment they are to receive. Their cooperation and participation in that service is often monitored, and decisions about subsequent treatment (including release from treatment) are partially based on their observed attitudes and progress. This creates some pressure on the clients to treat the referral seriously.

One example of the use of involuntary referral of clients is the case of child abuse. The decision to allow a child to remain in or return to a home may be contingent on agreement by one or both parents to receive counseling services. For another example, the juvenile court may order involuntary services for first offenders. Depending on the crime and the circumstances, judges often sentence juveniles to receive counseling, to perform tasks in the social services, or to assume other responsibilities related to their crimes. A third example involves individuals incarcerated for crimes. Much of their time in prison is programmed by others, and they have little say over their treatment.

Involuntary clients and voluntary clients may feel very differently about human services. Someone else has decided that the involuntary clients need assistance; they have not admitted that they need help and probably would not have chosen the human services they are receiving if they had decided to seek help on their own. They are often embarrassed or angry that someone else has decided what they need and has sent them to receive the services in question. Because they have not chosen the assistance, they may also feel trapped. Their alternatives are much more limited than those of voluntary clients. If they do not like the treatment or the worker, they may have little ability to change the helping situation.

INADVERTENT SERVICES

Another way of entering the human service system is to be part of a larger population that is targeted for services. In this situation, receipt of services does not depend on the individual's need or ability to qualify for the services, and the client does not have to ask for them. Although inadvertent services can often help the client, they also have their limitations. Ideally, before services are provided to a large population, the consumers using the services are consulted. However, some of the clients receiving the services may not have had any input about the type of service provided or the manner in which it is delivered. In such cases, the services provided may seem useless to the client. Services that clients receive inadvertently include the redevelopment of low-cost housing; neighborhood crime watch programs; shelters for the homeless, AIDS victims, or the elderly; and emergency help for disaster areas.

Barriers to Seeking Help

Many clients who need help do not receive the services they need, and they do not seek the services for a variety of reasons. Gross and McMullen (1982) discussed this phenomenon in terms of the "cost" to the individual client of seeking help, as represented by barriers to clients attempting to involve themselves in the human service system. Barriers that clients experience are discussed next, including how they view the problem, the cost of the resources, and the reluctance to use friends as helpers (Gross & McMullen, 1982; "One-Stop Shopping," 1992). Reading a description of these barriers may be frustrating, because the problems are presented from the client's point of view, without any discussion of how helpers can overcome such client barriers. We have chosen to separate client barriers from helper responses to retain the focus

Mental Health Facts

WHAT TO WATCH FOR

Even when you try your best, you will still experience periods of frustration and unhappiness. Usually, with time, you will overcome your distress. But you should learn to recognize when your problems—or those of your loved ones—are too much to handle alone. You can help yourself, your family, and your friends by knowing when to ask for professional help. Some of the warning signs include these:

Undue, prolonged anxiety. This is an anxiety out of proportion to any identifiable reason or cause. Of course, all of us experience problems that make us tense and anxious. But a deep, continuing anxiety—a state of constant tension and fear that fastens itself to one cause after another—is a signal that help is needed. Unrelieved anxiety not only causes mental anguish but can also lead to physical problems.

Prolonged or severe depression. Depression strongly affects thinking, feelings, and behavior. Feelings of inadequacy, helplessness, hopelessness, undue pessimism, and loss of confidence are symptomatic of depression. Changes in behavior patterns are a key sign that depression may be getting out of hand and help should be sought.

Depressed individuals often withdraw from friends they normally enjoy, from loved ones, and from the usual occupation and hobbies that give pleasure. Their eating and sleeping habits change. Some suffer from loss of appetite and insomnia; others seek solace in overeating and sleeping.

Other symptoms of depression include low energy; chronic fatigue; decreased effectiveness at school, work, or home; and loss of sexual interest. Depressed individuals are those most likely to think of suicide as a solution, although people with other mental and emotional disturbances may also be suicidal. During periods of crisis, people should be with others, avoiding isolation.

Abrupt changes in mood and behavior. These changes do not include deliberate steps a person adopts for self-improvement. They refer to changes in mood and behavior that reflect serious alterations in an individual's normal habits or ways of thinking. For example, the exceptionally frugal man or woman who suddenly begins gambling away large sums of money may be experiencing emotional problems.

on the client. Subsequent chapters will provide a human service response to such barriers.

BARRIERS TO PROFESSIONAL HELP

In discussing barriers, one of the first factors to consider is how the client views the problem. If the client considers the problem too difficult to solve, too

Tension-caused physical symptoms. Some bodily ailments and complaints have no physical cause, such as a daily headache, a migraine induced by tension, nausea, pains, and other complaints. These symptoms, including pain, are very real. But only a physician is qualified to determine whether they are caused by distress rather than physical malfunctioning. Because medical tests may reveal an organic cause, any persistent physical ailment should be checked by a doctor.

If any warning signs are severe or long lasting, professional help may be needed. If the true cause of the problem can be identified, often the symptoms can be relieved.

HOW TO FIND HELP

There are many services available to persons experiencing mental and emotional problems:

- Mental health associations provide information about mental health resources available in your community.
- Professional associations usually have state or local chapters that can help in finding an appropriate professional in the community. These include the state psychological and psychiatric associations or medical societies.
- Family service agencies provide information, referrals, and counseling for individuals and families.
- Self-help organizations, such as the National Alliance for the Mentally Ill, Recovery, Inc., and Alcoholics Anonymous, can provide assistance.
- State and local departments of social services, city or county health departments, or county medical associations and others, including Veterans Administration hospitals, school counseling programs, and private clinics, can also provide help.

TWO IMPORTANT TIPS

How much you are helped depends on the "fit" between your personality and that of the therapist. It pays to seek help from another if you feel dissatisfied or unaided by a particular therapist.

If you have a mental or emotional problem from time to time or over a long period, try not to be unduly discouraged. Most of us experience some symptoms of stress in the course of living. When stress or its symptoms seem more severe than usual, help should be sought. *Remember, you are not alone.*

SOURCE: National Institute of Mental Health, 1985.

overwhelming to consider, or too embarrassing to admit, then he or she is less likely to seek help. Clients who perceive the problem this way may consider seeking help a burden or a waste of time. From the client's perspective, the problem cannot be solved even by experts.

If the client is embarrassed at having the problem, seeking help means admitting to others that there is a problem. The very nature of many problems

Getting Help: One Client's Perspective

I needed help, and I had mixed feelings. I felt guilty needing help. It probably had something to do with the way I was raised. If you're strong enough, you shouldn't be having emotional problems. The barriers to getting help were mostly internal. I didn't feel like it was okay to be as angry or depressed as I was. I felt I should just snap out of it. There's a family history of breakdowns. I really don't know if it's hereditary. Some people thought that was an excuse.

I really didn't have any contact with a human service worker until the second time I was hospitalized, and I think that she was the one who was instrumental in getting me the help I needed to get out. She was the first one who told me there was even any way out at all, that I might be able to get an education. I think she was helpful because she had been through a divorce and had a child, so she knew firsthand what it was like—the fear of being alone, providing for children, and the hurt that you go through in a divorce. She understood. And while she was very helpful, on the other hand, I got to where I didn't look forward to talking with her because our sessions turned into discussions of the things she had experienced. So it was good on one hand, and then again, I wanted to back away after a while.

I also had one doctor who put me on so many medications, I gained weight until I weighed over 200 pounds, which was just making me more depressed. I had to go for a physical, and the doctor said one of those medications shouldn't even be mixed with the others. That added to the depression, so I took myself off everything and I lay down to die. And my husband would have allowed it. It seemed like the depression was in cycles, too. I'd be depressed and I'd want to die, and then I'd get angry. When I got angry the last time, I was the one who called the doctor and said I needed help.

in living involves a reluctance to admit to having problems. Spouses in troubled marriages may be reluctant to talk about their difficulties because parents and significant others have warned them about the trouble this could cause them. Abused children, spouses, and parents keep the abuse quiet because making an accusation would cause great disruption and because they, the abused, feel that the situation is ultimately their fault. Men in this society are less likely to seek help than women experiencing similar problems because men are socialized to solve problems on their own.

Another barrier is the individual's perception of the human service professional. Such workers are viewed as strangers and experts—two categories that establish immediate barriers for those in need. The helping process requires the individual in need to talk about personal issues and concerns with someone unknown. For many individuals in our society, the "stranger" evokes distrust and suspicion. The expert commands respect but also fear. The client initially sees the expert as an "accomplished" person who has little in common with individuals who have overwhelming problems. Fears of the stranger and the expert are barriers that prevent individual clients from seeking services and from trusting workers in the initial stages of the helping process.

Three barriers are directly related to available client resources: money to pay for the services, transportation to reach the place of service delivery, and the time and distance involved in traveling to receive the services. For the disabled, architectural barriers may present additional problems. Many clients may be ready and willing to seek assistance but cannot determine a way to surmount the problems of paying for services or of finding time and transportation to receive them. One solution to the inability to pay is to provide services to poorer clients on a realistic sliding scale. Transportation is a difficult problem for rural clients who live miles from the nearest population center. Equally vulnerable are clients who live in smaller cities without mass transportation or in larger cities with expensive mass transportation. Other clients cannot use services because they work long hours or are caring for children or an elderly parent. Unless service hours are extended and house care relief is provided, services may be inaccessible (from the client's perspective) even if they are affordable and nearby. What makes these barriers particularly frustrating for the clients is that they add one more set of problems to an already troubled situation.

The psychological costs of seeking help are also serious barriers. Some clients view help as effecting an immediate loss of their freedom; they fear that helpers will demand changes in their behavior, lifestyle, and work habits. They do not want to lose what little freedom they have. Clients also fear that they will ultimately have to assume responsibility for their problems, and this may frighten them. When clients admit that they need help and seek assistance, they are also afraid that they will be considered inadequate. When a person seeks help, it is a signal to others that the individual cannot solve problems alone and that his or her efforts have failed. To admit such "failure" is very difficult. Sometimes there is considerable pressure from peers not to seek help, especially if the peers see themselves as having a similar problem. Finally, clients resist seeking help because they fear being indebted to a human service worker or agency. Asking for and receiving help means giving the worker the power of a caregiver. Clients feel pressed to live up to the worker's expectations and fear disappointing the worker if little or no change takes place in their lives.

BARRIERS TO FRIENDS AS HELPERS

The barriers are very real to individuals who are experiencing problems in living and choose not to seek help. Besides being reluctant to seek the help of professional workers, such individuals often hesitate to seek out informal help from family and friends. This reluctance stems from their own fears and fear of the reactions of others. Some of the barriers to seeking help from significant others are similar to the barriers to seeking professional services. Telling friends about their problems may cause a loss of face; reputations and good appearances may suffer if others know about the problems. People want others to think well of them. It is a common worry that once others know about their problems, the individuals will lose friendships or respect. People also fear that the disclosure will be a burden to those who have been told—that the problems might upset the listener or place him or her in an uncomfortable situation. To impose on friends might violate the "rules" of the friendship.

Another reason individuals do not ask their friends for help is that they do not find them helpful. Many friends do not know how to respond appropriately, offering only advice, authoritarian "shoulds," and cliches. Also, many friends cannot be trusted. What the individual experiencing problems considers confidential may be considered public information by the friend. Most potential clients do not want their problems to be common knowledge in their own environment.

THE RELUCTANT CLIENT

Reluctance, in its many forms, may have its positive characteristics, although many experienced helpers believe that establishing a bond with a client is easier if the client wants and seeks help (Vriend & Dyer, 1973). Brammer (1995) acknowledged that client reluctance is to be respected. Reluctance is often self-protective, designed to maintain personal integrity. Part of the helping process requires clients to admit there is a problem, sharing information about themselves and their environment, and engaging with the helper to change their behaviors and evaluate the change. This process requires an inner strength that potential clients may lack at the beginning of the process.

The Client's Perspective

Once individuals have decided to use the human service system to seek solutions to their problems, they become voluntary clients, categorized by Perlman (1975) in three ways. *Buffeted* clients are those with multiple problems, who come often for services and use them to address their various problems. *Problem solvers* are those clients who use the services less often but for a range of different problems. *Resource seekers* are those clients who do not use the services often and come to the human service system for the resolution of just one problem. Buffeted clients and resource seekers perceive the nature of problems and the nature of services differently. Buffeted people see the human service system as a place to get help with their many problems. They perceive the system as equipped to handle a variety of the problems they experience. Resource seekers, in contrast, see the human service system as available on a more limited basis for assistance with one specific kind of problem.

Client Expectations

To understand the client, we must know what he or she expects from the human service system and the human service professional and how he or she perceives that same system after receiving help. Today's clients are focusing more than ever on the quality of care they will receive. The following discussion of client perceptions before and after receiving services is based on the results of several studies of client perception of the juvenile justice system, family services, protective services, and services to unmarried mothers. Although the information was collected from clients requiring different services, the results are surprisingly similar.

First, many clients imagine that the helper will have an unbiased attitude toward the client and will have experience in working with the problems the client is experiencing. The helper will understand the problems because he or she will have the client's point of view. The potential clients studied also expect the helper to listen, help them decide what to do, and help them do whatever needs to be done. Clients also expect the helper to assist them in dealing directly with the environment (Craig & Hennessy, 1989; Mayer & Timms, 1969).

Clients also have clear expectations of how the helper should behave (Pohlman, 1986). According to a survey, clients expect helpers to tell them what they should do. Helping professionals should be able to understand what clients say, provide them with necessary information, and offer an opinion of their own if it differs from the clients' opinions. In other words, the helper is expected to take a very active role in the helping process.

Clients also have ideas about what they expect from the helping process. These expectations fall into three categories (Franklin, 1995; Kenny, 1995; Maluccio, 1979; Toczek-McPeake & Matthews, 1995). First, the clients want to find a cure or straighten out a situation. They are looking for quick solutions and quick answers. If they want change, they define results as change in self and change in others. Their ideas about what changes should occur are concrete rather than general or abstract.

When asked about the problems they were experiencing and what services they needed, the clients again answered in concrete terms (Kenny, 1995; Mayer & Timms, 1969; Morse, Calsyn, Allen, & Kenny, 1994; Toczek-McPeake & Matthews, 1995). For clients, the lack of resources and the need for tangible goods and services were the most important. Of secondary importance was the need to solve intrapersonal and interpersonal problems. Clients defined problems in practical terms and were reluctant to define something as a problem if they thought it could not be resolved.

Client Evaluations of Services

Clients today are much more sophisticated in the area of client satisfaction. They are acquainted with issues of access and quality of services, and many of them provide feedback to agencies and service providers by filling out satisfaction surveys and questionnaires after they have received services. Because of the current climate of accountability, clients are more vocal about what they expect and what will satisfy them.

The clients' views of services after the process were consistent with their prior expectations. The most positive outcomes, in their view, were the practical

A Client Speaks

ABOUT BEING A CLIENT

When I chose to be a client, I didn't think there was any hope for me as far as my disease of alcoholism was concerned. I thought that I didn't have a choice, that I would end up one day dying as an alcoholic. And I didn't know anything about AA or about treatment centers. One day I stumbled on this information from another alcoholic who was still practicing his disease, and he told me they had a treatment program for veterans. At that point, I was in school, I was trying to get some education to better myself, and I was sick and tired of trying to fight this disease on my own. I wasn't getting anywhere with it. I might go two or three days, but then the next thing I know I'm back out there again. When exams came around, I got test anxiety, and just to relieve that pressure I would take a drink, saying to myself, "I'm just gonna take a couple of drinks." But I would drink until I'd get sick. And I decided that it was time for me to try something, 'cause what I was doing was not helping. So I called the hospital and they set up an appointment. I really didn't know what to expect when I got there. I was kind of fearful. I thought it was a place where you go to dry out and get back on your feet and then they send you back out. But it was not that way. They educated us about the disease of alcoholism and that people were beginning to accept it as a disease, and that there was hope for the alcoholic. I started to feel a little better, because until then I didn't think there was any hope for me. And I found out that I had a choice. I had a choice to drink, or to go to AA meetings to get help.

ABOUT THE FIRST DAY IN THE HOSPITAL

What stands out for me the first day I went to the hospital was that I was not alone. I thought I was the Lone Ranger, and I saw that I was not the only person suffering with this disease. I felt a sense of hope. Because everybody I talked to said, "I understand how you feel. You should have seen me three weeks ago. I was worse than you." So, my first day, my first week there, I started seeing other people coming in like I came in, and some of them were worse than I was, some were not, but when you see them that first day, you say, "Man, that was me two weeks ago." Then when they leave, you look at them, and there is no comparison. They begin to look like human beings—not just drunks that have low self-esteem and no future. The biggest thing that stood out was that I wasn't alone. For years I thought I was the only one out there.

ABOUT BARRIERS TO GETTING HELP

I think the biggest barrier is myself. I don't think it's anything out there, because wherever I go, there I am, and I still have those same problems. The world is not gonna change; you can't change other people, places, and things.

ABOUT HUMAN SERVICE WORKERS

The majority of the workers are compassionate people and are very understanding. The ones that I find are not understanding are the ones that have not experienced this disease. They don't know what alcoholism is all about. The last time that I went in treatment, I had a doctor who told me about will power, and he did not want to admit me to the hospital on a Sunday evening. He told me to go downtown and get a motel and come in Monday to be admitted. The secretary, however, said, "We will make an appointment with you Monday, and if you think that you won't be able to make it, detox is open 24 hours a day. You can come up there, and we'll admit you in detox." But the doctor was being real tough. I think that if he had been an alcoholic, he would have admitted me, because they had beds. I even walked over to the unit and talked to the nurse on duty. She said that she had two or three beds available, but he told me that he was not gonna admit me. At first he said he was. He said, "I have to call over there and find out if they have any beds, and if they do, then we'll see what we can do for you." I don't know if he called or not, but he didn't admit me. But getting back to what I was saying, people who have been through alcoholism understand and they can see through all your cunning, manipulative ways.

ABOUT GETTING HELP

I think the biggest thing for any person seeking help, or anyone who is in an institution, is to break out of the denial stage. I think that is the biggest downfall for everybody, for any client. That was my biggest problem for years. I knew I had a problem, but I would not admit it. I always said, "No, it was just circumstances, I was at the wrong place at the wrong time," or "I just had one beer too many." I was in denial for a long time. And today sometimes I'm in denial about certain things, but the key to that is awareness; today I'm aware of what my downfalls are, and what I need to do to make life better. If you really and truly want to do something about your problem, you have to be totally honest with yourself, because you can't be honest with other people until you start being honest with yourself. And once you start being honest, you got to be open-minded, be able to take criticism from other people, and in my case, I needed to stop being passive and start being assertive and not letting people control my feelings.

ABOUT BEING A VIETNAM VETERAN

I was over there for a period of 90 days in Saigon, Thailand, and Korea. I was in the air force and I didn't have a rifle, I had an IBM computer. Life centered around the NCO club. That's where I started my drinking. I had a lot of fear when I went over there, a fear of dying. The first place I went was Da Nang in 1970. Every day we had rockets coming in, and I was afraid all the time that I was over there, and I first started drinking to relieve all of my fears—the nervousness and the worry that the

(continued)

(continued)

next one was gonna hit this barracks. When I first went over there, every time that siren would go off, I would take cover. After a period of time, I got into drinking, and any time that siren would go off, we'd sit there and continue to drink. It's a part of my life sometimes I really don't like to talk about. We have a veterans' group at the hospital, and I told them that I didn't think that I was qualified to sit in with those who were out there in the field and are now suffering from posttraumatic stress syndrome. Every time they see a Vietnamese, something just goes off and all they see is just that person, and they're ready to fight, ready to kill them right here in America today. I'm fortunate that I don't have to go through that. But coming back here to the United States and saying that you're a veteran, putting on your veteran's cap, and feeling proud that you served your country, and then someone spits in your face and calls you a baby killer when we were over there taking orders, I don't know what this world's coming to. It makes me angry, it makes me angry.

improvements in their lives, such as better living conditions, food, and clothing, as well as intangible improvements, such as increased self-confidence, assumption of new roles, acquisition of new skills, and solution of their problems in living. Helper activities that they viewed as particularly helpful were the ones that went beyond talking to them. They praised workers for helping them get something, taking them somewhere, talking to someone for them, seeing someone with them, and referring them. Most clients considered the outcomes of the helping experience to be very positive, viewed the workers as helpful and fair, and felt that things were better for them after the service than before. Most perceived at least some improvement or the potential for improvement in their situations.

Several research studies have examined the factors that are linked to client satisfaction and client dissatisfaction. The following description of those factors represents a summary of this research (Franklin, 1995; Gariti, Alterman, Holub-Beyer, & Volpicelli, 1995; Kenny, 1995; Mayer & Timms, 1969; Morse, Calsyn, Allen, & Kenny, 1994; Toczek-McPeake, 1995; Winefield & Barlow, 1995). The factors are related to client expectations before services, as described above.

SATISFACTION

1. The client's satisfaction is linked to the client's perceptions of the helper. Specifically, the clients were more satisfied with the services they received if they perceived the worker as having similar values, if the helper accurately perceived their needs, and if they perceived the worker as an expert with experience in the problem area.
2. The clients also wanted to have a good relationship with their human service professional. For them that meant that the helper spent time with them, listened to their problems, and provided emotional support.

This also included being called prior to appointments and receiving follow-up contacts.

3. The clients wanted to participate in the process of helping, especially if they were long-term clients. They wanted to have input into the decisions about their treatment. They also based their satisfaction on the amount and accuracy of the information that they received.
4. Satisfaction is also linked to the helper's ability to solve problems and the amount of change the clients felt occurred during the helping process. Clients also expressed a willingness to return for help if the need were to arise. They measured their satisfaction based on the number of outcomes that were met and the ways in which their treatment plan was followed.
5. These clients also stated that their environment had been supportive and that they themselves were independent and proactive in seeking solutions to their problems.

Conversely, those clients who expressed dissatisfaction can be described as follows:

DISSATISFACTION

1. Dissatisfaction arose when clients wanted material assistance from the helper, but the helper wanted to focus on personal and interpersonal problems. There was a clash between the helpers' and the clients' expectations.
2. The clients who were dissatisfied received unwanted advice and help. They also felt that the helper did not have the skills to assist them with their problems, that the helper was inaccessible, and that the helper never understood their problems.
3. Clients were also dissatisfied when they were not clear about their problems and their treatment plan—that is, they could not articulate precisely what the problem was or what intervention was proposed to resolve it.

✧ Things to Remember

1. Understanding the client is critical to any study of human services. The term *client* includes more than just individuals; a client may be a small group, such as a family, or a larger population, such as the residents of a geographic area.

2. Definitions of problem suggest that "problems in living" can have two components: a description of the problem and a course of action for resolving the problem.

3. A way of defining human problems is to identify basic human needs and ask, "Which of these are not being met?" Abraham Maslow developed a hierarchy of needs, which begins with the most basic of physical human needs and ends with the need of individuals to become self-actualized.

4. Human beings experience similar problems, not just because of their individual needs but also as a result of rapid social changes, the breakdown of many traditional forms of society, and conflicts between old and new values.
5. Individuals can become involved with the human service delivery system in several ways, including self-referral or referral by other professionals. Self-referral occurs when individuals have tried every way they know to cope, to no avail, and have no other ideas about how to address the problem.
6. Ministers, physicians, mental health workers, and other helping professionals often see an individual who needs assistance for problems beyond their expertise. The referring professional first assesses the client's complex situation and then refers the client to one or more additional human service agencies.
7. Client expectations fall into three categories. The clients want to find a cure or straighten out a situation. If they want change, they define results as change in themselves and change in others. Their ideas about what changes should occur are concrete rather than general or abstract.
8. From the clients' perspective, positive outcomes were the practical improvements in their lives, such as better living conditions, food, and clothing, and intangible improvements, including increased self-confidence, assumption of new roles, acquisition of new skills, and solution of their problems in living.
9. The client's satisfaction is linked to his or her perceptions of the helping professional and of the relationship. Satisfaction is also linked to the worker's ability to solve problems and the amount of change the clients felt occurred during the helping process.
10. Conversely, clients who expressed dissatisfaction did so for two reasons. First, some clients wanted material assistance from the helper, but the helper wanted to focus on personal and interpersonal problems. Second, the clients were dissatisfied because they received unwanted advice and help.

Additional Readings: Focus on Clients

Dash, L. (1996). *Rosa Lee: A mother and her family in urban America.* New York: Basic Books.

For four years the author followed Rosa Lee Cunningham, her eight children, and five grandchildren, in an effort to capture life in the growing black underclass.

Knapp, C. (1996). *Drinking: A love story.* New York: Dial Press.

The author began drinking at age 14 and drank for years until a series of personal crises forced her to confront her alcoholism.

Kotlowitz, A. (1991). *There are no children here: The story of two boys growing up in the other America.* New York: Anchor Books.

This portrait of two boys who live in a Chicago housing project chronicles their struggles with school, the lure of gangs, and the death of friends. The realities of urban poverty are described through their eyes.

Sheehan, S. (1993). *Life for me ain't been no crystal stair.* New York: Pantheon Books.
This account of 14-year-old mother, Crystal Taylor, describes the emotional consequences of foster care—of being moved from one home to another, from foster family to institution and back.

Swados, E. (1991). *The four of us: The story of a family.* New York: Farrar, Straus & Giroux.
The book describes the experiences of an upper-middle-class family in Buffalo as they cope with one member's descent into madness. It is the story of a family's disintegration fueled by a combination of anguish, guilt, denial, and anger.

Williams, D. (1992). *Nobody nowhere: The extraordinary autobiography of an autistic.* New York: Times Books/Random House.
The author maps the closed world of the autistic in this tale of her lifelong struggle with autism. Decoding the language and behavior of autism provides new insights into this condition.

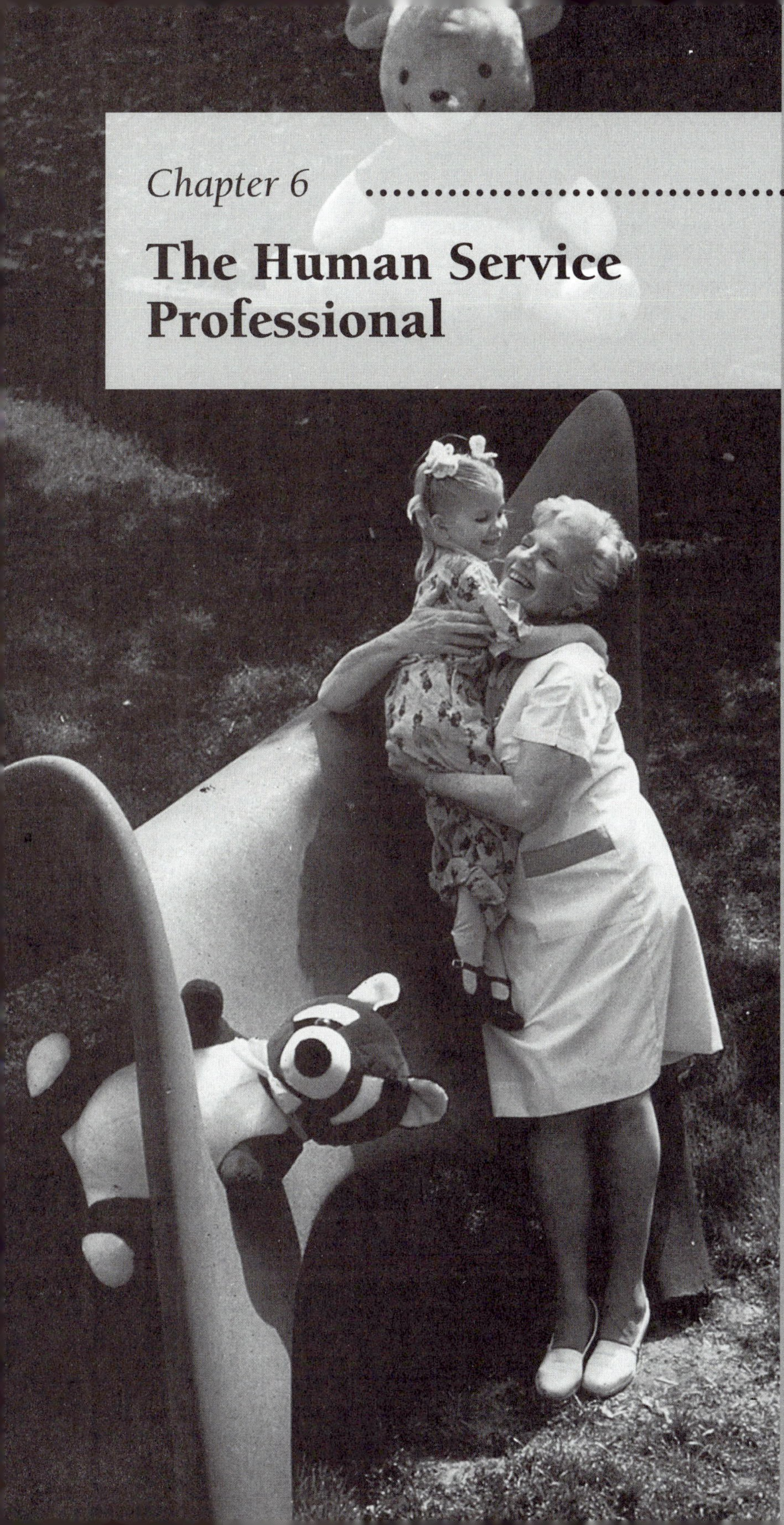

Chapter 6

The Human Service Professional

Helping means assisting other people to understand, overcome, or cope with problems. The *helper* is the person who offers this assistance. This chapter's discussion of the motivations for choosing a helping profession, the values and philosophies of helpers, and the special characteristics and traits helpers have will assist in establishing an identity for the helper. We also define workers as human service professionals, as well as introduce other professionals with whom they may interact.

This chapter also focuses on how one becomes a human service professional—by examining characteristics as well as transition issues that may be encountered by a student entering the profession. Among the issues explored are the frustrations of working with a bureaucracy, difficulties that arise from a strong desire to help, and problems involved in the change from the role of student to the role of professional. The topics discussed in this chapter should help you understand who the human service professional is.

Who Is the Helper?

In human services, the helper is an individual who assists others. This very broad definition includes professional helpers with extensive training, such as psychiatrists and psychologists, as well as those who have minimal training, such as volunteers and other nonprofessional helpers. Regardless of the length or intensity of the helper's training, his or her basic focus is to assist clients "to understand, overcome, or deal with external or internal problems" (Okun, 1997, p. 7), "to reach goals that are important to them" (Brammer, 1977, p. 303), to provide a "link between the traditional professional and the client" (Epstein, 1981, p. 33), or all these functions.

The human service worker is a helper who can be described in many different ways. For example, Hutchins and Cole Vaught (1997) suggested that effective helpers are people who are "together"—that is, whose thoughts, feelings, and actions are congruent. Such a helper, believing that each client is a unique individual different from all other clients, will greet each one by name, with a handshake and a smile. Others view a helping person as an individual whose life experiences most closely match those of the person to be helped (Lyon & Duke, 1981). The recovering alcoholic working with substance abusers is an example of this perspective. Still another view of the helper, and the one you are most familiar with from your reading of this text, is the generalist human service worker who brings together knowledge and skills from a variety of disciplines to work with the client as a whole person.

Your understanding of the human service worker as a professional helper will become clearer as this section examines the reasons individuals choose this type of work, the traits and characteristics they share, and the different categories of their actual job functions.

Motivations for Choosing a Helping Profession

Work is an important part of life in the United States. It is a valued activity that provides many individuals with a sense of identity as well as a livelihood. It is also a means for individuals to experience satisfying relationships with others, under agreeable conditions.

Understanding vocational choice is as complex and difficult a process as actually choosing a vocation. Factors that have been found to influence career choice include individuals' needs, their aptitudes and interests, and their self-concepts. Special personal or social experiences also influence the choice of a career (Kantor, 1960). There have been attempts to establish a relationship between vocational choice and certain factors such as interests, values, and attitudes, but it is generally agreed that no one factor can explain or predict a person's vocational choice.

My Work as a Human Service Professional

Thom Prassa, a case manager at a community health agency, describes his work and the skills necessary to be effective.

> In my job, I am a strong advocate for children, which means that I listen, communicate, sell, and monitor. Once a child is remanded to state custody, we must complete an assessment and a plan of services for the child. This requires that we work with the child, the family, the court, and other agencies and professionals in the community.
>
> Adeptness at placements is critical. Which service providers in the community are good and which are not? Who is going to be able to work effectively with these children? Case managers must have their finger on the pulse when it comes to getting these kids in the right place at the right time. Communication is also important. Being diplomatic in the sense of getting together people who are dysfunctional. Trying to develop a creative plan of care for the child sometimes means that it is necessary to tell parents or custodial designees what their responsibilities are. What must the parents do to get the child back? In a staffing, all the participants are present, they learn what their responsibilities are, and they agree to a plan of care. Then you must sell the plan to the child, explaining what is going to happen and how the child will benefit.
>
> Sometimes I feel like much that I do is responding to crises. We put out fires all the time. We have disruptions, suicide attempts, children who need different levels of care, decisions about what to do, and communications with the custodial designee about a child. We also talk with parents, report to foster care review boards, and make progress reports to the community. This is all an incredible responsibility but I know we make a difference in the lives of children here.
>
> There are a number of approaches to a job like mine. I have survived the past two and a half years because of my relationship with my team members. The camaraderie in the office is excellent and we support each other. You also have to have a life outside of work—hobbies, education, and friends. Strong supervisors and co-workers who respond to your needs are also helpful. (Thom Prassa, personal communication, July 10, 1994)

Donald Super, one of the leaders in vocational development theory, believes that the vocational development process is one of implementing a self-concept. This occurs through the interaction of social and individual factors, the opportunity to try various roles, and the perceived amount of approval from peers and supervisors for the roles assumed. There are many other views of this process, but most theorists agree that vocational choice is a developmental process.

How do people choose helping professions as careers? Research in this area tells us that the choice is influenced by direct work experience, college courses and instructors, and the involvement of friends, acquaintances, or relatives in helping professions (Pins, 1963). Money or salary is actually a small concern compared with the goals and functions of the work itself. In other words, for individuals who choose helping as their life's work, the kind of work they will do is more important than the pay they will receive.

There are several reasons people choose a helping profession. It is important to be aware of these motivations because each may have positive and negative aspects. One of the primary reasons individuals choose helping professions (and the reason that most will admit) is the desire to help others. To feel worthwhile as a result of contributing to another's growth is exciting. However, helpers must also ask themselves the following questions: To what extent am I meeting my own needs? Even more important, do my needs to feel worthwhile and to be a caring person take precedence over the client's needs?

Related to this primary motivation is the desire for self-exploration. The wish to find out more about themselves as thinking, feeling individuals leads some people to major in psychology, sociology, or human services. This is a positive factor, because these people will most likely be concerned with gaining insights into their own behaviors and improving their knowledge and skills. After employment, it may become a negative factor if the helper's needs for self-exploration or self-development take precedence over the client's needs. When this happens, either the helper becomes the client and the client the helper, or there are two clients, neither of whose needs are met. This situation can be avoided when the helper is aware that self-exploration is a personal motivation and can be fulfilled more appropriately outside the worker-client relationship.

Another strong motivation for pursuing a career in helping is the desire to exert control. For those who admit to this motivation, administrative or managerial positions in helping professions are the goal. This desire may become a problem, however, if helpers seek to control or dominate clients, with the intent of making them dependent or having them conform to some standard.

For many people, the experience of being helped provides a strong demonstration of the value of helping. Such people often wish to be like those who helped them when they were clients. This appears to be especially true for the fields of teaching and medicine. Unfortunately, this noble motivation may create unrealistic expectations of what being a helper will be like. For example, unsuccessful clients do not become helpers; rather, those who have had a positive helping experience are the ones who will choose this type of profession. Because they were cooperative, motivated clients, they may expect all clients to be like they were, and they may also expect all helpers to be as competent and caring as their helper was. Such expectations of both helpers and clients are unrealistic and may leave the helper frustrated and angry.

Values and Philosophy

Values are important to the practice of human services because they are the criteria by which helpers and clients make choices. Every individual has a set of values. Both human service workers and clients have sets of values. Sometimes they are similar, but often they differ; in some situations, they conflict. Human service workers should know something about values and how they influence the relationship between the worker and the client.

Where do our values come from? Culture helps establish some values and standards of behavior (Brill, 1995). As we grow and learn through our different experiences, general guides to behavior emerge. These guides are *values,* and they give direction to our lives (Raths, Harmin, & Simon, 1978). Because different experiences lead to different values, individuals do not have the same value systems. Also, as individuals experience more, their values may change.

What exactly are values? Values are statements of what is desirable—of the way we would like the world to be. They are not statements of fact. Three processes determine whether something is a value; collectively, they define *valuing,* the process that results in values. The three categories are explained by Raths, Harmin, and Simon (1978, p. 28):

CHOOSING

1. Freely
2. From alternatives
3. After thoughtful consideration of the consequences of each alternative

PRIZING

4. Cherishing, being happy with the choice
5. Enough to be willing to affirm the choice to others

ACTING

6. Or doing something with the choice
7. Repeatedly, in some pattern of life

Values provide a basis for choice. It is important for human service professionals to know what their own values are and how they influence relationships with co-workers and the delivery of services to clients. For example, professionals who value truth will give the client as much feedback as possible from the results of an employment check or a home visitation report.

Because human service delivery is a team effort in many agencies and communities, there have to be some common values that will assist helpers in working together effectively. According to Austin, Skelding, and Smith (1977), the following are the most commonly held values in human services: acceptance, tolerance, individuality, self-determination, and confidentiality.

The next paragraph introduces Beth Bruce, a human service professional with a variety of experiences. In this section, her experiences are used to illustrate the values that are important to the human service profession.

INTERNATIONAL FOCUS
A Peace Corps Experience

I am a Rural Health Education volunteer. I am currently trying to determine what the population of Gouessesso (my village of 600 people) think their primary health problem is. I am a replacement volunteer, meaning that there was a volunteer here before me for two years. The Peace Corps often has two volunteers and sometimes three in the same site consecutively, depending on the programs under way. I am the third volunteer in Gouessesso. I am going from courtyard to courtyard with the village animatrice (an educator who does health talks, helps with weekly vaccinations, etc.) who is fluent in the local language, Yakouba. Also, there is a health committee here so I'll be meeting with them next week. They will have input on the priority problem and will also be able to put their feelers out. Once I determine the priority health problem, I, along with a nurse, will develop a program to educate the population about the problem and work on a solution.

The priority problem the previous volunteer focused on was malaria. When I ask people about malaria, they have all the information they need to prevent it. They know causes, symptoms, treatments, and prevention techniques.

I think the biggest health problem is the lack of latrines and the fact that all garbage gets tossed in the woods. Some of the houses here have inside toilets, but most don't have toilets or electricity. Many of those with inside toilets (none have running water inside) have to be bucket flushed because they are broken. Building latrines or somehow organizing the garbage (maybe having just two places for dumping or building a garbage collection site and arranging for pickups) are ambitious projects.

AIDS is also a problem here in Cote D'Ivoire, in general. The previous volunteer did lots of AIDS work, too. He got the two boutiques to start selling condoms and did lots of educational presentations. I may have to keep up the pressure on that, as far as getting programs in schools, etc. There are no conservatives here when it comes to AIDS—just lots of parents, teachers, and governmental officials who want to keep people alive and know that people must be educated before making any choices.

That is one cultural lesson I have learned. Bodily functions here are nothing to be embarrassed about. People burp, pass gas, pick their noses, etc., like it's nothing. Once I burped unexpectedly and immediately covered my mouth and said "Excuse me." People stopped talking and looked at me. "It's nothing," "No problem," "It's good," they said. "Oh, okay," I said. I'm still not comfortable with all that but I am much less noticeable about noticing it than I was when I got here.

Melinda Bridges
Peace Corps Volunteer and Human Service Graduate
September 1996

Beth Bruce is a human service professional in the Estes Mental Health Center, a comprehensive center serving seven counties. She has been a case manager at Estes for the past eight months and has really enjoyed her first year's work in mental health. Her first job was as a social service provider in a local nursing home, where she worked for two years. She then worked with adolescents as a teacher/counselor at a local mental health institution before joining the Estes staff. Let's see how human service values relate to Beth's experience as a human service professional.

Acceptance is the ability of the worker to be receptive to the client regardless of the way a client is dressed or what the client may have done. Workers act on the value of acceptance when they are able to maintain an attitude of goodwill toward clients and to refrain from judging them by factors such as the way they live or whether they have likable personalities.

One of the most important values that Beth holds is accepting her clients for who they are. She has worked with the elderly, teenagers, and now persons with mental illness. These populations are different, but they retain one important quality for her: They are all human beings. Her acceptance of all clients has been put to the test. She had a male client in the nursing home who had once been tried for murder and found guilty. Because Beth believed that no circumstance justifies the killing of another, she had difficulty accepting that man as a worthwhile human being.

The second value of human service work is *tolerance:* the helper's ability to be patient and fair toward each client rather than judging, blaming, or punishing the client for prior behavior. A helper who embodies this value will work with the client to plan for the future, rather than continually focusing on the client's past mistakes.

Beth works with a friend and co-worker who is not very tolerant of persons with mental illness. Several times, this co-worker's intolerance of client behavior has caused problems for the client. Just yesterday, a problem arose with Ms. Mendoza, a 26-year-old schizophrenic who is currently receiving day treatment and lives in a group home. She refused to see her parents when they came to see her at the day treatment center. Mr. Martin, Beth's co-worker, forced Ms. Mendoza to see them because he believes that family is very important and that parents have a right to see their children. Now the parents are upset because Ms. Mendoza threw a chair at them. Ms. Mendoza is upset with Mr. Martin for making her see her parents, and Mr. Martin is angry with his client because he feels he was right to insist that she see them.

Individuality is expressed in the qualities or characteristics that make each person unique, distinctive from all other persons. An individual's lifestyle, assets, problems, previous life experiences, and feelings are some of the areas that make him or her different. Recognizing and treating each person individually rather than stereotypically is how workers put this value into practice.

When Beth first started working with the elderly, she had had little contact with older individuals. What she knew about them she had learned from her grandparents. She thought of the elderly as lively and quick-witted like her grandmother or quiet and shy, living in the past, like her grandfather. During her first months at the nursing home, the clients she encountered continually surprised her. They represented a broad range of human attitudes, behaviors, and experiences. She learned to distinguish between the generalizations she had made about the elderly and the information she now possessed based on her experiences at the nursing home.

Deciding for oneself on a course of action or the resolution to a problem is *self-determination.* The helper allows clients to make up their own minds regarding a decision to be made or an action to be taken. The helper facilitates this action by objectively assisting clients to investigate alternatives and by remembering that the decision is theirs. In some cases, clients are limited by their situations or their choices. For example, a prison inmate may have restricted alternatives from which to choose recreational activities. However, it is the inmate's right to choose from the available alternatives.

When Beth worked with teenagers, she was constantly aware that although these clients were not of legal age, they needed to feel they had some control over their own lives. She often helped them sort out alternatives, but she constantly resisted when they asked her to give advice or to make their choices for them. She believed that they should be responsible in most situations.

The last human service value is *confidentiality.* This is the helper's assurance to clients that the helper will not discuss their cases with other people—that what they discuss between them will not be the subject of conversation with the helper's friends, family, or other clients. The exception to this is the sharing of information with supervisors or in staff meetings where the client's best interests are being served.

A speech that Beth learned early when she was working with the elderly still applies in her work with clients in community mental health. When clients ask if she will keep information confidential, she responds, "Most informa-

tion that you give me I will keep to myself. I do keep records about my discussions with you to share with other colleagues who need the information. But at any time, if you tell me of your plans to hurt yourself or others, I will need to tell the appropriate people." This speech reminds Beth of the practical application of this important value.

You should consider the following questions as you think about the meaning of these values in your own life and practice.

- What kinds of client behaviors would be the most difficult for you to accept? How would you meet the challenge of working with these clients?
- When was the last time you felt uncomfortable sharing information about another person? How did you resolve the situation?
- As you think about these five values in relation to yourself as a future human service professional, consider the possibility of working with many different clients. As you think about the clients listed below, place a check beside those clients who would be difficult for *you* to work with. Which values might present problems or conflicts for you? Try to respond honestly, not what you think would be socially or professionally desirable.

_______ a man with fundamental religious beliefs who refuses treatment for a life-threatening illness

_______ a same-sex couple who wants to resolve some conflicts they are having in their relationship

_______ a man who wants to leave his wife and two children to have sexual adventures with other women

_______ a young woman who wants an abortion but is seeking your help in making the decision

_______ a person who has severe burn scars on the face, shoulders, arms, and hands

_______ a man or woman from a Middle Eastern culture where the male is dominant and the female submissive

_______ a person who does not want to work

_______ a man who strongly believes the only way to bring up his children is by punishing them severely

_______ a woman who wants to leave her husband and children in order to have a career and independence, but is afraid to do it

_______ a person who is so physically attractive that you can't concentrate on what the person is saying

Values are the groundwork for creating a philosophy of helping, which, in turn, provides a basis for working with people. A philosophy of helping embodies beliefs about human nature, the nature of change, and the process of helping. As individuals grow and develop and as their values change, their helping philosophy and style also develop. An example is the way Beth's values

The Task of Philosophy

Whether we recognize it or not, all facets of our behavior, the way we treat other people, our choices and decisions, our reactions, our values, our responsibilities or lack of it, are embedded in a philosophical base. Whether or not we are philosophically aware, we function one way or another depending on what we believe. Our philosophical beliefs are more often than not only vaguely sensed, more shadow than substance. Asked to delineate our philosophical tenets, most of us would deny ever having considered the subject. And yet our philosophical beliefs determine our response to our environment and to the individuals who people it.

Consider, for example, how one would react if he believed on the one hand that man is essentially good, or on the other, that man is essentially evil; if he were an idealist or a pragmatist; if he believed man to be a rational being or a nonrational being; if he believed in free will and freedom of choice or if he believed in determinism and predestination; if he operated from a scientific base or from a religious one.

Man is essentially good.	Trust in man, individually and collectively.
Man is essentially evil.	Distrust.
Idealist	Search for the absolute, the perfect in terms of goodness, truth, etc.
Pragmatist	Concentration on the present; "what works is good, useful."
Man is a rational being.	If man has the facts, he will solve his problems and work through to a logical conclusion,
Man is a nonrational being.	Emotions play a major role in man's decisions; information alone won't guarantee a solution and an end to problems.
Free will	Man has freedom to make choices, and can be the major architect of his future.
Determinism	Man is a victim of his environment, has no choices, and is the victim rather than the master of fate.
Scientific orientation	Concern with objectivity, logic, and empiricism.
Religious orientation	Concern with subjectivity, faith, and inspiration.

SOURCE: Excerpt from *Barriers and Hazards in Counseling,* by D. E. Johnson and M. J. Vestermark, pp. 39–42. Copyright © 1970 by Houghton Mifflin Company. Adapted with permission.

translate into her philosophy of helping, which influences her human service practice.

Beth believes that all human beings are good and that all behavior is directed to the good. She thinks that violence to others, cruelty, and self-abuse are all behaviors that the perpetrators consider to be positive ways to meet their personal needs. She also believes that people have the capacity to change, if only they believe they can change. Hence, the helper's responsibility is to develop clients' belief in themselves and help provide alternatives for change, practical assistance, and support. Because of these views, Beth has high hopes for her clients, and she believes that her major responsibility is to motivate them. She is frustrated when she works with clients who have tried to hurt others, and she is puzzled when those clients do not want to change. In spite of her frustration, she has maintained her belief in the goodness of human beings.

Characteristics of the Helper

To be an effective helper demands the use of the helper's whole self, not just a professional segment of it. This requirement creates difficulty when one tries to generalize about the values and characteristics that helpers ought to have. Ideas differ widely about what helpers should be like and what they bring to their work with others. In this section, you will read about some of these ideas. You will also be encouraged to think about the qualities you possess that might be important to your work as a helping professional, as well as qualities you may want to develop more fully to increase your effectiveness.

Brill (1995) believes that individuals learn attitudes and behaviors as they respond to their circumstances. Some responses may even be unconscious. Through the learning process, a person internalizes these attitudes and behaviors and they become a pattern in his or her life. A major influence on how an individual reacts to these needs is culture. Families, schools, and peers are among the agents that communicate ways of behaving and help determine what an individual considers to be acceptable and unacceptable behavior in different situations.

An increasing body of research supports the concept that the personal characteristics of helpers are largely responsible for the success or failure of their helping (Brown & Srebalus, 1995). In fact, Brammer (1995) concluded from numerous studies that these personal characteristics are as significant in helping as the methods helpers use. A number of researchers have examined these characteristics, and we studied this work to identify the traits that seem to be universal in effective helpers.

Eriksen (1981) began by stating what the helping person should be able to do: "listen with understanding and act with skill, experience, information, and self-awareness" (p. 128). To do this, the helper should be self-aware, objective, professionally competent, and actively involved in the enabling process.

Okun (1997) reviewed a number of research studies and concluded that certain qualities, behaviors, and knowledge on the part of the helper most influence the behaviors, attitudes, and feelings of clients. Self-awareness, honesty, congruence, the ability to communicate, knowledge, and ethical integrity are included in her list.

Brown and Srebalus (1995) also reviewed the literature and found a consensus that effective helpers have definite traits. One way to discuss what these are is to use a framework based on the work of Brammer (1995) and Combs (1969), which suggests two sets of attitudes: one related to self and one related to how one treats another person. The traits they consider important are personal congruence, empathy, cultural sensitivity, genuineness, respect, and communication.

All the characteristics mentioned are important ones for helpers. Many other perspectives can be studied, but this brief discussion shows that certain characteristics tend to be common to most studies. In preparing this text, we have reviewed a number of perspectives. Our guiding question was, "What characteristics are important for the beginning human service professional?" We identified the following qualities as important: self-awareness, the ability to communicate, empathy, and professional commitment. Each of these is discussed in depth to help you form an understanding of what the quality is and why it is important for entry-level practice.

SELF-AWARENESS

Most authorities in the helping professions agree that helpers must know who they are because this self-knowledge affects what they do. Developing self-awareness is a lifelong process of learning about oneself by continually examining one's beliefs, attitudes, values, and behaviors. Recognizing stereotypes, biases, and cultural and gender differences are part of the self-awareness process. It is a particularly critical process for helpers because it assists them in understanding and changing their attitudes and feelings that may hinder helping. The importance of self-acceptance is underscored by the helper's use of self in the helping process.

ABILITY TO COMMUNICATE

Helpers' effectiveness depends in part on their ability to communicate to the client an understanding of the client's feelings and behaviors (Okun, 1997). Listening, a critical helping skill, is the beginning of helping and is necessary for establishing trust, building rapport, and identifying the problem. Careful listening means being "tuned in" to all the nuances of the client's message, including verbal and nonverbal aspects of what is said as well as what is not said. Such focused listening enables the helper to respond with thoughts and feelings to the client's whole message.

EMPATHY

Empathy is acceptance of another person. This quality allows the helper to see a situation or experience a feeling from the client's perspective. This may be

Maslow's View of Helping

Abraham Maslow, a man of vision, described life by taking into account "its highest aspirations." He was dedicated to encouraging development of human potential. This enthusiasm led Maslow to make statements on how people can help each other more effectively. The following written statement demonstrates his creativity and his sensitivity toward helping.

Helping? Well, I have a label for it (labels are good, they are useful for me), I call it the Bodhisattvic Version (Path). We have no good word in English for *helper*; it carries too many surplus connotations with it. I've used the Eastern conception of the Bodhisattva and transformed it a little bit for our purposes. Do you know what the word means?

There are two Buddhistic legends. In one the Buddha sat under a tree and had the great revelation he saw the truth. It's very Socratic. He saw the truth, the truth was revealed to him, and then he ascended to heaven, so to speak, to Nirvana. In another version, the Bodhisattvic Version, the Buddha sat under the tree, had a great illumination, saw the truth, ascended to the gates of heaven, and there, out of compassion for mankind, could not bear to selfishly enter heaven and came back to earth to help—on the assumption that nobody could go to heaven unless we all go to heaven.

So this is a beautiful legend, and what it means for us, I think, is to recognize that helping in the first place is a very, very hard job and the helper can be a clumsy fool—the helper can be a hurter. Very frequently it would be best to be Taoistic about helping; to keep your damn hands off is frequently the best way to help. To know when to be available and when not is to think of the helper as being available, being the consultant, rather than being the manipulator, controller,

easier for helpers who have had experiences similar to those of their clients. For example, this may explain the understanding that recovering alcoholics have for other alcoholics, widows for the recently bereaved, and parolees for the incarcerated. It does not mean, however, that helpers whose experiences are different cannot express the unconditional acceptance of the client that is a characteristic of empathy.

RESPONSIBILITY/COMMITMENT

Feeling a responsibility or commitment to improve the well-being of others is an important attribute of human service professionals. This includes attending to the needs of clients first and foremost. It also means a commitment to delivering high-quality services. In other words, workers act in the best interests of clients and do so to the best of their ability. One way that workers do this is by following a code of ethics or a set of ethical standards that guide professional behavior or conduct. Among other things, codes of ethics in the helping interferer, giving orders and telling people what to do, which is our choice and which is very Western. The helper comes. The helper is very frequently just a plain god-damn nuisance—as, for instance, anybody in the ghettos can tell you. Why should it be that the social workers, who want to help, who devote their lives to helping, should be so frequently despised and hated?

I've supposed that the Bodhisattvic kind of helping is a reliance on the self-choice of the person with you the helper being available at the wish of the other, rather than you the helper taking control of the situation and telling people what to do. This implies a kind of humility, also, because in effect what I'm asking here is that the helper become a perfect person. This is a very hard thing to do—that is, to know when to keep your hands off and when you help and when to be available and so on—especially with our young children, where frequently we do have to interfere.

What is implied, therefore, is that one of the paths to being a helper is to become a better and better person, in the psychotherapeutic sense, in the sense of maturing, evolving, becoming more fully human, and so on. If you want to help others best, improve yourself. Cure yourself. To the extent that you're neurotic when you try to help them. To the extent that you can be democratic, accepting, Taoistic, to that extent you are more likely to help better them. But this is a paradox, because one of the paths to becoming a person is by being selfish, by being within your own skin. So this paradox has to be resolved; it's kind of like the hen and the egg thing, of simultaneously, if you want to be the better helper, improving yourself and being helpful the best way you can—but doing it in the spirit of humility and of modesty rather than in the spirit of taking control.

SOURCE: Excerpt from *Abraham H. Maslow: A Memorial Volume, an International Study Project,* pp. 39–42.

profession spell out what the client has a right to expect from the helper. Honesty may be one expectation of the client—a belief that the worker will be honest in answering questions or practicing only what he or she is trained to do.

Typology of Human Service Workers

Besides understanding who the human service professional is in terms of characteristics, values, and philosophy of helping, the student of human services should also know the professional categories that describe such workers. The human service profession includes several levels of workers, which may be classified in a variety of ways. Two considerations present in most categorizations are educational preparation or training and competence. The next subsection discusses categories of professional work developed by three professional educators.

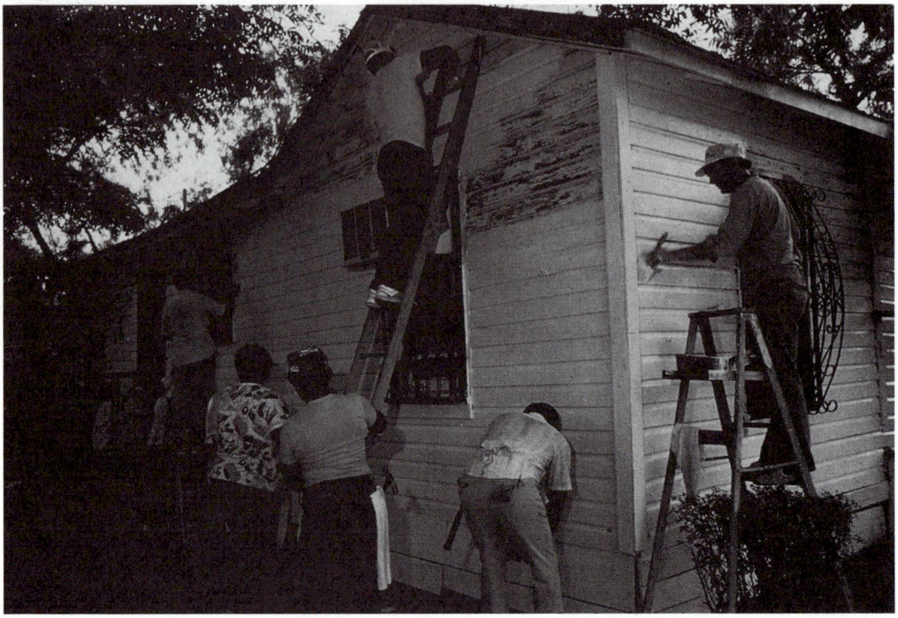

Volunteers contribute to the community in many ways.

Categories of Workers

The Southern Regional Education Board (SREB) identified four levels of competence in its publication *Staff Roles for Mental Health Personnel: A History and a Rationale* (1979). Level 1 is an *entry-level* category that includes those workers who have a few weeks or months of instruction and some inservice training. These individuals may have little actual on-the-job experience. Level 2, the *technical/apprentice* level, includes those who have one to two years of formal training or experience. Sometimes these helpers have earned an associate in arts degree. Level 3, the *associate professional* level, includes those helpers with formal training or experience, usually at the baccalaureate level. Helpers with master's or doctoral degrees are in Level 4, the *professional/specialist* level.

Another way of categorizing helpers is to divide them into two classes (Brammer, 1995). The first includes helpers who offer unstructured assistance through friendships, family relations, and community and general human concern. The second category, that of structured helping, is the one in which we are interested. It is further divided into three categories of workers: *professional helpers, paraprofessionals,* and *volunteers* and *peers.* Professional helpers are characterized by certification from professional groups, licenses by governing bodies, and degrees from educational institutions. Examples of professionals in this category are social workers, nurses, ministers, and counselors. The second group consists of paraprofessional helpers who perform some of the traditional counseling functions but also engage in broader roles, such as those of advocate and mobilizer. What distinguishes each group is the amount of formal training its members have had, their level of responsibility, and their degree of participation in policy formation. In addition, members of the professional group possess research skills, a wider theoretical background, and clinical judgment, a result of their clinical training and supervision. Tension may occur between paraprofessionals and professionals, in part because of increasing evidence that each group may be as effective as the other in delivering services.

A third way to categorize helpers, similar to Brammer's system, is one proposed by Okun (1997), who categorizes workers as *professional helpers, generalist human service workers,* and *nonprofessional helpers.* Workers who are trained specialists with graduate-level training in helping theory and skills and who often have supervised clinical experience are classified as professional helpers, even though their training and credentials may vary. These professional helpers may work with generalist human service workers as part of a team, as supervisors, or as consultants. Generalist human service workers have education and training at the undergraduate level and job titles such as psychiatric technicians or aides, youth street workers, day care staff, probation officers, and church workers. Okun's third category, nonprofessional helpers, includes workers with some training in helping and little agency responsibility. They use communication skills to develop helping relationships with those people they are assisting. Included here are volunteers who work for no pay and peer helpers, who may be similar in age and experience to the clients.

The Human Service Professional

As a result of an unmet need for trained, educated workers in human services, the 1992–1993 edition of the *Occupational Outlook Handbook* included an entry on the human service worker. The latest edition continues to highlight the diversity of job titles, duties, client groups, and employment settings found in the human service profession. For example, the list of possible settings in which such workers may be employed includes "offices, group homes, shelters, day programs, sheltered workshops, hospitals, clinics, and in the field visiting clients" (p. 129). Examples of the variety of job titles are "social service assistant, case management aide, social work assistant, residential counselor, community support worker, alcohol or drug abuse counselor, mental health technician, child-care worker, community outreach worker, life skills counselor, and gerontology aide" (p. 129).

According to the *Occupational Outlook Handbook,* human service workers are generally under the direction of professionals who have advanced training or degrees. However, the degree of supervision they receive and the amount of responsibility they have vary a great deal, depending on their education and training, job duties, and client groups. "Some are on their own most of the time and have little direct supervision; others work under close direction" (p. 128). Those with a high school education are likely to perform clerical tasks, and those with a college degree may engage in counseling, service coordination, or management. The attainment of a bachelor's or master's degree is necessary for supervisory positions that involve greater responsibilities.

In 1994, human service workers held about 168,000 jobs. State and local governments employed about one-fourth in public welfare agencies and facilities for mentally disabled and developmentally delayed individuals. Another fourth were employed by private social or human service agencies offering a variety of services, including adult day care, group meals, crisis intervention, and counseling. Many supervised residents of group homes and halfway houses. They also worked in clinics, detoxification units, community mental health centers, psychiatric hospitals, day treatment programs, and sheltered workshops.

The following excerpt from the *Occupational Outlook Handbook* (1996–1997) illustrates the diversity of settings, client groups served, and job duties (pp. 128–129):

> Human services workers provide direct and indirect client services. They assess clients' needs, establish their eligibility for benefits and services, and help clients obtain them. They examine financial documents such as rent receipts and tax returns to determine whether the client is eligible for food stamps, Medicaid, welfare, and other human service programs. They also arrange for transportation and escorts, if necessary, and provide emotional support. Human services workers monitor and keep case records on clients and report progress to supervisors.
>
> Human services workers may transport or accompany clients to group meal sites, adult daycare programs, or doctors' offices; telephone or visit clients' homes to make sure services are being received; or help resolve disagreements, such as those between tenants and landlords.
>
> Human services workers play a variety of roles in community settings. They may organize and lead group activities, assist clients in need of counseling or crisis intervention, or administer a food bank or emergency fuel program. In halfway houses, group homes and government-supported housing programs, they assist adult residents who need supervision in personal hygiene and daily living skills. They review clients' records, ensure they take correct doses of medication, talk with their families, and confer with medical personnel to gain better insight into clients' backgrounds and needs. They also provide emotional support and help clients become involved in community recreation programs and other activities.
>
> In psychiatric hospitals, rehabilitation programs, and outpatient clinics, they may help clients master everyday living skills and teach them how to communicate more effectively and get along better with others. They support the client's participation in the treatment plan, such as individual or group counseling and occupational therapy.

The job outlook for human service workers is excellent. Projections are that the number of workers will grow much faster than the average for all occupations between 1994 and 2005, making it one of the most rapidly growing occupations.

The rapid growth in the demand for services coupled with slower growth in resources to provide services means that employers will rely increasingly on human service workers rather than higher paid occupations.

Other Professional Helpers

As a human service professional, you will be working with a variety of other professional helpers. This section, adapted from the 1996–1997 *Occupational Outlook Handbook,* identifies the nature of the work and the training of these individuals so you will be familiar with them.

PHYSICIANS

Physicians perform medical examinations, diagnose illnesses, treat injured or diseased people, and advise patients on maintaining good health. They may be general practitioners or specialists in a particular field of medicine.

Physicians are required by all states to be licensed. It usually takes about 11 years to become a physician: 4 years of undergraduate school, 4 years of medical school, and 3 years of residency. Those who choose to specialize usually spend 3 to 5 years in training and another 2 years in preparation for practice in a specialty area.

One example of a specialist with whom you will likely be in contact is a *psychiatrist.* Concerned with the diagnosis, treatment, and prevention of mental illness, psychiatrists may be found in private offices and institutional settings, courtrooms, community-centered care facilities, and specialized medical areas such as coronary and intensive care units. They frequently act as consultants to other agencies. Psychiatrists are medical doctors who have an additional five years or more of psychiatric training and experience and are qualified to use the full range of medical techniques in treating clients. These include drugs, shock, and surgery, in addition to counseling and behavior modification techniques.

PSYCHOLOGISTS

Although their training and the kinds of treatment they use are different, psychologists are sometimes confused with psychiatrists. Psychologists study human behavior and mental processes to understand and explain people's actions.

An individual may specialize in any of several areas within psychology, including clinical, counseling, developmental, industrial-organizational, school, and social psychology. Each specialty focuses on a different aspect of human behavior. For example, the developmental psychologist is concerned with the behavioral changes people experience as they progress through life. Clinical psychologists, on the other hand, may work in hospitals, clinics, or private practice to help mentally or emotionally disturbed individuals adjust to life and to help medical and surgical patients deal with their illnesses and injuries. They may use interviews, diagnostic tests, and psychotherapy in their work.

Psychologists may practice with a master's degree or a doctoral degree. A master's degree prepares the person to administer and interpret tests, conduct research, and counsel patients. The doctoral degree usually requires five to seven years of graduate study and is often required for employment as a psychologist. A doctorate in psychology and two years of professional experience are generally required for licensure or certification; although requirements may vary from state to state, certification is necessary for private practice.

SOCIAL WORKERS

The focus of social workers is helping individuals, families, and groups cope with a wide variety of problems. The nature of the problem and the time and resources available determine the methods used, which may include counseling, advocacy, and referral. Social workers also function at the community level to combat social problems. For example, they may coordinate existing programs, organize fund-raising, and develop new community services.

Social workers may also specialize in various areas. Medical social workers are trained to help patients and their families cope with problems that accompany illness or rehabilitation. Those who specialize in family services counsel individuals to strengthen personal and family relationships. Corrections and child welfare are other popular areas of study and employment.

Preparation for the field of social work occurs at two levels. The baccalaureate level (B.S.W.) is the minimum requirement, followed by the master's in social work (M.S.W), which is usually required for positions in mental health and for administrative or research positions. Training generally includes courses of study focusing on social work practice, social welfare policies, human behavior, and the social environment. Supervised field experiences are also necessary.

The National Association of Social Workers (NASW) awards certification in the form of the title ACSW, which stands for the Academy of Certified Social Workers. Licensing or registration laws have also been passed by many states to regulate social work practice.

COUNSELORS

One of the largest categories of professional helpers is counselors. Although their exact duties depend on the individuals or groups with whom they work and the agencies or settings in which they are employed, counselors help people deal with a variety of problems, including personal, social, educational, and career concerns. Examples of the different types of counselors are school and college counselors, rehabilitation counselors, employment counselors, and mental health counselors. Two that you may interact with as a human service professional are mental health counselors and rehabilitation counselors.

The *mental health counselor* works with individuals who are dealing with problems such as drug and alcohol abuse, family conflicts, suicidal thoughts and feelings, stress management, problems with self-esteem, issues associated with aging, job and career concerns, educational decisions, and issues of mental and emotional health. Their work is not limited to individuals, however; it may involve the family of the individual. These counselors often work closely with other specialists such as psychiatrists, psychologists, clinical social workers, and psychiatric nurses.

The rehabilitation counselor helps people deal with the personal, social, and vocational effects of their disabilities. Disabilities may be social, mental, emotional, or physical, calling for the services of counseling, evaluation, medical care, occupational training, and job placement. Rehabilitation counselors also work with the family of the individual when necessary and frequently with other professionals such as physicians, psychologists, and occupational therapists.

Positions as a counselor usually require a master's degree in a counseling discipline or a related area. This preparation frequently includes a year or two of graduate study and a supervised counseling experience. Licensure and certification are available; requirements vary, depending on the specialty. The National Board for Certified Counselors (NBCC), the Commission on Rehabilitation Counselor Certification (CRCC), and the National Academy of Certified Clinical Mental Health Counselors (NACCMHC) are three national certifying bodies.

Human service workers could assume the responsibilities of social workers or counselors, or be given this title, even though they might not be specifically certified as such. The variation in the needs of agencies and the competencies of individual workers makes it difficult to establish rigid categories for function or title. However, having the title or performing the job of a mental health counselor is definitely not the same thing as being nationally certified. Some states and agencies will only hire workers with national certification, whereas other sites have more flexible hiring categories.

Becoming a Professional

Human service professionals are helpers who meet the criteria established for that group (Barber, 1965). First, such professionals have a high degree of generalized systematic training in the knowledge, skills, and values of the profession. The training may encompass specialized training for child care, criminal justice, or other specific areas of work, or it may include more generic training designed to prepare workers to perform entry-level roles in various social service settings. Second, human service professionals' primary focus is the client. Trained to understand that their primary responsibility is to clients, they believe in the importance of the client perspective. Third, human service professionals are regulated by and follow a personal and professional code of ethics, which specifically guides the workers' respect for the client perspective. The personal and professional values of acceptance, individuality, tolerance, self-determination, and confidentiality, discussed earlier as crucial to the professionals' value system, provide the foundation for this code. Ethical considerations also guide helpers' actions in the work setting, with co-workers, and with other professionals. Fourth, there is a system of rewards for work achievement although not always in a structured or well-defined form. Often the intrinsic rewards of "helping others," "being part of a team," and "working for the common good" foster feelings of professional accomplishment. More extrinsic rewards for effective professional performance include recognition from the community for outstanding work and recognition by the bureaucracy in the form of raises, additional benefits, and promotions.

The Transition from Student to Professional

The early development of the beginning professional is characterized by a growing sense of professionalism. One of the first changes human service students undergo is the shift from thinking of themselves as students to thinking of themselves as professionals. There are many differences between the two roles. Students who do not demonstrate commitment usually experience the consequences directly, in the form of poor grades. Human service professionals, however, are part of a team of professionals who depend on high-quality performance. If the professionals are not committed, the clients may suffer the consequences. Another difference between students and professionals is the structure of the experience. In a classroom, the student is expected to work within the guidelines of an instructor's outline or syllabus and may not deviate from these expectations. Workers, although expected to follow the rules and regulations of the agency, are constantly in situations that require creativity, initiative, and judgment. Not all actions are predetermined (especially those involving clients), and not all decisions that need to be made are clear-cut. A third difference between the roles of students and professionals is in the evaluations each receives. At the end of a term, students receive evaluations that reflect their individual performances. Evaluations of job performance are more varied. For one thing, the professional works as a member of a team. Also, success with clients is difficult to measure, as clients often disappear before service is complete or receive services for only a short time. Gauging the long-term effects of services is difficult in many cases. Success as a team member, a member of the organization, and a participant in the social service community is equally difficult to evaluate. In short, the evaluation of professionals is very different from the evaluation of students.

One factor that assists individuals in the transition from student to helper is the experience of actually working as a human service professional. During these early work experiences, developing professionals have the opportunity to observe other respected professionals. As beginning helpers model their behavior on that of people working around them, they constantly modify what they see to fit their own personalities and understanding of professional behavior.

Another phenomenon critical to the development of new helpers is for others to treat them like professionals. Early in their professional experiences, they may be amazed that others have confidence in them, seek their advice, and give them problems and cases to handle, as if they knew exactly what they were doing. As others treat them as professionals, they begin to see themselves that way.

It is typical for entry-level professionals to be totally consumed by their jobs, spending long hours at work and worrying about their clients during their off-time. It is also common for beginning professionals to start work with high job satisfaction, which decreases when realistic assessments of the work replace their earlier dreams of what the job would be. If the transition is successful, beginning professionals emerge with a more stable sense of professionalism. For some entry-level professionals, the discovery of reality is less positive. Their self-esteem may decline, and they may feel that if they were better, more committed workers, they would have more success with clients and would be more satisfied with their jobs.

Characteristics of the Beginning Professional

Beginning human service professionals are particularly vulnerable when developing their sense of professionalism (Cherniss, 1980). As discussed in the next section, working within a bureaucracy can be difficult and can retard professional growth. Another difficulty beginning helpers face is rooted in their motivations for choosing human services as a profession. Some have made the choice because of a personal commitment to assisting other people in making their lives better; underlying such workers' expectations and dreams is an idealized view of their role as helpers. Beginning professionals imagine all the important work they must perform if they are going to help needy individuals, and they are excited about all they may contribute to this important task.

This idealism is not the only emotion beginning professionals feel strongly about. They are also plagued by a fear of being incompetent, of not being able to do what will be asked of them in helping situations, such as relating to clients and acting as advocates for clients in the complex human service system. In essence, professionals fear that they will be unable to make a difference. Accompanying this fear of incompetence is the burden of being responsible for others. Entry-level professionals feel deeply committed to helping people in need, and they feel that clients depend on them. This burden, combined with their commitment to make a difference, may contribute to feelings of guilt if helpers do not meet their goals. Entry-level professionals may feel that whatever they do is not enough.

One last factor that makes the job of beginning professionals so frustrating is that not all clients are motivated or appreciative of services. That clients may do little or nothing to help themselves can come as quite a shock to professionals, who spend their time and energy working with and worrying about clients. When clients are not very motivated, beginning professionals often take the lack of motivation as a personal affront and rejection. For them, offering help is comparable to offering a handshake and friendship; professionals extend their hands and themselves, and the clients refuse to greet or work with them. Of course, the workers probably understand intellectually that not all clients will be motivated. They may even have encountered unmotivated clients during their field experiences. However, the reality of working with clients who refuse to accept responsibility for helping themselves is very difficult for many to accept.

Working in a Bureaucracy

Despite the professionalism that prevails in human services, becoming a professional does not occur automatically the day a degree is granted or the first day a person is employed as a human service professional. Professionalism evolves through actual work experience and the gradual acceptance of oneself as a beginning professional. For many new human service workers, developing a sense of professionalism is difficult and takes time. One difficulty in establishing this new identity is that human service professionals perform their jobs in a bureaucracy that does not always support professional development. Three factors related to working within a bureaucracy seem to cause many of the problems beginning professionals encounter: the tension between ability and authority, the formal impersonality of the bureaucratic structure, and the bureaucracy's resistance to change (Neugeboren, 1991).

In a bureaucracy, there is often tension between the individuals who provide direct services to clients and the individuals who administer the program or agency; each has a special perspective on the workplace. In a large organization, administrators make decisions from a broad institutional perspective. Tensions arise because helpers have a different perspective. They have much more information about particular situations and a more focused understanding of the organization. Helpers become frustrated because they do not understand how administrative decisions can be made with such little apparent regard for the helpers' or the clients' points of view. For entry-level professionals, this frustration can be harmful. They begin to see a division between supervisors or administrators and workers, drawing a distinction between "us" and "them." Once helpers make this distinction, they have more difficulty feeling part of the organization, and they are less likely to use the organization for support. Helpers who see issues in terms of "us" and "them" may feel alienated, powerless, and even isolated.

Also frustrating to the entry-level professional in a large bureaucracy is a sense of formal impersonality when working with clients and colleagues. The system formalizes relationships in two ways: with regard to clients and in terms of professional responsibilities. First, needy individuals must meet specific criteria before becoming clients. Forms must be completed and procedures followed before clients can receive the attention they so desperately need. Some clients who appear needy may not be helped by the organization because they do not meet the specific criteria to receive services, do not have the resources to pay for the services, or need the services sooner than can be provided. In these cases, the needs and rules of the bureaucratic structure appear to take precedence over client needs. New professionals may resent the bureaucracy's treatment of the client, seeing the organization as insensitive to client needs. Such workers feel that they are betraying their clients when they objectively enforce the regulations of the organization.

Another form of impersonality occurs as the bureaucracy defines the roles of the professional. The work of an organization is divided into the roles and responsibilities of human service professionals. There are formal lines of communication and formal procedures for clients to use while receiving services. For a complex system to work effectively, the helpers and the clients must follow these procedures and use the appropriate channels of communication. Helpers often feel limited by these formal procedures. The procedures may seem to inconvenience clients or restrict the workers' role or responsibility with the clients (Neugeboren, 1991). Often, the roles and rules must be followed so that clients do not get lost in the system or so that clients may be best served by the system. However, understanding the rationale for the formal structure is difficult for beginning professionals. They become frustrated, because, from their point of view, their clients are being treated unfairly. They also feel that formal procedures stifle their own creativity and initiative. This frustration may lead to anger against the system or apathy concerning the system and what it is trying to accomplish.

One of the most difficult bureaucratic characteristics for beginning professionals to accept is the bureaucracy's resistance to change. This is a reality with which even the best and most professional helpers struggle long after they have shed the label of "beginning professional." Slow change is especially frustrating when there are flaws in human service systems, especially in complex systems with limited resources. A difficult problem for beginning professionals is determining what can be changed, what cannot be changed, and how to accomplish the targeted change. Unfortunately, few people are able to have a major impact on a large organization in a short period of time. Human service professionals who make no impact on the bureaucratic structure are likely to feel frustrated and helpless.

Even though working within a human service bureaucracy does have its frustrations for beginning professionals, they may follow guidelines that will ease their transition (Neugeboren, 1991). First, becoming a good bureaucrat requires devoting time and energy to studying the system's structure and the place of clients and helpers within it. To understand the system, helpers need information about it; they need to know the barriers for both clients and helpers, and the procedures and regulations that work efficiently and effectively. One way to understand the bureaucracy is to read the available written information about the organization and to study organizational charts and descriptions of each position's responsibilities. The flow of paper in the system and the ways decisions are made and evaluated are also important pieces of information to have. Another way to learn about the system is to identify people who appear to get things done for the bureaucracy and for their clients. Watch how they do their jobs and ask them questions about how to handle certain situations.

Second, entry-level human service professionals who are not paralyzed by the bureaucracy and who use their initiative and creativity can avoid some of the barriers. To be good bureaucrats, new professionals need not always submit to the will of the system, but they may have to study the system and find ways of working within it. If beginning human service professionals make an effort to find a place within the organization and believe in their power to influence the system, they are more likely to feel a sense of belonging and less alienation. Systematic study of the organization may help workers be active agents within their bureaucracy, rather than victims. Entry-level professionals will then develop their own personal styles.

Conclusion

The following case study provides an excellent example of a human service professional involved with many of the issues helpers encounter. As you read the case study, consider the helper's roles, values, and characteristics. Are there any potential sources of frustration for the worker? What are her expectations?

Carmen Rodriguez has worked as a vocational evaluator for a state agency in the southwestern United States for the past four years. She considers herself a human service professional; with most of her clients, the focus of her work is much broader than just vocational counseling. She describes her job as follows.

> I have been a work evaluator for the past four years. In my position, I work with clients to assist them in preparing for and finding gainful employment. One of the requirements for eligibility for services at my agency is that the individual must have a mental, physical, or emotional disability that is a handicap to employment. There must also be a reasonable expectation that the person can be gainfully employed after receiving services.
>
> One of the aspects of my work that I like a lot is the variety of clients I encounter. They are of different ages and from varied backgrounds. I work with many Mexican Americans and Native Americans. My clients are both males and females and, as I said, they have various disabilities. Usually I work with a client every day for a period of six to eight weeks. Because of this close contact, I feel that I get to know my clients well.
>
> Clients come first with me. I constantly think about what I can do for them, and I want to help them in any way I can. Sometimes their circumstances seem so poor, but I know that if I work hard enough I can make their lives better.
>
> Another rewarding part of my job is working with other professionals. We are all committed to meeting client needs, although at times we are limited by the purposes of our various agencies. We've found that we are much more successful working together. In fact, ten of us from different agencies meet monthly for lunch to talk about our work and find out about other services that may be available. It's also a good time to find out about new legislation and regulations and the ways agencies are dealing with funding problems or new grants.
>
> Another part of my work that I find particularly challenging is consulting with a variety of specialists, including psychologists, psychiatrists, and other medical specialists. It's important that I be able to speak their language to a certain extent so that I can tell them what we

want them to evaluate and the kinds of information they can provide to assist us in our evaluation of the client. It's also helpful to know some of the terminology so that I can understand their reports. It does make me nervous to talk to these professionals, because their training is different from mine. It is easier now than when I first began working here.

I guess it's pretty obvious how I feel about my work. It's rewarding and challenging, and I feel as if I learn something new each day. It may seem as if it's the perfect job, but it really isn't. There are some negative aspects to it, and probably the most frustrating is that in a bureaucracy things never seem to move as quickly as I want them to. For example, there is quite a bit of paperwork. To receive an authorization for services, I have to go through several channels. This sometimes takes days, and since I work with the client on a daily basis, I get as impatient as the client.

The other aspect of my job that I sometimes find frustrating is that clients often do not do what I would like them to do. When you work with people, it's important to realize that you don't tell them what to do. Actually, we try to teach them to take responsibility for their actions, and this involves making decisions for themselves. When they make a decision that is not in their best interest or may lead to problems or failure, it's very difficult for me not to intervene. I want so much for my clients to succeed, but I've learned that they are independent individuals who must live their own lives. In spite of the frustrations, I hope to keep this job for several years. It offers many opportunities for professional growth and gives me a chance to make a difference.

✧ Things to Remember

1. Helping means assisting people to understand, overcome, or cope with problems. A helper is one who offers such assistance.
2. The primary reason that individuals choose helping professions (and the reason that most will admit) is the desire to help others. Related to this is the desire for self-exploration.
3. Values are important to the practice of human services, because they are the criteria by which human service professionals and clients make choices. Acceptance, tolerance, individuality, self-determination, and confidentiality are important values for human service professionals.
4. Characteristics that are important for the entry-level human service professional are self-awareness, the ability to communicate, empathy, and professional commitment.
5. One way of categorizing helping professionals is a three-level system: professional helpers, entry-level professionals, and nonprofessionals.
6. Human service professionals work with other professionals, including physicians, psychologists, social workers, and counselors.

7. The broad range of job titles, duties, client groups, and employment settings in human services supports the generic focus of the profession.
8. The transition from student to human service professional is often difficult, because the expectations and responsibilities for each role differ.
9. Working in a bureaucracy as a beginning human service professional can be problematic unless the worker learns to operate in the system by identifying the barriers for both clients and workers and finding out which procedures and regulations work best.
10. Beginning professionals can become frustrated by the contrast between the imagined ideal job (and ideal clients) and the realities of everyday human service work. As a result of these frustrations, they may become closed to learning about clients and the work, or they may experience burnout.

Additional Readings: Focus on Helpers

Freedman, S. G. (1990). *Small victories: The real world of a teacher, her students, and their high school.* New York: Harper Perennial.
The author, a former reporter for the *New York Times,* spent a year at Seward Park on the Lower East Side to discover why 80 of its graduates are continuing their education. Seward Park is ranked as one of the worst high schools in the state.

Goldsmith, S. (1993). *A city year: On the streets and in the neighborhoods with twelve young community service volunteers.* New York: New Press.
This account of a young Harvard-educated reporter's year with City Year, the Boston-based community service program, describes renovating a building for the homeless, tutoring schoolchildren, reclaiming a community garden from drug dealers, and organizing a community street-cleaning.

Hilfiker, D. (1994). *Not all of us are saints: A doctor's journey with the poor.* New York: Hill and Wang.
This is the story of a physician's move from a practice in rural Minnesota to an inner-city neighborhood in Washington, D.C., and the world of poverty medicine.

Humes, E. (1996). *No matter how loud I shout: A year in the life of juvenile court.* New York: Simon & Schuster.
The author takes readers to the street with probation officers fighting to keep kids alive, into the courthouses where hope and hopelessness collide daily in epic struggles, and past the triple-steel doors of Los Angeles's Central Juvenile Hall.

Minuchin, S., & Nichols, M. P. (1993). *Family healing: Tales of hope and renewal from family therapy.* Riverside, NJ: Macmillan.
This autobiographical account of Minuchin's distinguished career provides an introduction to the theory and practice of structural family therapy. Case histories and vignettes illustrate his experiences during his years of clinical practice.

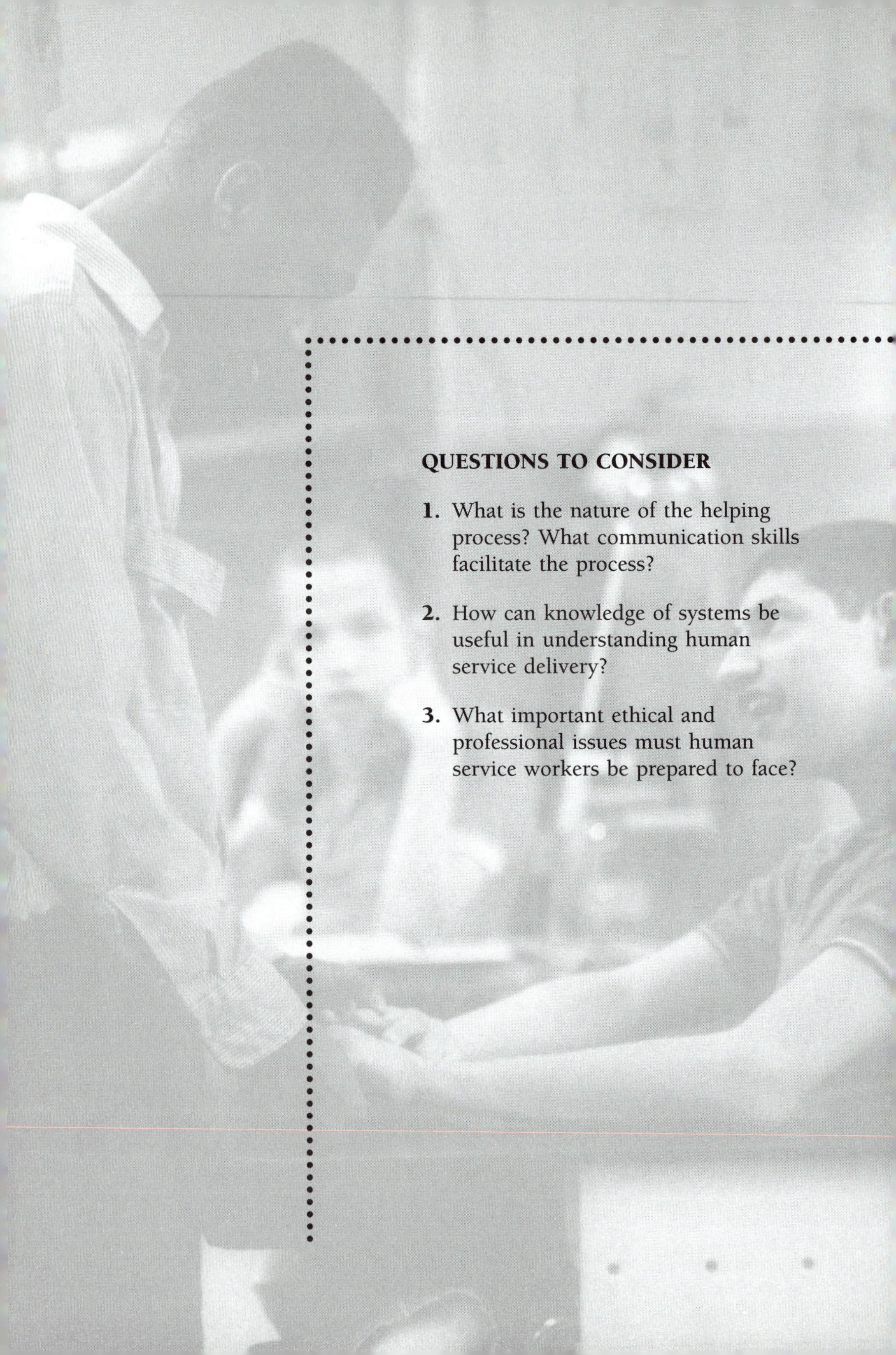

QUESTIONS TO CONSIDER

1. What is the nature of the helping process? What communication skills facilitate the process?
2. How can knowledge of systems be useful in understanding human service delivery?
3. What important ethical and professional issues must human service workers be prepared to face?

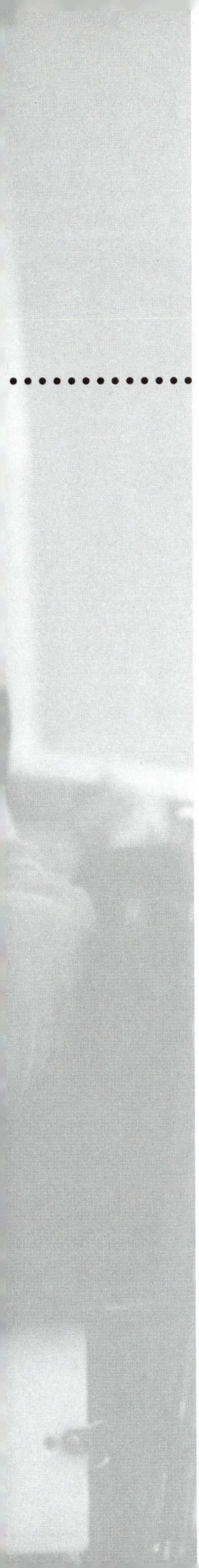

PART THREE

The Practice of Human Services

Part Three focuses on the practice of human services and the context in which helping occurs. Chapter 7 explores the helping process, including the different roles human service professionals play and the skills helpers need to do their jobs well. The chapter concludes with a section on crisis intervention. Chapter 8 addresses the environment of the human service system. It begins with an examination of systems theory and its application to the helping process. The chapter then covers the referral process and ways of using the system to assist clients and the community at large. Part Three concludes with Chapter 9, "Professional Concerns." This chapter presents ethical considerations for the human service professional and describes practical applications of ethical principles. Other professional issues are then discussed: the professional status of human service workers, the career ladder, the dangers of encapsulation and burnout, and professional development in the field of human services. The purpose of Part Three is to refine the definition of human services (developed in Parts One and Two) by examining the helping process in actual practice. As you read the chapters in Part Three, think about the questions on page 216.

Chapter 7

The Helping Process

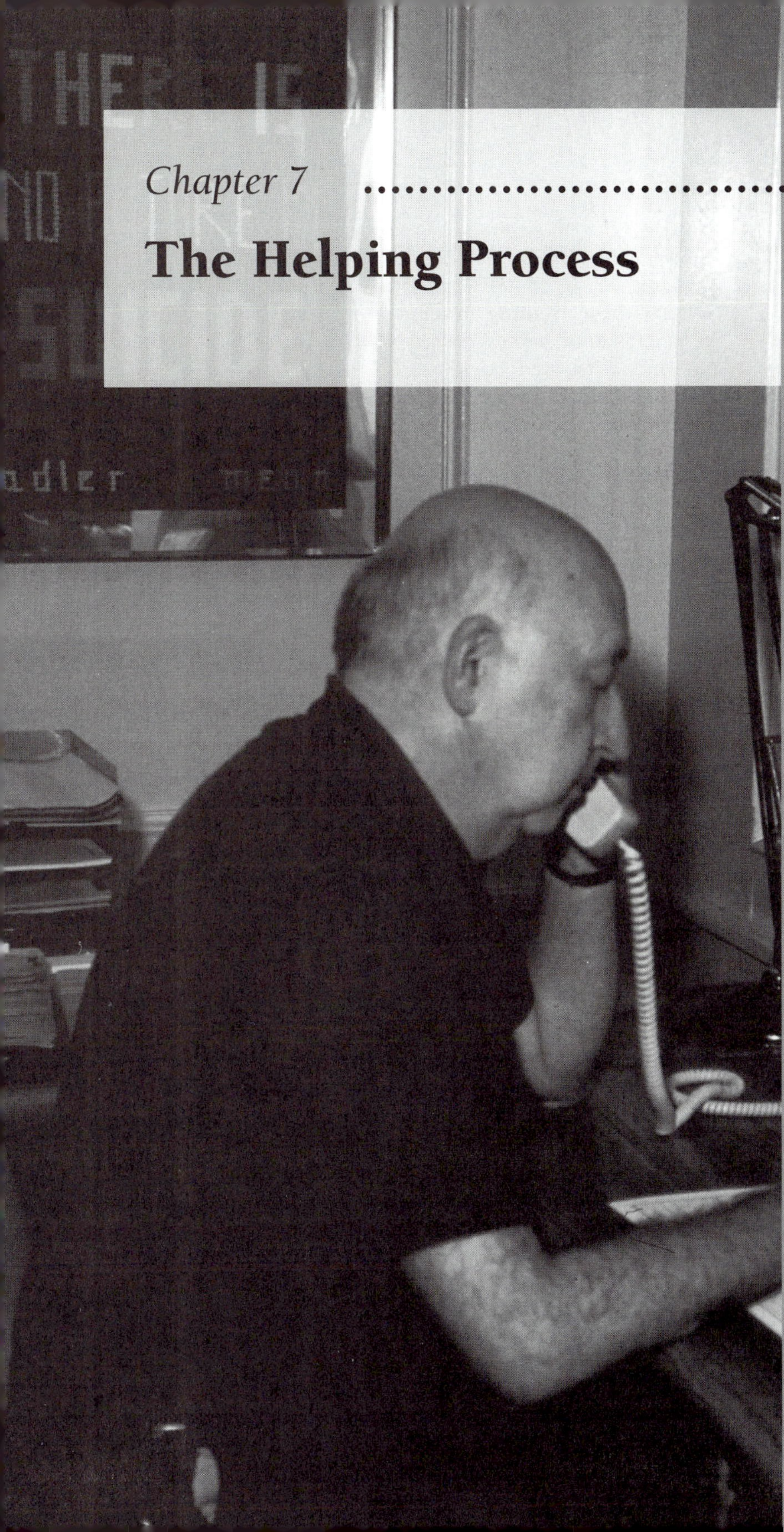

Helping can take many forms: "requesting information, soliciting support, making a decision, and sharing feelings" (Brammer, 1978, p. 476). Yet it is always guided by two questions: (1) What is helpful? (2) How can the needs of the client be met? In human services, assistance to the client occurs through *the helping process*. As they engage in this process, human service professionals must remember that clients are responsible for themselves and make their own decisions. Giving advice or telling someone what to do does not encourage responsibility or promote self-help, which are goals of the helping process.

The effectiveness of the helping process depends greatly on the skills of the helper, the focus of this chapter. The helper's ability to communicate an understanding of the client's feelings, clarify what the problem is, and provide appropriate assistance to resolve the problem contributes to the effectiveness of the process. The roles of human service professionals, the nature of the helping process, the skills of helping, and the challenge of difficult clients will be investigated in this chapter. A look at a special human service, crisis intervention, will provide an overview of the helping process and the various roles that a worker may play.

The Roles of the Human Service Professional

The roles human service professionals play provide the framework for the helping process. In performing the various roles, the worker is continuously focused on the client; this client focus provides the common thread connecting the roles.

Although the roles of human service professionals are constantly evolving, the helper remains a "Jack or Jill of all trades," or, in human service terms, a generalist. The generalist knows a wide range of skills, strategies, and client groups and is able to work effectively in a number of different settings. Engaging in a variety of roles enables the human service professional to meet many client needs. What exactly do these helpers do?

Many professionals have attempted to answer this question. The Southern Regional Education Board (SREB) conducted a study in the late 1960s to define the roles and functions of human service professionals. Making use of the developmental approach, SREB recognized that professions emerge in response to client needs. To reexamine the needs and problems that originally brought the profession into being, SREB asked the following questions:

- Are the needs still the same?
- What are they?
- What tasks must be carried out to meet them?

As a result of this analysis, SREB identified 13 roles that human service workers could engage in to meet the needs of their clients, agencies, or communities (SREB, 1969). These 13 roles include administrator, advocate, assistant to specialist, behavior changer, broker, caregiver, community planner, consultant, data manager, evaluator, mobilizer, outreach worker, and teacher/educator.

In a more recent study the U.S. Department of Education funded a Community Support Skills Standards Project to define the skills that human service personnel need to work in the field. The result of the work was a set of 12 broad, functional themes of human service work. These emerged from a job analysis and are reflected in their report as competency areas. The areas are as follows: participant empowerment; communication; assessment; community and service networking; facilitation of services; community living skills and supports; education, training, and self-development; advocacy; vocational, educational, and career support; crisis intervention; organizational participation; and documentation (Taylor, Bradley, & Warren, 1996).

To better understand the varied roles that are assumed by the human service professional we used the results of these two studies to categorize three areas of responsibility: providing direct service; performing administrative work; and working with the community. Next, we examine these three categories and the roles that represent each area of responsibility.

Providing direct service to clients is a responsibility with which many beginning professionals are familiar. This work represents the development of the helping relationship and the work that helpers do in their face-to-face encounters with their clients. Many roles, such as behavior changer, caregiver, communicator, crisis intervener, participant empowerer, and teacher/educator, are included in the category of direct services. The following illustrate many of these roles and how human service professionals perform them.

Behavior changer—carries out a range of activities planned primarily to change clients' behavior, ranging from coaching and counseling to casework, psychotherapy, and behavior therapy.

Sun Lee Kim is a substance abuse counselor at a drug and alcohol inpatient clinic at a local hospital. Sun Lee, one of the staff group leaders, facilitates a reality therapy group each day. The purpose of this group is to encourage participants to change their communication behavior, first in the group and later in the wider context of the facility. Peer support and pressure are used to facilitate this behavior change.

Caregiver—provides services for people who need ongoing support of some kind, such as financial assistance, day care, social support, and 24-hour care.

Jim Gray works in foster care. His major responsibility is to provide support to families with foster children. One of his favorite activities is to visit foster homes to determine the success of the foster care situation and provide emotional and practical assistance to the families.

Communicator—is able to express and exchange ideas and establish relationships with a variety of individuals and groups, including clients, families, colleagues, administrators, and the public.

Dal Lam works with AIDS patients in a self-help center established by a regional hospital in a rural desert area. His responsibilities require him to communicate with different populations that include individuals testing HIV-positive, individuals with AIDS, medical staff, insurance providers, families, and community groups. He spends much of his time in prevention work that takes him to the elementary schools, local high schools, civic meetings, and churches. His approach is always the same: clear, articulate, compassionate, and confident.

Crisis intervener—provides services for individuals, families, and communities who are experiencing a disruption in their lives with which they cannot cope. This intervention is short term, focused, and concrete.

Christy Haslam works in a sexual assault crisis center and is a victim advocate. She receives four or five new clients a week, mostly women, who are dealing with issues of sexual assault, attempted rape, or rape. Some of her clients call through the hotline immediately after being assaulted, others are referred through the emergency room at the hospital, and others call to ask for help many years after the crisis.

Participant empowerer—shares with clients the responsibility for the helping relationship and the development and implementation of a plan of action. This helper ultimately encourages clients to care for themselves.

Judy Colin is a case manager for developmentally disabled young adults. In the program, First Steps, she works with clients to move from group home living to apartment living. She coordinates daily living training, vocational assessment and training, and first employment. Her clients participate fully in the case management process and are called "co-case managers." There is a graduation ceremony when these clients become their own "case managers."

Teacher/educator—performs a range of instructional activities, from simple coaching to teaching highly technical content, directed at individuals or groups.

Dr. Washington Lee, a physician, and Ned Wanek, a human service professional, work in a family planning clinic. They spend two mornings a week teaching classes to women and men about the reproductive system and alternative methods of family planning. In addition, they counsel individuals, provide physical exams, plan educational media, and talk to schools and community groups about family planning.

Performing administrative work is also another important responsibility for many human service professionals. In addition to providing direct services to clients, many helpers are involved in managerial activities as they supervise or oversee processes or projects. As they work with clients, they assume administrative responsibilities such as planning, linking clients to services, allocating resources, and evaluating. The specific administrative roles are broker, data manager, evaluator, facilitator of services, planner, report writer (documentation), and resource allocator.

Broker—helps people get to the existing services and helps make the services more accessible to clients.

Marta Giovanni's caseload at the Office for Student Services consists primarily of students with physical disabilities. One of her functions is to make sure these students have their classes scheduled in accessible buildings on campus and are able to get around campus to their classes and events. To achieve this goal, Marta may have to help students reschedule classes or arrange for parking. She is also "on call" to assist these students in getting other services they might need.

Data manager—gathers, tabulates, analyzes, and synthesizes data and evaluates programs and plans.

Roosevelt Thompson is part of the staff of a local day care center. Although he assists the child care staff when needed, his actual responsibilities are business oriented. The day care center is privately owned but partially funded by the city. Its clients include children referred to the center from the courts for temporary care as well as children of working parents. His concern is to see that the center maintains an appropriate balance between referred and regular paying clients to maintain its financial stability. He continually gathers information and projects the financial needs of the day care center.

Evaluator—assesses client or community needs and problems, whether medical, psychiatric, social, or educational.

Karen Tubbs leads a community planning organization established to assess the community's needs in relation to the problems of AIDS. Its meetings are part of a complex process of planning for and developing resources to begin providing human services for this client group.

Facilitator of services—brokers (links the client to services) and then monitors the progress the client makes with the various helping professionals. This helper also uses the problem-solving process when services are deficient or inappropriate.

Louisa Gonzales works in a group home for young children who need a short-term safe haven. During the time the children are in the home, Louisa spends many hours coordinating their care with schools, child care agencies, the health department, and the welfare department. Many times, without her services, these children would get lost in the system and would receive substandard care.

Planner—engages in making plans with both short-term or long-term clients in order to define accurately their problems and needs, develops strategies to meet the needs, and monitors the helping process.

Ruth Marlin works with families who are planning for the long-term care of aging parents. This requires careful attention to the needs and priorities of all involved. She has better luck with her families when she uses a very structured planning and decision-making model. With this model, everyone in the family has a clear understanding of the problems and the goals and can monitor the success of the plan.

Report writer (documentation)—records the activities of the agency work. This can include intake interview reports, social histories, detailed treatment plans, daily entries into case notes, requests for resources, rationale and justification for treatment for managed care, and periodic reports for managed care.

Lisa Wilhiem is a social worker in a local hospital emergency room. She is the intermediary for clients who will potentially need longer-term care. It is her responsibility to coordinate the initial requests for services to the managed care organizations or insurance companies. Although she spends several hours of her day with patients and the medical care staff, a majority of her time is spent documenting how the patient entered the health care system and what the current needs of the patient are.

Resource allocator—makes recommendations on how resources are to be spent to support the needs of the client. These recommendations are made once priorities are set and prices for services are determined.

The substance abuse center is developing a new program that will individualize the treatment of its clients. In the past, there was a standard treatment for all clients regardless of their substance abuse difficulties. Because of the pressures from managed care and the limited resources available for the center, the decision has been made to ask each client's case managers to establish priorities and determine how the resources per client are to be spent. The case manager will submit a plan that will be approved by the supervisor and then submitted to the managed care organization for review and final approval.

Many professionals are also very involved with their community as they develop collegial networks and work on behalf of their clients to create and improve services within the local area and beyond. The roles of advocate, community and service networker, community planner, consultant, mobilizer, and outreach worker are all roles in which the helper assumes responsibility in the community context.

Advocate—pleads and fights for services, policies, rules, regulations, and laws on behalf of clients.

Jose Cervantes is a lawyer for a legal aid clinic in an urban area. His clients, referred by the courts, are individuals who need legal services but cannot pay for them. Most of his cases involve marital separation, divorce, custody of children, and spouse and child support. Besides handling individual cases, Jose works with politicians, judges, and other lawyers to develop a legal system that is sensitive to the needs of his clients.

Community and service networker—works actively to connect with other helpers and agencies to plan for providing better services to the community and to clients, share information, support education and training efforts, and facilitate linking clients to the services they need.

Cameron DeBusk has been working for the public schools for the past 20 years. Early in his career he worked with in-school suspension programs and today he supervises school counselors in 15 high schools, 12 middle schools, and 32 elementary schools. One of his responsibilities is to help his counselors find the services their students need. Cameron has colleagues within the criminal justice system, child welfare services, health department, and vocational rehabilitation agency, to name just a few. Each day he spends time on the phone and on the road helping those in his network and also asking them to help his counselors and their students.

Community planner—works with community boards and committees to ensure that community services promote mental health and self-actualization, or at least minimize emotional stress on people.

Hector Gomez is director of the local department of human services. As director, part of his responsibility is to provide leadership in human services to the city and county. He spends many evenings attending board meetings with other members of the community, discussing funding and future planning for human services.

Consultant—works with other professions and agencies regarding their handling of problems, needs, and programs.

Three members of a pediatric language lab serving young children with communication disorders have formed a consulting service as part of their job responsibilities with the lab. The focus of the service is to educate teachers and day care staff about communication disorders and help them work with children in their own facilities. The consulting activity will enable the lab to expand the impact of its services.

Mobilizer—helps to get new resources for clients and communities.

Just last week Jimmy Owen, a psychiatric social worker at the research hospital, discovered that the funding for the newly formed hospice service was not being renewed. The support services provided to family members of dying patients will be difficult to replace. Jimmy has decided to schedule a meeting with hospital staff and members of local churches to assist him in thinking about alternative support for these family members.

Outreach worker—reaches out to identify people with problems, refer them to appropriate services, and follow up to make sure they continue to their maximum rehabilitation.

Greg Jones from the local mental health center travels into rural sections of a three-county area to follow up on patients who have been released from the regional mental health facility. His primary responsibilities are to provide supportive counseling, assess current progress, and make appropriate referrals.

Each human service job represents a unique combination of roles and responsibilities. The following list shows the way in which roles and responsibilities can be configured.

HOME HEALTH CARE COORDINATOR
Broker
Data manager
Evaluator
Facilitator of services
Report writer (documentation)

PAROLE OFFICER
Broker
Data manager
Planner
Report writer (documentation)

MENTAL HEALTH CASE MANAGER
Behavior changer
Caregiver
Crisis intervener
Data manager
Evaluator
Facilitator of services
Report writer (documentation)
Resource allocator

CHILD CARE PROFESSIONAL
Advocate
Behavior changer
Communicator
Report writer (documentation)
Teacher/educator

FOOD BANK ORGANIZER
Communicator
Community and service networker
Community planner
Mobilizer
Outreach worker

As you learn more about human services and meet human service professionals, try to determine the roles they are performing and the responsibilities they assume as they work with clients, their colleagues, and the community.

Front-Line Worker or Administrator

Workers may generally be categorized as having either front-line or administrative responsibilities. Using only these two categories may oversimplify the actual responsibilities of a given helper, but the categorization is useful when you are visualizing what human service professionals actually do. The schedules that follow outline the typical day of a front-line worker and an administrator.

FRONT-LINE WORKER: WOMEN'S CASE COORDINATOR (SHELTER FOR BATTERED WOMEN AND THEIR CHILDREN)

8:00 A.M. Use this time to finish what needs to be completed from the previous day, if planned activities were interrupted by an emergency with a client. Read the progress notes in the case files. See clients at about 8:30—have the appointments set up a day in advance. See each client two or three times each week, depending on what is going on with them. Be prepared for a crisis and a new client.

10:00 A.M. Go to court for orders of protection. This can last all day, depending on how many cases are on the docket. Go to court with a client for her hearing or to file for an order of protection.

11:00 A.M. If back from court, see clients or do paperwork.

12:00 noon Go to the dining room to eat with the clients.
1:00 P.M. Run errands with clients, going to their homes for clothing or important documents. Get a police escort for entering the home.
3:00 P.M. Attend staff meetings once a week (usually lasting a couple of hours). During these meetings, discuss each case and service issues.
4:00 P.M. Update case notes. Set up appointments for the next day.

ADMINISTRATOR: DIRECTOR, SOCIAL SERVICES
8:00 A.M. Attend morning meetings to coordinate staff activities. Prioritize week's projects.
9:00 A.M. Check client vacancies; plan for number of admissions. Make phone calls. Gather information, review referrals, schedule meetings and follow-up activities.
10:00 A.M. Meet with families, phone hospitals for possible admissions, meet with clients.
11:00 A.M. Meet with head administrator. Make plans, revise schedule for afternoon.
12:00 noon Eat at desk or with clients. Catch up on mail, read reports, write letters.
1:00 P.M. Discharge planning for clients. Meet with part-time staff. Repri-oritize based on morning's activities.
2:00 P.M. Meet with other professionals, such as bookkeepers and nurses; contact services outside agency for information, planning, and referrals.
3:00 P.M. Complete referral book and complaint log. Make sure all tasks and written correspondence are completed. Be available to see clients and families.
4:00 P.M. Answer phone calls. Finish reports due that day. Visit with clients and families.
5:00 P.M. Complete paperwork. Plan for the next day. Answer phone calls, call people at home.
Evening visit with family or client in hospital, read mail, work on big projects to improve services, attend professional meetings.

As you can see by reading these examples, both professionals perform more than one role. Although front-line workers and administrators sometimes have similar responsibilities, each has a different focus. The front-line worker focuses on caring for the client; the administrator's primary focus is on planning and organizing services. Both have valuable responsibilities in human service delivery and share the ultimate goal of helping clients.

The Nature of the Helping Process

The helping process occurs in both formal and informal settings. *Informal helping* is usually unstructured and may occur in any place. Whatever help is offered is secondary to another, already established relationship. This sort of help may occur in hair salons or neighborhood bars. *Formal helping,* on the

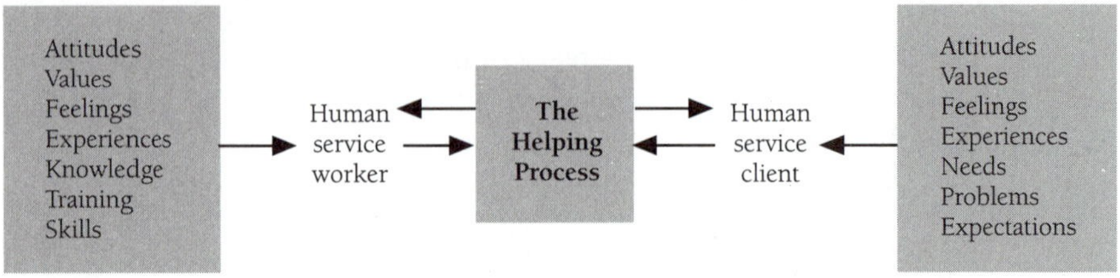

Figure 7-1 ✦ The helping process

other hand, takes place in human service organizations and agencies. The helper and the client are distinct, in that the helper has some specialized knowledge and skills with which to provide assistance. The relationship between the two parties is solely for the purpose of helping.

As noted in Chapter 5, the term *client* can mean an individual, a group such as a family, or a geographic population such as a neighborhood. Helpers can also vary in types as well as numbers. A client may work with only one professional or a team of professionals from the same agency or from different agencies. The length of involvement may vary, depending on the problem, the agency, and the client.

The Helping Relationship

The cornerstone of helping, the medium through which help is offered, is the helping relationship. The helping process takes place within the context of a relationship that differs from others in that one person sets aside his or her own needs to focus on the needs of the other (or others), refraining from expressing opinions or giving advice.

Each participant brings to the relationship different perspectives and experiences. (See Figure 7-1.) Both the client and the helper bring attitudes, values, feelings, and experiences, which may be similar or may be very different. In addition, the client brings needs, problems, and expectations about what will happen, whereas the helper comes with knowledge, training, and skills to assist with the problems of the client. Matching clients with helpers is often random, but there is considerable evidence that compatibility between the two is important for an effective helping relationship.

Because the helper has the knowledge and expertise that the client is seeking, much of the initial responsibility for establishing the relationship rests with the helper. The importance of the characteristics, values, and philosophy of the helper are discussed in Chapter 6. As mentioned there, a growing body of research shows their importance in establishing and maintaining the helping relationship. The following questions (adapted from Rogers, 1958) may help you increase your self-awareness in relation to your own helping skills:

Can I be perceived as trustworthy, dependable, and consistent?
Can I express myself well enough that the client understands what I am saying?

Can I experience attitudes of warmth, caring, liking, interest, and respect for the client?
Can I separate my needs from those of the client?
Am I secure enough myself to allow the client to be separate and independent from me?
Am I able to see the world as the client does?
Can I accept the client as he or she is?

As you begin to grasp the concept of the helping relationship and its importance to human service delivery, you may be asking yourself how it differs from other relationships. Several characteristics help make it unique (Perlman, 1979). First, helping relationships are formed for a recognized and agreed-on purpose; they are goal-oriented. Second, a helping relationship is time-bound. This means that it usually occurs over several sessions (depending, of course, on the nature of the problem); the relationship ends when the purpose has been accomplished. Third, the helping relationship carries authority. In this sense, the word *authority* has a very different meaning from the one with which you are probably familiar. The helper's authority consists of the knowledge and skills that enable him or her to work with the client toward resolving the problem. Finally, this relationship is for the client. The focus is always on the client's problems and concerns.

Stages of the Helping Process

Usually the agency or organization with which a helper works shapes the focus, the services, and the duration of the helping process. For example, vocational rehabilitation agencies are concerned with the work histories of clients, any disabilities that may prevent them from being employed, and their vocational capabilities and aspirations. Finding low-income housing, arranging adoptions, and processing applications for food stamps are not part of their services. Regardless of the focus of an agency and its services, you will find that the stages of the helping process are similar. They will include components of the problem-solving process such as identifying the problem, setting goals to resolve the problem, and determining and applying strategies designed to help the client reach those goals.

PREPARATION

Before the client arrives, the helper will want to attend to several matters. One is the *physical setting*. Are there any barriers that will prevent or make it difficult to establish a relationship with the client? For example, many clients will perceive a desk as a symbol of authority, which may seem a barrier to them when the helper sits behind it. It may also be unwise to seat the client facing a window. Activities outside may distract clients and prevent them from focusing on what is happening in the office. Does the physical setting ensure confidentiality? To promise the client that all matters discussed will remain between the two of you means nothing if the setting is such that any discussion may be overheard by others.

INTERNATIONAL FOCUS
Mother Teresa and the Missionaries of Charity

Mother Teresa received God's call to serve the poorest of the poor in 1946. Her work began in Calcutta in a small way by caring for one sick and dying person she found on the streets of Calcutta. Until March of 1997, she was head of the Missionaries of Charity, a religious order she formed with the Vatican's blessing in 1950. The numbers of sisters and brothers in this order now total more than 4,000 worldwide. They live what they teach, not owning more than the poor they serve. Mother Teresa has won many awards, including the Nobel Peace Prize. She has founded hundreds of homes throughout the world, including four in Calcutta: Shishu Bhavan (the children's home); Prem Nivas (the center for leprosy patients in Titagarh); Nirmal Hriday (the home for the dying and destitute); and Prem Dam (the home for TB sufferers and patients with mental disabilities).

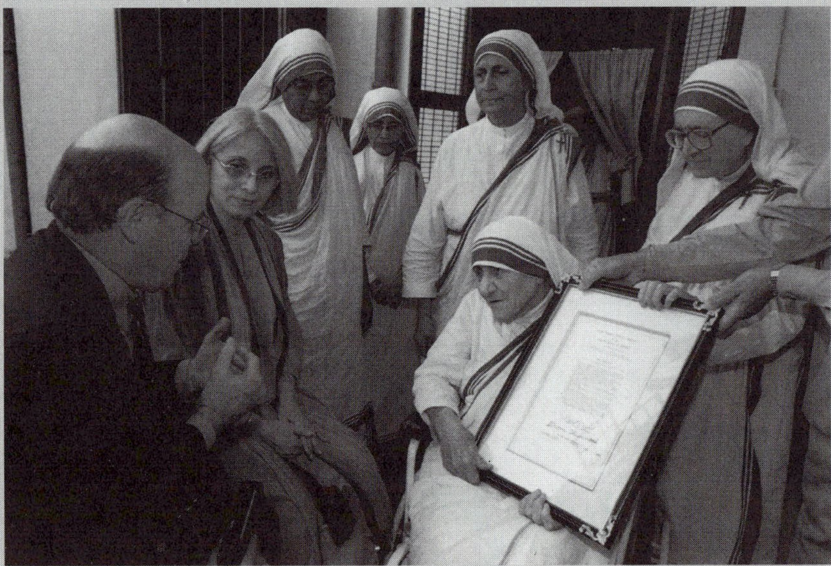

Mother Teresa accepting honorary U.S. citizenship in 1996

Most agencies require extensive paperwork on clients. How will you handle note taking, filling out forms, and recording information? These decisions are best made before the client arrives. They can be handled in several ways; each helper must choose the method that works best for him or her. For example, some helpers prefer taking notes while interviewing the client because it enables them to get all the facts while the client is present. Others say that taking notes

During the summer of 1995, Larry Coleman, a professor at the University of Tennessee, was with a Fulbright Hays group who visited the Mother House and three institutions in Calcutta run by the Missionaries of Charity. His account of the visit to Nirmal Hriday follows.

> Noah, a Dartmouth student who volunteers with Mother Teresa, was our guide. We went to the Mother House of the Missionaries of Charity, then to Shishu Bhavan, then on to Prem Dam, and finally to the house of the dying, Nirmal Hriday. At the last place I began to shudder as one does before sobbing. I managed to accept the feeling, thereby reducing the emotional overload. Seeing children and adults in such trying circumstances and the love and caring of the sisters and volunteers to ease their suffering is a life-affirming and a life-questioning experience.
>
> Nirmal Hriday was the original mission. It adjoins a Kali temple. Apparently, Mother Teresa took care of a monk whom no one else would care for, so she was given the house. It holds about 50 beds. As one approaches the mission, it is indistinguishable to me from other buildings in a busy shopping area. We enter through a door between two shops. Inside, a row of cots with sick and dying men is to the left on two levels. To the right is the medical and food dispensary. Volunteers were talking to the men. A blackboard provided a tally of the men, the women, the dismissed, and the dead. A short staircase descended opposite the dispensary and a long staircase went up to the roof.
>
> Down the steps we see stone sinks in the floor, a cooking area with bright coals heating water and oil for cooking. Mounds of vegetables are evident. Separating the washing area from the food area is a narrow shelf (step) leading through a partially opened louvered door into a room with two parallel shelves. I am looking at the empty morgue. Noah commented that it is a powerfully moving experience to carry someone you know into the morgue.
>
> Up the long staircase on the roof, sheets and clothes are drying. Volunteers are resting, either sitting on the roof in the shade or lying on the top of the outer walls of the building. Through the clothes lines and up three steps to a flat section, one could walk over to the spires of the Kali temple. At that moment I felt overwhelmed by what I had witnessed that morning. Before leaving, we met Sister Dolores who runs the house. Outside the sun was shining, people were yelling, selling, sitting, etc.; inside it was quiet, softly lighted and the talking was subdued. Always contrasts in India.

while the client is talking is too difficult for them. They find that they miss important gestures and facial expressions.

The same is true of filling out forms. Some agencies require forms to be completed before the client sees a human service professional. In such cases, the helper may have little choice. If there is no such policy, the worker may choose to have the client complete necessary forms before their meeting, or he or she may wish to assist the client in completing the forms, using this opportunity to establish rapport with the client and begin developing a helping relationship.

Finally, before the client arrives, the worker reviews the information about the client that is already accessible. What records are available? Is additional information needed? Based on the information available, what is the best way to approach the client? Has the helper made arrangements to have uninterrupted time with the client?

What follows is one client's description of an initial visit to a Social Security office. As you read it, pay attention to the physical setting, the workers, and the climate. What messages do those seeking services receive?

> The first thing I noticed when I entered the double glass doors of the Social Security office was the back of everyone's head. I mean that there were rows of people sitting in metal folding chairs facing a blank white wall that had a door in the middle of it. All kinds of people were there—young, old, white, black, a couple of mothers with babies, some disabled. On the left side of the room was a counter with a glass partition. Three women were behind the counter. I watched the person who entered in front of me. He approached the counter and one woman told him, in a rather loud voice I thought, to take a number and sit down to wait his turn. I took number 38 before she could yell at me. As I sat there facing the blank white wall, I had a chance to observe how the agency operated. As each worker was ready for a client, she simply yelled out the number. The person then approached the counter, and there was an exchange of information, which I could plainly hear. In some cases, the individual then approached the door in the middle of the blank white wall. A buzzer sounded, unlocking the door, and the person entered. I suppose there were other workers behind the door, but I only made it to the counter. When number 38 was called, I found out I needed to write a letter to the regional office. The local office could not help me with my problem.

THE CLIENT ARRIVES

When the client enters the office, a climate of respect and acceptance is established if the client is greeted with a smile, a handshake, and an introduction. Remember that clients come with problems, feeling vulnerable, and sometimes in pain or discomfort. A helper who takes charge of the initial meeting will help the client feel at ease by giving the client time to adjust to the new situation. The use of "ice breakers" or "door openers" allows the client to become accustomed to the setting and the helper: "Did you have any trouble finding the office?" or "Parking is sometimes a problem here. I hope it wasn't for you."

Since the helping relationship is time-bound and goal-oriented, the helper will at some point need to inquire about the client's problem. Many clients will be eager to share their problems. Others will be reticent about discussing problems that are personal and painful; they may test the helper by sharing less important problems first. The helper can initiate problem identification in a number of ways: "Let's talk about why you're here," "Tell me what's going on," "I'm wondering what's on your mind." These are relatively nonthreatening ways of focusing on the client and the problem. Another way to do this is to have focused dialogue. After greeting the client, the helper and client can fill out the intake form together. This is a humanizing way to complete the form, and it does not require asking so many questions.

During this initial stage, the helper can provide the client with information about the agency. For example, the client may want to know exactly what services the agency can provide. Other questions might concern the cost of the services, the criteria for eligibility to receive services, and the responsibilities of clients. In turn, the helper will probably have additional questions for the client. Does the client have any insurance? How did the client hear about the agency? Did someone refer him or her? What expectations does the client have for the agency and the helper?

EXPLORING THE PROBLEM

In Chapter 5, different perspectives on client problems were discussed. As the helper and the client begin to explore the problem, the helper should keep those perspectives in mind. The human service concepts of the whole person and the multidimensionality of problems will also guide this phase of the helping process. Once the problems are identified, it is time to move to the next stage.

INTERVENTION STRATEGIES

During this stage, the helper and the client set goals and determine how those goals will be reached to resolve the problem. Should the helper find that the client's problem calls for expertise or experience that the helper does not have, he or she should refer the client to another professional who has the necessary knowledge and skills. Another reason for referral at this point arises if, once the problem has been identified, the helper has such strong feelings or biases about the situation that he or she is unable to work objectively with the client. Referral will be discussed in detail in Chapter 8.

Depending on the problem, strategies may be as simple as providing a one-time service such as pregnancy testing or as complex as working with a client who has been injured in a car wreck and is permanently disabled. In the latter case, problems may include the client's loss of ability to work at his or her previous job, difficulties of the client and the family in adjusting to the client's disability, and barriers in the home to the client's mobility. All these must be addressed if the client is to adjust to his or her new reality.

TERMINATION

The final stage of the helping process is termination. The relationship between the helper and the client may end in several ways. The most positive conclusion is when the services needed are provided and both participants are satisfied that

Carl Rogers and Client-Centered Therapy

Carl Rogers, American psychologist and educator, was born on January 8, 1902, in Oak Park, Illinois. He attended the University of Wisconsin and graduated in 1924 with a degree in history. He then attended Union Theological Seminary in New York City and began to study for the ministry. He soon became influenced by a number of psychologists affiliated with Columbia University and transferred there to receive both his master's and doctoral degrees.

Rogers was initially concerned with environmental and institutional solutions to the problems of children, which he described in *The Clinical Treatment of the Problem Child* (1939). Later, he became interested in the psychotherapeutic process and gradually formulated the approach associated with his name—client-centered therapy. Client-centered therapy, or nondirective counseling, had a controversial beginning but proved to be a successful psychotherapeutic model. In *Counseling and Psychotherapy* (1942), Rogers maintained that the client knows better than anyone else what the problem is; with the help of a permissive, caring counselor, the client can find a solution to the problem. In client-centered therapy, the helper does not direct, give advice, or offer solutions and interpretations. The primary technique is "reflection of feelings." When the client speaks or acts, the helper responds by communicating perceptions of what the client means and feels. Through this "mirroring," the client can think more clearly about problems and feelings.

Rogers recognized the importance of the helper's self-awareness. He believed that the counselor's attitudes are more important than technique. Rogers considered three conditions necessary to facilitate a healthy personality change in a client. The counselor must have congruence (or genuineness); empathy (or understanding of the world as the client sees it); and unconditional positive regard or respect for the client, no matter how antisocial the client may be.

In 1942, Rogers became the first person to record, transcribe and publish verbatim a complete psychotherapy case. Recording of counseling sessions is now a common practice and an accepted part of the profession. It was largely due to the success of his book *On Becoming a Person* (1961) that the work of Carl Rogers began to attract the attention of a wider audience. Rogers has proved to be one of the most important trend setters in the field of psychotherapy. He died February 4, 1987.

SOURCE: From Taylor (1985).

the objectives have been reached. Unfortunately, not all terminations are so positive; services may be interrupted by either the helper or the client before the objectives have been reached. For example, the client moves from the area; the helper is transferred, promoted, or leaves the agency; or the client refuses to return for services.

The case study that follows provides an example of a human service professional who fills a variety of roles. It also illustrates how she deals with many of the concepts discussed in this section. The helper is Carmen Rodriguez, the vocational evaluator who was introduced in the concluding section of Chapter 6.

One aspect of my work that makes it challenging is that I perform a variety of functions. For example, I always begin my work with a client with an interview. During this initial contact with the client, I try to establish rapport. I explain what we will be doing together for the next six weeks and what the schedule is like at our facility. It also helps clients to know what is expected of them. One of the best ways I've found to get this relationship off on the right foot is to talk to the client as someone I really want to get to know. I do have some background information on the client (usually an intake form, a medical evaluation, and a financial statement), and I briefly skim it before I see the client. When I meet with the client the first time, I always stand up and invite him or her in with a handshake and a smile. I leave the folder in a drawer, because I can concentrate on the client totally if I'm not distracted by reports.

After the initial meeting, I read the client's folder carefully. At that point, I usually ask myself the following questions: What do I know about this client? Does this client have a documented disability that is a handicap to employment? What evaluative information do I need to determine whether there is a reasonable expectation that this client can eventually be gainfully employed? Has this client been evaluated previously? Finally, what additional information would be helpful to best serve this client?

During the period of time that I work with the client on a daily basis, the goal is to determine what types of work the client would like to perform and what types the client is capable of performing. Sometimes these are similar, but often they are not. Staff members administer vocational tests, do some vocational counseling, and arrange for the client to try working as an employee in two or three different job settings. In most cases, I find myself going beyond these tasks. For example, many of the clients do not know about personal hygiene, so it is up to staff members to teach them about taking showers and using deodorant. Also, they may not know about proper work behavior. To succeed at a job, they must learn appropriate work habits such as being at work on time, taking limited breaks, dealing with conflicts, and getting along with other workers.

I've also discovered over the past four years that our clients often have multiple problems. Although the primary concern of our agency is vocational, clients come with other problems that affect their vocational evaluation. For example, a client may be having difficulty with a parent or guardian who is too protective. Or perhaps the client is not receiving a disability check that is due. Sometimes, clients have needs or problems that call for services from other agencies. My agency is limited to providing vocational evaluation, so if a client needs clothes or dental care, we must contact other agencies.

This leads me to one of the more rewarding parts of my job: working with other professionals. All of us are committed to meeting client needs, and we've found that we are much more successful when we work together. Another challenging part of my work is consulting with specialists such as psychologists, psychiatrists, and other medical specialists. Different specialists are consulted, depending on client needs. Frequently, it's left to me to make that decision. In that sense, I tend to function independently, although we operate as a team at our facility, consulting one another both formally and informally.

For the protection of the client, the agency, and the human service professional, it is necessary to maintain written case notes and documentation of services. This can be very time-consuming. I've noticed that each worker handles this task differently. What works for me is reserving the last 30 minutes of the day for updating files. I realize that these notes are important—the client may be transferred, I may change jobs, or I may be out sick—but some days it's a real chore to pull all the files and condense what's necessary into two or three sentences.

I hope to continue in my job for several more years, but eventually I would like to go back to school for further training. I want to develop my counseling skills to work with clients as individuals or groups in a more specialized way. My position as a case manager gives me practical experience and allows me to explore my career options by filling a variety of roles and working with other professionals.

An Introduction to Helping Skills

Communication is the foundation for all interpersonal relationships. Exchanging messages to understand another's perceptions, ideas, and experiences is especially important in helping relationships. Helping others will be difficult if we don't understand their problems or concerns.

In this section, basic helping skills are introduced. We begin by focusing on the client's message. This means perceiving both the verbal and the nonverbal messages of the client. Next, we focus on the helper's communication by identifying the skills necessary for effective listening and responding. Finally, we discuss what the helper needs to know about cultural differences.

One person's sending a message to another person with the conscious intent of affecting the receiver's behavior is *communication* (Johnson, 1993). This process is illustrated in Figure 7-2. When the receiver interprets the message the way the sender intended, *effective communication* has taken place. When one person interprets the message differently from the way it was intended, the result is communication failure, the most common source of misunderstandings in interpersonal relationships.

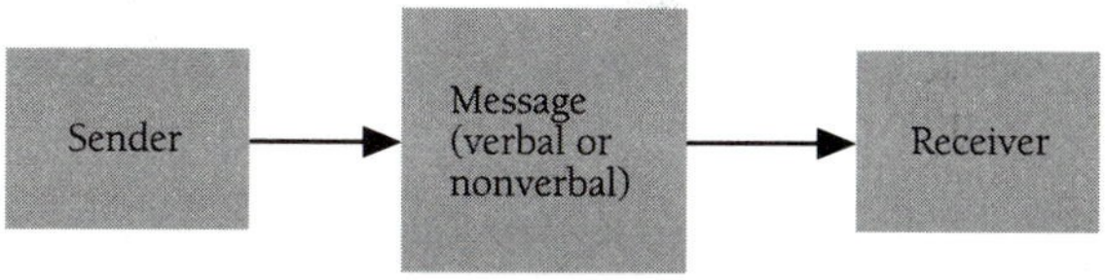

Figure 7-2 ✦ Communication

The message that a person sends can be verbal or nonverbal. The most common example of a verbal message is the spoken word: "Hello, how are you today?" The smile and handshake or the hug accompanying that verbal greeting are nonverbal messages. The skillful helper is able to "hear" the client's behavior (the nonverbal message), as well as what is actually said (the verbal message), and to respond verbally and nonverbally to these messages (Okun, 1997). It sounds complicated, and it takes practice to communicate effectively. A good beginning is through an introduction to each component of the communication process.

Nonverbal Messages

Nonverbal behaviors (body language) include a person's posture, tone of voice, gestures, eye contact, and touch. Everyone communicates nonverbally. Each of us engages in some nonverbal behavior that we are aware of and perform intentionally. For example, when meeting someone for the first time, most of us want to make a positive first impression, so we deliberately greet that person with a smile or some other pleasant facial expression. However, we also communicate unconsciously in a nonverbal fashion. You may recall a time when you visited the doctor's office for shots and afterward wondered at the soreness in your muscles. The tension, fear, or hurt you experienced during the visit caused you to tense your muscles.

In a normal two-person conversation, more than 65% of the meaning is carried nonverbally. This fact emphasizes the importance of nonverbal communication in a helping situation. Frequently, you may find that a client's nonverbal message will provide you with valuable clues about what the client is thinking or feeling—important ideas that the client is unable to verbalize. Table 7-1 lists some common nonverbal cues and their meanings.

Another area in which nonverbal cues are important is the expression of feelings. Feelings are most often communicated nonverbally, particularly by facial expressions and tone of voice. One difficulty with "hearing" the nonverbal expression of feelings is the ambiguity of the nonverbal message. A nonverbal behavior such as crying could be interpreted in various ways; one cannot determine just from the tears on a person's face whether the person is sad, hurt, or disappointed. In fact, the person may be scared or even very happy.

Thus, we may think that nonverbal communication is a fairly straightforward process of sending and receiving messages, but it is actually a complicated mode of communication. Although they provide us with important cues about the person with whom we are conversing, nonverbal messages should be interpreted with caution.

TABLE 7-1 ✦ SOME NONVERBAL CUES AND THEIR MEANINGS

Cue	*Meaning*
Lifting an eyebrow	Disbelief
Lowering eyebrows	Uneasiness, suspicion
Lifting both eyebrows	Surprise
Eye contact	Interest, confidence
Winking an eye	Intimacy
Slapping forehead	Forgetfulness
Rubbing the nose	Puzzlement
Turning up corners of mouth	Happiness
Cocking head to one side	Friendly, human
Little or no head and/or hand movements	Cool, no emotion
Raised shoulders	Fear
Retracted shoulders	Suppressed anger
Square shoulders	Responsibility
Bowed shoulders	Carrying a burden
Shrugging shoulders	Indifference
Sitting with arms and legs crossed	Withdrawal, resistance
Clasping arms	Protection
Tapping fingers	Impatience
Fondling and touching inanimate objects	Loneliness
Leaning forward in a chair	Interest
Leaning back, arms uncrossed	Open to suggestion
Leaning back, arms crossed	Not open to suggestion
Postural change—facing away	Finished with interaction

Try this exercise: At some point today, select two people who are communicating with each other. (You may be in the library, a food service area, or anywhere you choose.) For 10 minutes, observe the nonverbal communication of one of the participants. What behaviors do you observe? What possible interpretations can you make about the meanings of the behaviors?

Verbal Messages

Verbal messages consist of words spoken by a person. Such messages can be divided into a cognitive component and an affective component. The cognitive component consists of the facts of a message and reflects the person's thinking processes. This is the realm in which we are most comfortable. A cognitive message addresses such matters as who, what, where, when, and why. Consider the following statements by a co-worker and try to pick out the cognitive messages:

> I left work at 5:00 P.M. today. The last client I saw was Raphael Santini, and I just can't seem to get him off my mind. He is making such an effort to find a job, but he's had no luck. I couldn't believe it when he showed up today. I hardly recognized him, and I guess he could tell I was surprised, because I couldn't think of anything to say for a moment. He looked great. His hair was clean and neatly combed, and his clothes were new. He was so proud of himself, and I was proud of him too. I told him I was so pleased with the changes. I also felt good about myself, because some of my hard work with this client has paid off. I'm going to make some phone calls first thing in the morning to see what assistance I can find to help him locate a job. There's just got to be help for a motivated client like Raphael.

Some of the cognitive messages you probably identified were the speaker's leaving work at 5:00; the appointment with Raphael Santini, who is trying to find a job; and the description of his neat, clean appearance. In the cognitive realm, facts are the focus.

The affective component, the feeling part of the message, may be expressed directly or indirectly. Many clients who are unsure about what they are feeling, or who are simply uncomfortable talking about feelings, may choose to express their feelings indirectly. This means that the individual may not name the feeling at all ("Stop driving so fast!"), or they may describe it by telling what they feel like doing ("I feel like punching him in the nose"). One of the helper's main tasks may be to encourage the client to become aware of feelings and to learn to express feelings appropriately and directly: "I'm scared when you drive so fast," or "I'm angry at you for spoiling the surprise."

Review the statements about Raphael Santini. What feelings are expressed directly? In fact, there are very few, but they do include feeling "proud," "surprised," and "good." These feelings are named, and the reader clearly understands how the helper feels. Read the excerpt again, and consider the feelings that are being expressed indirectly. (It might be helpful to read it aloud.) You might identify such feelings as discouragement at Raphael's lack of success, exasperation at the job situation, disbelief at his appearance, and determination to find some type of assistance for Raphael. Determining exactly what the client (or, in this case, the helper) is feeling may be more difficult when feelings are expressed indirectly.

Listening and Responding

The way we listen and respond to the client is crucial in building a helping relationship. The first thing a helper must do before making any response to the client is to listen carefully to what the client is expressing, both verbally and nonverbally. Even though listening takes up more of a person's waking hours than any other activity, and many people consider themselves good listeners, few of us actually are. This section will introduce listening behaviors and some helper responses that promote effective helping. (See Table 7-2.)

TABLE 7-2 ✦ SOME HELPFUL BEHAVIORS IN COMMUNICATING

Verbal	*Nonverbal*
Mirroring feelings	Making eye contact
Clarifying	Listening
Showing a sense of humor	Smiling
Providing support	Nodding one's head
Providing information that client needs	Leaning forward
Explaining helper's role	Maintaining a relaxed posture
Sharing information about oneself	Facing the client
Being nonjudgmental	Displaying facial expression
Asking few questions	Being punctual
	Occasionally making appropriate use of gestures and touching
	Maintaining a moderate rate of speech

THE HELPER LISTENS

The kind of listening that helpers engage in is called *responsive listening* or *active listening*. These terms describe the behaviors of helpers as they attend to both the verbal and the nonverbal communication of the client. What makes this type of listening special or different from other listening behaviors is that helpers also attend to what is not said—that is, to the underlying thoughts and feelings of the client, which are not expressed in words. Two ways of considering responsive or active listening as helping behaviors are presented here.

Egan (1994, pp. 91–92) suggested several things a helper can do to communicate to the client that he or she is listening. These five behaviors are presented as a set of guidelines a helper can follow to let the client know the helper is physically present and actively involved in the helping relationship. They can be easily remembered by thinking of the acronym SOLER.

S—Face the client *squarely*. This is a posture of involvement. To face away from the client or even at an angle lessens the degree of involvement.

O—Adopt an *open posture*. This is usually perceived as nondefensive. Crossing arms or legs may not communicate openness or availability.

L—*Lean toward* the other person. A natural sign of involvement, this posture is a slight forward inclination. Moving forward or backward can frighten a client or communicate lessened involvement.

E—Maintain *eye contact*. This is normal behavior for two individuals who are involved in conversation. It is different from staring.

R—Try to be *relaxed*. This means avoiding nervous habits such as fidgeting or tapping a pencil. Behaviors such as these can distract the client.

Remember that these are only guidelines. A helper's physical behavior may vary in accordance with the cultural identity of the client or what is comfortable for that particular helper.

Ivey (1994, p. 24) described *attending behavior* as another way to let the client know the helper is listening. The goal of attending behavior is to encourage the client to talk about and examine issues, problems, or concerns. Attending behavior has four dimensions: three nonverbal components and one verbal component.

1. *Eye contact.* If you are going to talk to people, look at them.
2. *Attentive body language.* In general, clients know you are interested in them if you face them squarely and have a slight forward trunk lean, have an expressive face, and use facilitative, encouraging gestures.
3. *Vocal qualities.* Your vocal tone and speech rate indicate much of how you feel about another person. Think of how many ways you can say, "I am really interested in what you say," just by your vocal tone and speech rate.
4. *Verbal tracking.* The client has come to you with a topic of interest; don't change the subject. Keep to the topic initiated by the client. If you change the topic, be aware that you did and realize the purpose of your change.

Engaging in these behaviors encourages the client to talk, reducing the amount of talk from the helper. Benefits include communicating interest and concern to the client and increasing the worker's awareness of the client's ability to pay attention. Attending behaviors also allow the helper to modify helping behaviors to work effectively with clients who may be racially, culturally, or sexually different.

THE HELPER'S RESPONSE

Once the helper has heard the verbal and nonverbal messages of the client, it is time for the helper to speak. Remember that helpers' responses must be purposeful. Think about the characteristics of the helping relationship. This is not a casual conversation between two people, but a goal-directed exchange. Therefore, the helper must know his or her intent before speaking.

The helper has several options at this point. For example, did the helper understand what the client said? Was the message clear? Does the helper need further information to grasp the message correctly? Questions such as these will assist the helper in determining the intent of his or her response. Let's examine some of these options.

First, suppose the helper does understand the client's message and decides that the most helpful response would be one that lets the client know this. To communicate that intent, the helper may choose to *paraphrase*—to make a statement that is interchangeable with the client's own words.

CLIENT: I've been able to complete five tasks today that were on my list.

HELPER: You've had a productive day today.

The helper may determine that more than a simple paraphrase is needed to help the client become aware of or clarify feelings. In this case, a helper statement that reflects both the feeling (or affective component) and the facts (or cognitive component) is helpful. For example:

HELPER: You're really pleased that you were able to accomplish what you set out to do today.

If the helper is confused about what the client said, perhaps because the client was relating a complicated incident, the helper should ask the client for clarification. To attempt a response that will make little sense to the client and will let the client know that the helper did not understand what was said is not helpful. Responses such as "I'm not sure I understand . . ." or "I'm confused about . . ." are appropriate at this point. They also let the client know that the helper is interested enough to want to get the story right in order to be able to help.

Beginning helpers sometimes encounter situations in which clients are asking questions or seeking information that the helper does not know. Many helpers believe they should know everything and may feel embarrassed about being asked something they do not know. Unfortunately, they may attempt to answer off the tops of their heads or give an answer they believe may be correct. A better response in situations like this would be, "I do not have that information, but I do know where we can find it; let me check on that for you," or "I'm not sure about the eligibility requirements for that type of assistance, but I can refer you to someone who knows." Helpers are not supposed to have all the answers. The effective helper who wants to maintain a relationship with the client will enrich that relationship by being honest with the client.

ASKING QUESTIONS

Another technique that beginning helpers should be wary of is *questioning.* Most of us consider ourselves skilled at asking questions and find it a natural form of communication in everyday life—particularly questions that begin with the words *who, what, where, why,* and *when.* For the beginning helper, the question is the most common method of eliciting information from the client, and many helpers find themselves resorting to questions frequently. Unfortunately, one question seems to lead to another, and too many questions can interfere with the helping relationship, causing the client to feel like a witness. An overreliance on questioning, neglecting other kinds of responses, hinders the helping process. It also creates a dependent client who has no role other than answering questions. Most questions can be rephrased as statements that elicit the same information. For example, the question "What was the last grade completed in school?" can be rephrased as "Tell me about your school experiences." In addition to discovering the final grade completed, the helper may learn how the client felt about school, whether he or she enjoyed learning, and what circumstances surrounded the end of the client's educational experience.

Now that you have been alerted to the pitfalls of questioning, let's explore when asking questions is appropriate and how one asks good questions. Long,

Paradise, and Long (1981) suggested several situations in which a question is helpful. One is to begin the interview. "How would you like to begin?" or "Could you tell me a little about yourself?" are examples. A second situation occurs when specific information is needed. Asking for information to clarify ("How long have you been ill?") or to elicit examples of specific behavior ("How does that make you feel?") can provide the additional information necessary for complete understanding. Finally, questions can be useful to focus the client's attention. For example, a client who is digressing or rambling on about several problems may need the helper's assistance to focus. Such assistance can be provided by statements such as the following:

> "You've mentioned several concerns that you have about your daughter. You're afraid she is using drugs, and you suspect she is not doing well in school. I guess I hear you expressing the most concern, though, about your inability to talk with her. Let's focus on that. What happens when you do try to talk with her?"

Thus, there are times in a helping relationship when asking questions is appropriate and beneficial. How does one ask good questions? Egan (1994) suggested that the helper might first want to consider how the question will relate to and promote the helping relationship. Having specific objectives in mind before asking the question will help in formulating a good question.

Both closed and open questions can facilitate the development of the helping relationship when the helper has specific intentions. *Closed* questions are those that elicit facts necessary to facilitate the helping process. "How old were you when your father died?" and "How many brothers and sisters do you have?" may provide important information regarding the client's family situation if he or she is having difficulties at home. Closed questions that require a "yes" or "no" answer should usually be avoided, because they lead the beginning helper to ask more and more questions.

Open questions, on the other hand, are broader, allowing the client to express thoughts, feelings, or ideas. They contribute to building rapport with the client and also assist him or her in exploring a situation, a problem, or an interaction. For example, "How did you feel after talking it over with your parents?" asks for the client's view. On the other hand, "Did you feel better after talking with your parents?" can be answered with a simple "yes" or "no," which does not enhance the helping process.

In summary, questions can be useful tools in the helping process. As with other types of responses, the key to effective questioning is knowing the intent of the question before posing it to the client. Are you seeking factual information or asking the client to offer thoughts or opinions about the topic of discussion? Considering how the question will promote the helping relationship will assist the helper in determining the appropriate strategy.

What you have read in this section is a brief introduction to helping skills. As you pursue your education and training in preparation for work in the human services, you will increase your knowledge about these skills and refine your use of them so that you become an effective helper. There is another matter to consider before concluding the discussion of skills: working with clients from different cultures.

Culturally Different Clients

A recent Census Bureau report projects profound shifts in America's population that should make the country far more ethnically diverse than ever before (Friedman, 1996). By 2050, immigration patterns and differences in birth rates, combined with an overall slowdown in the growth of the country's population, will produce a United States in which 53% of the people will be non-Latino whites, down from 74% today. Latinos and Asians will grow fastest, whereas African Americans will nearly double in numbers by 2050.

As these population shifts occur, it is increasingly likely that human service professionals will encounter clients whose cultural backgrounds differ from their own. The key to working with culturally different clients is awareness of and sensitivity to cultural differences. In Tucson, Arizona, for example, Suzy Bourque at the Family Counseling Agency emphasizes the need to hire workers who appreciate different cultures. Their client population is about 30% Latino and 10% African American. Native Americans are underrepresented because they tend to take care of their own. She is constantly looking for staff who are bilingual, bicultural, and/or African American (personal communication, October 7, 1994). For the case workers at Casita Maria Settlement House in the Bronx, sometimes getting people to accept help is difficult because accepting outside help is not part of their culture (personal communication, May 4, 1994). Instead of saying to a Latino client, "You need counseling," they find that a more acceptable phrase is "Maybe you need someone to talk with." Because many of their clients are Latino, they find that they can no longer refer to them as Hispanic or Latino. Now, it is important to recognize that Latino include people from Puerto Rico, Nicaragua, Colombia, and Honduras. And they are all different. Even human service providers from Knoxville, Tennessee, must be culturally sensitive as they work with clients from rural areas as well as Appalachia (personal communication, July 10, 1994).

Helpers must realize that culture shapes body language. Few gestures and body movements have universal meaning. For example, Arabs tend to cling or huddle together, whereas Americans like their space. Postures also vary by culture. The posture of the German male is stiffer than that of the American male, whereas the French male exhibits greater body limpness (Sielski, 1979). The direct eye contact that is so critical to standard American helping behavior may be offensive to people from Native American and Latino cultures. A helper with no knowledge of this may intend to communicate complete attention but be perceived by the culturally different client as disrespectful.

The beginning helper is cautioned against assigning too much meaning to a single gesture; instead, all means of expression—the verbal, postural, facial, and cultural—should be considered. It is also wise not to generalize about cultural traits. Some Asian Americans may not like direct eye contact, yet some might.

Axelson (1985, p. 17) suggested that a multicultural approach to counseling should start with four steps to conceptualize the culturally different client:

1. Recognize that all human beings possess the like capacity for thought, feeling, and behavior.
2. Be knowledgeable in several cultures; study both differences and similarities among people of different groups and their special needs and problems.
3. Gain an understanding of how the individual relates to important objects of motivation, what his or her personal constructs are, and how they coalesce to form his or her worldview.
4. Blend steps 1, 2, and 3 into an integrated picture of the distinctive person as experienced during the counseling process.

The following account, written by Michiko, a foreign student from Japan, may help you to begin thinking about culturally different clients in light of the preceding four steps.

I am a foreign student from Japan who is studying at an American university. It has been more than a month since I arrived in the States, and still I am not making American friends. I usually hang around with my Japanese buddies, so that does not help either. I hardly have any time for socializing because of all of the assignments I have to do for class. I am tense and timid around people and feel uncomfortable most of the time because I do not know how to act in pleasing, acceptable ways. I miss my friends and family and often cry when I am alone.

I have two great needs. One is to feel accepted among Americans and to adjust to the American culture. The other need is for academic excellence, since I did not come all the way from Japan just to fool around. I would like to have American friends with whom I can talk and share experiences, who will like me the way I am. I find most of my classes large and impersonal and have hardly any hope of finding a friend there. I need someone who is interested enough to get past the language barrier to get to know me. As for the academics, my professors know that I am a foreign student and they will go out of their way to help me with any difficulties I might be facing. I appreciate the attention, but that is not enough. I need help with the report assignments because I am unfamiliar with formats in English writing. I also need to be advised on study skills, because even if I prepare well in advance for a test, the grades I get are C's and D's.

I have many fears. I am afraid being Japanese, a racial minority, makes me less desirable as a person worth knowing in the eyes of an American. I am in constant fear of saying wrong things at the wrong moments and acting weird in front of people. My language problem still persists. Conversational English is something I find difficult, and people must speak slowly and clearly for me. I am afraid this makes me boring to talk to and hard to discuss complex subjects with. The greatest fear of all is having to go back to Japan because I could not make it academically and socially at an American university.

The young woman in this case study is one among many culturally different clients. Axelson's four steps are useful in understanding Michiko as a unique, worthwhile individual. Michiko definitely has the capacity for thought, feeling, and behavior as she attempts to function successfully in a culture foreign to her. A helper would need to learn about the Japanese culture and the ways in which it differs from and resembles American culture. Michiko has established personal goals that focus on academic and social success and is frustrated by the barriers she is experiencing. To engage effectively in the helping process with Michiko, the helper would need to explore the relevant differences between American and Japanese cultures. For example, many Asian cultures are collectivist—the individual is less important than the group. Michiko may be fearful of not succeeding academically and socially because of the disgrace it would bring to her family.

The helper would also want to adjust his or her helping behaviors to the individual of a different culture and to assess appropriate strategies of intervention. In American culture, the individual is perceived as autonomous and separate from groups. Even though a person can be a member of many groups, no one group determines identity completely. In collectivist societies, however, the individual belongs to fewer groups, but the attachment is stronger; often the individual is defined by membership in a group. Taking this information into account, the helper would choose an intervention that would focus on Michiko in relation to her group rather than an intervention designed to promote independence.

Challenging Clients

Ideally, all human service clients would be motivated, cooperative, and responsible. It is one of the challenges of human service practice that not all clients fit that description. In your experience as a helper, you will likely meet the resistant client, the silent client, the overly demanding client, and the unmotivated client. In this section, such clients are referred to as *challenging* clients.

You need to know something about these client groups because they often elicit in the helper feelings of uncertainty, hostility, and resentment. They are particularly difficult for many beginning helpers to work with, and it is important to realize that the client's behavior is not necessarily the helper's fault.

THE RELUCTANT OR RESISTANT CLIENT

There are some distinctions between reluctant and resistant clients, but the principles for working with them are similar. The *reluctant* client is one who does not want to come in for help in the first place and is more or less forced to come. Such clients may be found in schools, correctional settings, court-related settings, and employment agencies (Egan, 1994). The *resistant* client may come more or less willingly but fail to carry through or participate actively in the helping process. Some of the causes of clients' reluctance and resistance are having negative attitudes about help, seeing no benefits in changing, feeling that getting help means admitting weakness or failure, and seeing no reason for going for help in the first place.

Reluctant clients may be embarrassed or angry that they are there for help. In many cases, they are there only because the court or some other authority has said they must be. These feelings are compounded by their unfamiliarity with the agency or the process. To attempt to lessen the reluctance, the helper can explain the process to the client (Ritchie, 1986). Discussing matters such as confidentiality, time limits, and expectations (for the client as well as the helper) can help demystify the process. Also, the manner in which the helper relates this can allow the client to see him or her in a role other than that of interrogator or advice giver.

Resistance is slightly different from reluctance, because resistance can occur at any time in the helping process. Clients who come to the attention of human service agencies may initially feel threatened by the referral and application procedures. Resistance may also arise later in the helping process if the client feels threatened by the subject being discussed, by the helper, or even by the helping relationship.

What is resistant behavior? Missing appointments, rejecting the helper, and inattentiveness are examples of such behavior. Clients may try to protect themselves by denying the existence of a problem, claiming it is caused by other people or situations, or distancing themselves from it.

The helper can use several strategies when working with a resistant client. First, recognizing and accepting the antagonism may defuse the situation. This type of action is very different from what the client might expect; a statement such as "You probably don't want to see anyone like me" may minimize the threat to the client. Second, asking for the client's perceptions of the problem will communicate support for the client's feelings. This does not mean that the helper must accept or believe everything the client says, but it does communicate support and respect. Asking what the client wants to happen in this situation is a third strategy. It engages the client in the helping process and also emphasizes the worker's support and respect for the individual. In addition, it can provide the client with some sense of control over his or her life. Finally, for resistance that occurs later in the relationship, changing the pace or the topic may temporarily lessen feelings of threat.

THE SILENT CLIENT

Particularly difficult for the beginning helper is the silent client. The uncomfortable silence may cause the helper to believe that nothing is taking place; in fact, silence can have many different meanings. It is the helper's responsibility to evaluate what a silence means so he or she can decide how to respond.

Silence can mean that the client is waiting for direction from the helper. In this case, the client may feel that it is the helper's place to determine the topic of discussion or the direction in which the relationship should move. A second meaning of silence can be that the client is pondering what has been said. Resistance (discussed previously) may also manifest itself as silence; a change of pace or topic may be necessary until the client is ready to deal with what is happening.

THE OVERLY DEMANDING CLIENT

Calling the helper at home, monopolizing time in the office, and scheduling frequent and unnecessary appointments are behaviors of an overly demanding client. Sometimes such clients become so dependent that they may want to be told what to do. When the client makes demands, the helper may become resentful of the time the client takes up and frustrated with the unsuccessful nature of the helping process. For these reasons, the helper must deal appropriately with the client's behavior.

One strategy that may help with the overly demanding client is setting reasonable limits to decrease the client's dependence. Limiting client–helper contact to working hours only is one step toward decreasing dependence. A second strategy is to examine the helper's own need to be needed. Is the helper actually encouraging the demanding behavior of the client?

THE UNMOTIVATED CLIENT

Clients who are present because someone referred them or encouraged them to seek help may be unmotivated. They may not see the need for the service and may be showing up only because some authority such as their parents, the school, or the court is forcing them to attend. Unfortunately, the unmotivated client is often unwilling to change and only goes through the motions of the helping process. The helper may find that he or she is doing most of the work in the relationship and may come to feel resentful, frustrated, and even angry. Such clients may be classed as reluctant clients, and many of the same strategies previously suggested may be helpful in establishing rapport with them.

Crisis Intervention

Crisis intervention is a helping process that occurs at a much faster pace than other helping and incorporates many of the helping roles and skills that have been discussed in this chapter. You may find yourself engaged in crisis intervention when there is an emergency. For example, a crisis can be precipitated by suicide threats or attempts, the discovery of an unwanted pregnancy, abandonment, or natural disasters such as hurricanes or tornadoes. In this section, you will read a description of crisis intervention as a human service, including types of crises, the development of a crisis, the principles and skills of intervention, and the role of the human service professional providing this service.

Defining Crisis

Stressful events and emergencies are going to occur; an individual can probably handle some but may find himself or herself unable to cope with others. The inability to cope creates the potential for crisis. An individual's equilibrium is disrupted by pressures or upsets, and this imbalance results in stress so severe that he or she is unable to find relief by using coping skills that have worked before. The person is then experiencing a crisis. When identifying crises, we need to distinguish between the event or situation and the person's response. The crisis is the individual's emotional response to the threatening or hazardous situation rather than the situation itself.

Thus, the crisis lies in the individual's interpretation or perception of an event; the same event does not lead to crisis for all people. What one individual can handle may be a crisis for another person. For example, the houses of two neighbors were burglarized in the same afternoon by the same thief. In both burglaries, the door was kicked in, furniture overturned, and jewelry and radio and TV equipment stolen. Both neighbors discovered the damage when arriving home from work. Three weeks later, one neighbor has recovered from the event. She locks her doors at night, has marked her possessions, and has joined the neighborhood crime watch. The second neighbor has not recovered so well. She has yet to enjoy a good night's sleep, fears for her life each time she enters her empty house, and calls the police at least once a day. She says she is "as nervous as a cat."

Crises can be divided into two types: developmental and situational. A *developmental crisis* is an individual's response to a situation that is reasonably predictable in the life cycle. Chapter 5 explained that as a person grows and develops, there are periods of major transition such as childhood to puberty, puberty to adolescence, and adolescence to adulthood. Stresses can occur at each phase. For many people, the stresses are normal developmental problems with which they are able to cope. For those who cannot cope, the stresses of these stages can have destructive effects, such as suicide attempts, rejection of others, and depression. Such reactions constitute a developmental crisis in those circumstances.

Situational or *accidental crises* do not occur with any regularity. The sudden and unpredictable nature of this type of crisis makes any preparation or individual control impossible. Examples are fire or other natural disaster, fatal illness, relocation, unplanned pregnancy, and rape. Hazardous situations such as these may cause periods of psychological and behavioral upset. A crisis may result, depending on the individual's personal and social resources at the time of the event.

The skills and strategies that helpers use to provide immediate help for a person in crisis constitute *crisis intervention*. It is short-term therapy that focuses on solving the immediate problem and helping the individual to reestablish equilibrium (Aguilera & Messick, 1993). Common practice areas of crisis intervention are childhood and adolescence, mental health problems, marital and family conflicts, emergency hospitalization, and suicide prevention (Smith, 1977).

How a Crisis Develops

Even a sudden or short-lived crisis has identifiable components that create a pattern of development. The case study that follows examines crisis in terms of its development. You may want to make note of the different roles the worker plays.

Ben and Joan Matthews and their three children (ages 9 months, 2 years, and 5 years) left their trailer in rural Illinois to drive to Florida. Ben had lost his job because the factory where he worked for minimum wage closed down. He hoped to find a job in Florida working on some of the fruit farms. The Matthews were also hoping that the climate would improve the health of the children as well as the state of their marriage.

The hope for a job did not materialize in Florida, so they headed back to their trailer in Illinois and an uncertain future. The trip home seemed plagued with problems. Two of the children became ill, the car broke down twice, and Joan and Ben argued constantly about what they should do next. A couple of times, the arguments escalated into shouting matches that ended when Ben hit Joan.

By the time the Matthews arrived in Atlanta, they had no money for food, lodging, or gas. The children were hungry and crying, the car was making a funny noise again, Joan was complaining, and Ben had a raging headache. They stopped at a fast-food place so that everyone could use the bathroom and have a drink of water. Joan gathered the children together and headed into the restaurant. When they returned, Ben and the car were gone.

According to Caplan (1964), crisis development has four identifiable phases. In the first, the person reacts to a traumatic event with increased anxiety. The individual then responds with problem-solving mechanisms to reduce or eliminate stress. Here is Joan's initial response:

Joan thinks that Ben has gone to get gas, so she returns to the restaurant. Selecting an out-of-the-way booth, she and the children sit watching and waiting for his return. After an hour, Joan begins to feel desperate. She has no money and no identification since she left her purse in the car. The children are tired and hungry, and she is becoming uncomfortable with the looks from the people at the service counter. Joan fusses with the children and tries to look natural and unworried.

In the second phase, the individual's problem-solving ability fails. The stimulus that caused the initial rise in anxiety continues. In this case, the source of Joan's anxiety does not change: Ben is still missing. Her initial attempts to deal with the situation fail, and her anxiety continues to increase because she is worried about Ben and she is worried about herself.

Suicide Attempts

Suicide attempts, some of which result in actual suicide, are often responses to a crisis. There are common events which may occur to precipitate a suicide attempt, and one of the most common is an individual's reaction to a perceived loss.

Suicide prevention hotline
Although there is no single characteristic profile of a suicide, several demographic indicators of the suicide risk victim have been identified. . . .

1. *Sex.* Although more women attempt suicide, more men succeed.
2. *Age.* There is a positive correlation between suicide risk and age. Until the age of 35, the rate rises steadily for men. The rate does not level off for women until age 70.
3. *Race.* Overall, whites have a greater suicide risk than do non-whites; however, the rate for young black males is almost twice that for young white males.
4. *Socioeconomic status.* Suicide risk and socioeconomic status are inversely correlated.
5. *Marital status.* Single individuals are twice as likely as married individuals to commit suicide. The suicide rate is four to five times higher for divorced and widowed individuals than for married individuals.

SOURCE: Fujimura, Weis, & Cochran (1985), pp. 612–615.

At this point the manager approaches and asks if he can be of any assistance. By now the children are crying. They are still hungry, are tired of sitting, and sense their mother's tension. Feeling frightened and alone, but not wanting to upset the children, Joan explains to the manager that her husband went to get some gas and that he will be back soon to pick them up. She explains about the funny noise in the car, saying that this was probably being fixed, which accounted for her husband's delay. Joan thanks the manager for his concern and tells him that her husband will surely be there shortly.

Joan leaves the restaurant and begins to check the three nearby gas stations. She does not see their car but hopes it is inside the garage. At each station, she describes Ben and the car, each attendant gives her the same response—no one has seen Ben. Joan decides to return to the restaurant.

Joan's anxiety level is increasing, and all attempts at resolution have failed. In the third phase, the individual uses every resource available to solve the problem and to lessen his or her anxiety. Joan tries several alternatives.

During the next hour, Joan becomes more and more frightened that Ben is not coming back to the restaurant. The children are very hungry and tired. Perhaps sensing her anxiety and fear, they are whining, fighting among themselves, and clinging to her. She is losing patience and raises her voice several times to tell them to be quiet and sit still. She is aware that people are staring at them, and she is afraid the manager will ask them to leave the restaurant. Realizing that it is going to be dark soon, she decides to take the children and walk to the nearest gas station, again hoping against hope to find Ben.

There is no sign of Ben at the gas station, and the attendant still does not remember anyone fitting Ben's description. By this time, Joan is obviously very upset, and the attendant offers to let her come into the office to use the phone. She calls her mother collect in Illinois but gets a recorded message that the number is temporarily out of order. In desperation she then tries calling a neighbor of her mother's, but there is no answer. She really cannot think of anyone else to call, and she knows no one in this area.

At this point in phase three, the crisis may be prevented by redefining goals. Joan's original goal was to locate Ben or at least to wait for him to return to the restaurant. When she realizes that he is not returning, she attempts to resolve the situation by securing help from other known sources—informal helpers. The knowledge that she must get food for herself and the children as well as find shelter for the night prompts her to redefine her goal in terms of these needs.

She asks the attendant if he knows of a shelter or a church that might take them in for the night. He tells her that the shelter is on the other side of town and that he can't leave, since he is the only one at the gas station for the night. He suggests that she call the "welfare people," who might know how to get some transportation for her. She is reluctant to call them because she has heard that they take your kids away if you can't care for them. Besides, no one in her family has ever called welfare for anything. They have always been able to make it on their own.

The children are getting hungrier and more irritable, and Joan is feeling nauseous and on the verge of tears. She knows no one else to call. She doesn't want to call the welfare people, but she feels that she really has no other choice.

This is phase four. A state of crisis results when the problem remains unresolved and the tension and anxiety rise to an unbearable degree. Both social support and internal resources to deal with the situation are lacking. All attempts on the part of the individual have failed to lessen anxiety or change the situation.

The Helper's Role in Crisis Intervention

At this point in the case study, the human service professional becomes involved. To illustrate the steps, principles, skills, and possible outcomes of crisis intervention, the focus of the case study will shift to the perspective of the helper. Before that happens, however, let's review some of the *principles* and *skills* of crisis intervention so that you will understand what is happening in the case.

Crisis intervention is a time-limited service. It occurs with a minimum of delay and focuses on the individual's current life situation. The helper must quickly establish trust and rapport with the client and support the client's self-esteem and self-reliance. Usually, more than one helper is involved in providing services so the client will not become dependent on a single individual. Two strategies important to crisis intervention are referral for needed services and activation of a social network for support and assistance.

The successful crisis intervention worker is one who has mastered the skills of establishing a relationship quickly with the client. Remaining calm, using common sense, and projecting self-confidence are qualities that will help the worker in a crisis situation. Effective communication skills, particularly listening and responding, are also critical for establishing trust and rapport. Nonverbally, the use of physical gestures like holding hands or touching an arm will also facilitate the establishment of a relationship. Verbally, the worker helps the client to focus on available courses of action rather than past occurrences. These are the same skills necessary for effective communication in any helping process.

In some cases, clients may be reluctant, so the human service professional must initiate any direct action that is needed. Examples of such action are activating a support network, seeking medical help, notifying other family members or neighbors, and preventing clients from hurting themselves or others. People cannot remain in crisis forever; the duration is usually from a few days to a few weeks.

Caplan (1964) suggested several *possible outcomes* to a crisis. The first, a return to the precrisis state, is usually the result of effective problem solving. Both the internal strengths of the individual and the existence of social supports favor this outcome. A second possible outcome is a return to the precrisis state except that the individual acquires new skills or develops existing skills further as a result of the experience. Developing new resources and problem-solving skills are examples of ways the individual can grow. A third outcome would be behaviors such as excessive drinking, drug abuse, and blaming others. Clients may also become withdrawn, suspicious, or depressed. Extreme actions that may result are attempted or successful suicide or murder.

Returning to Joan's situation, it is now 8:00 P.M. and the office of the Department of Human Services is closed. Her call is automatically referred to the emergency child abuse line. The human service professional who is on duty frequently gets calls such as the one Joan is making, because few resources are available after 5:00 P.M. The first step in crisis intervention is to *assess* the nature of the precipitating event and the problem. A key question to ask in this assessment is "What level of danger does the person pose to himself or herself or to others?"

Shirley, the helper on duty, answers the call in a pleasant but businesslike voice and introduces herself, attempting to establish a climate for positive communication. Without knowing Joan's name or location, she listens as Joan describes her situation. Then Joan asks if the helper can do anything for her family. Shirley assures Joan that she has done the right thing by calling and explains that a number of options are available to her. Before she proceeds, however, the human service professional asks Joan if she is in a safe place. Feeling some relief that someone will help her and that something can be done, Joan tells Shirley about the gas station and the attendant who has been so helpful.

After noting the phone number of the gas station, Shirley tells Joan she will make some phone calls to the women's shelter, the mission, and to a short-term foster care facility to try to arrange housing. Thirty minutes later, Shirley calls her back. There is an opening at the women's shelter, and Joan and the children can take a cab there at the shelter's expense.

When Joan arrives at the shelter, assessment continues as the caseworker and the nurse on duty take over the case from Shirley. After they eat, the nurse completes a very basic physical assessment of Joan and each of the children. Since there are no signs of physical abuse or illness, the nurse listens to Joan's story and asks a few questions. The nurse postpones a more extensive physical assessment until the next day. Joan and the children are taken to their room, where the exhausted children fall asleep immediately. Although temporarily safe, fed, and sheltered, Joan is emotionally devastated by Ben's abandonment of the family and her lack of resources to return to Illinois.

Once the initial assessment is completed, the second step, *planning the intervention,* begins. The purpose of this step is to restore the person to a precrisis state. Factors considered during this phase are the amount of disruption the crisis has caused in the person's life, the amount of time that has passed since the event, the individual's strengths and coping skills, and the presence or absence of supports in the person's life.

In the morning, the family eats breakfast, and the children are allowed to go to the playroom with the other children at the shelter. Joan meets with the nurse and the caseworker in the private office next to the playroom. They are concerned about a bruise on Joan's face, which has developed where Ben hit her the day before. Joan assures them that Ben's action was an isolated incident, caused by frustration, and that he has never hit her before. Both the caseworker and the nurse pay close attention to Joan's nonverbal and verbal communication, paraphrasing and reflecting her responses. They notice that Joan keeps wringing her hands and running her fingers through her hair. She begins to cry and tells them how Ben has deserted her and the children and that she has no idea how she will get back to Illinois. The caseworker encourages Joan to express her fears and frustrations and is supportive of the huge task Joan has before her.

She takes Joan's hand as she assures her that she can stay at the shelter for as long as she needs to and tells her that the community has many resources that can help Joan get home as quickly as possible. As they begin to talk about Joan's situation, the caseworker is able to ascertain exactly what happened, when it happened, and how Joan has coped to this point. The caseworker finally decides that the primary problem is transportation home to Illinois. She also learns about Joan's mother and other family members in Illinois. Together she and Joan begin to explore some options. Joan wants to try to reach her mother's neighbor again in hopes of getting a message to her mother.

The third step in crisis intervention is *implementing the intervention.* In this case, it may involve only the phone call to the neighbor, who may be able to reach Joan's mother. In other cases, the intervention may be more complicated, relying on the skills, creativity, and flexibility of the worker (Aguilera & Messick, 1993). During this phase, the helper must focus on reality and identify the client's positive coping mechanisms and support systems. Allowing the client to express feelings about what has happened may also be important to reduce his or her tension. It may help clients deal with feelings that may have been suppressed (such as anger) or feelings that have been denied (such as grief).

The final step is the *resolution of the crisis,* in which the worker and the client plan for the future, reinforcing the new ways of coping. The worker also helps the client in planning for the future and preparing for any new crisis that may arise. Here is how Joan's situation is resolved.

Joan is able to reach her mother, who wires money for bus fare for Joan and the children. While they are waiting for the money to arrive, Joan is able to talk with the helper expressing her feelings about what happened and verbalizing her need for continued support. In response to Joan's need for support, the caseworker gets the necessary information to refer her to a free counseling service at a mental health center near her home in Illinois. The helper also gives her a list of sources of financial aid in Illinois for her to contact when she returns home.

As you reflect on the case study, what principles of intervention are illustrated? What roles did the helper play? What skills did the helper use in this situation? How would you describe the outcome? Finally, how is the helping process followed in this example?

INTERNATIONAL FOCUS
The Samaritans

The Samaritans, a British volunteer organization, was organized in 1953 to provide informal helping with crises and other problems. Present in most British communities, these volunteers befriend people with problems who are unwilling or unable to seek formal help. Having contributed to a dramatic reduction in Britain's suicide rate, The Samaritans are rapidly spreading to other countries. The seven principles and practices of the organization are as follows.

SEVEN PRINCIPLES

1. The primary aim of The Samaritans is to be available at any hour of the day or night to befriend those passing through personal crises and in imminent danger of taking their own lives.
2. The Samaritans also seek to alleviate human misery, loneliness, despair and depression by listening to and befriending those who feel that they have no one else to turn to who would understand and accept them.
3. A caller does not lose the freedom to make his own decisions, including the decision to take his own life, and is free to break contact at any time.
4. The fact that a person has asked the help of The Samaritans, together with everything he has said, is completely confidential within the organization unless permission is freely given by the caller for all or part of such information to be communicated to someone outside the Organization. A Samaritan volunteer is not permitted to accept confidences if a condition is made that not even the Director should be informed of them.
5. Samaritan volunteers in befriending callers will be guided and actively supported by experienced leaders who will have the advice, when required, of professional consultants.

The Team Approach

A new trend in crisis intervention is the team approach. Members of the team are selected on the basis of their knowledge and skills. Membership on the team may also vary according to the requirements of the agency and the geographic limits and socioeconomic needs of the community and the clients served. The human service worker may be a member of such a team, which may also include professionals such as psychiatrists, psychologists, nurses, and social workers. According to Aguilera and Messick (1993), tasks of the human service worker include doing initial assessments, observing behavioral changes, conducting interviews, and participating in various short-term therapies. The more intensive individual, family, or group therapy would be performed by the professionals on the team. At the conclusion of the crisis intervention, the client may need to continue with professional services. If the client shows little

6. In appropriate cases the caller will also be invited to consider seeking professional help in such fields as medicine and social work, and material help from other agencies.
7. Samaritan volunteers are forbidden to impose their own convictions or to influence callers in regard to politics, philosphy or religion.

SEVEN PRACTICES

1. Samaritan volunteers are carefully selected and prepared by the local Branch in which they are to serve.
2. The Samaritans are available at all hours to callers, and may be contacted (anonymously if desired) by telephone or personal visit, or by letter.
3. When a caller is believed to be in danger of suicidal action, the Samaritan is particularly encouraged to ask the caller's permission for contact to be maintained during the crisis.
4. Samaritans offer longer-term befriending of callers where appropriate, while recognizing that the Branch may from time to time have to set limits.
5. Samaritans listen to those concerned about the welfare of another person, and, if satisfied that the third person is despairing, depressed or suicidal, may discreetly offer befriending.
6. Samaritans are normally known to callers only by a forename and contacts by callers made only through the Branch Centre.
7. Samaritan Branches are banded together in a legally constituted Association whose Council of Management represents all the Branches and reserves to itself the appointment of the person in charge of each Branch.

SOURCE: Excerpt from "The Principles and Practices" of *The Samaritans* (1985). Reprinted by permission of The Samaritans, Slough, England.

progress after the crisis intervention, the team may recommend more traditional human service problem solving.

✧ Things to Remember

1. Helping is always guided by two questions: (1) What is helpful? (2) How can the needs of the client be met?
2. The effectiveness of the helping process depends greatly on the helper's ability to communicate an understanding of the client's feelings, clarify what the problem is, and provide appropriate assistance to resolve the problem.
3. Roles and responsibilities of human service professionals can be grouped into three categories: providing direct service, performing administrative work, and working with the community.

4. Formal helping takes place in human service organizations and agencies. The cornerstone of this helping, the medium through which help is offered, is the helping relationship.
5. Before the client arrives, the helper should attend to matters such as establishing the physical setting, deciding how to handle the paperwork, and determining how to gather information about the client.
6. During the helping process, the human service professional and the client set goals and determine how those goals will be reached to resolve the problem. The final stage of the helping process is termination.
7. Effective communication is especially important in helping relationships. The way a helper listens and responds to the client is crucial in building a helping relationship with that person.
8. The skillful helper is able to "hear" the client's behavior (the nonverbal message) as well as what is actually said (the verbal message) and to respond verbally and nonverbally to these messages.
9. Attending behavior is a way to let the client know that the helper is listening. There are four dimensions of attending behavior: eye contact, attentive body language, vocal qualities, and verbal tracking.
10. Once the helper has heard the verbal and nonverbal messages of the client, it is time for the helper to respond. The helper must determine his or her intent before speaking.
11. Beginning helpers should be wary of excessive questioning, which may hinder the helping process and make clients dependent.
12. The key to working with culturally different clients is awareness of and sensitivity to cultural differences.
13. Among the challenging aspects of human service practice is the reality that not all clients are cooperative and willing; helpers are likely to meet the resistant client, the silent client, the overly demanding client, and the unmotivated client.
14. Crisis intervention is a helping process that occurs at a very fast pace and incorporates many of the helping roles and skills. Crises can be divided into two types: developmental and situational.
15. The skills and strategies that helpers use to provide immediate help for a person in crisis constitute crisis intervention.

Additional Readings: Focus on Helping

Havens, L. (1989). *Safe place.* New York: Ballantine Books.

In a series of case studies, a psychiatrist shows that it takes more than theories to help people. Cases include a troubled student, a suicidal depressive, a schizophrenic, and a physician preoccupied by fears of death.

Meier, S. T., & Davis, S. R. (1997). *The elements of counseling.* Pacific Grove, CA: Brooks/Cole.

This book responds to the questions beginning helpers may have about the counseling process. It covers such fundamentals of counseling as explaining counseling to the client, noticing resistance, avoiding advice, listening for metaphors, and arranging the physical setting appropriately.

Verghese, A. (1994). *My own country.* New York: Vintage Books.

This author, an infectious disease specialist, recounts his life and experiences in an Appalachian town in East Tennessee as he becomes by necessity the local AIDS expert.

Chapter 8

Understanding the Environment

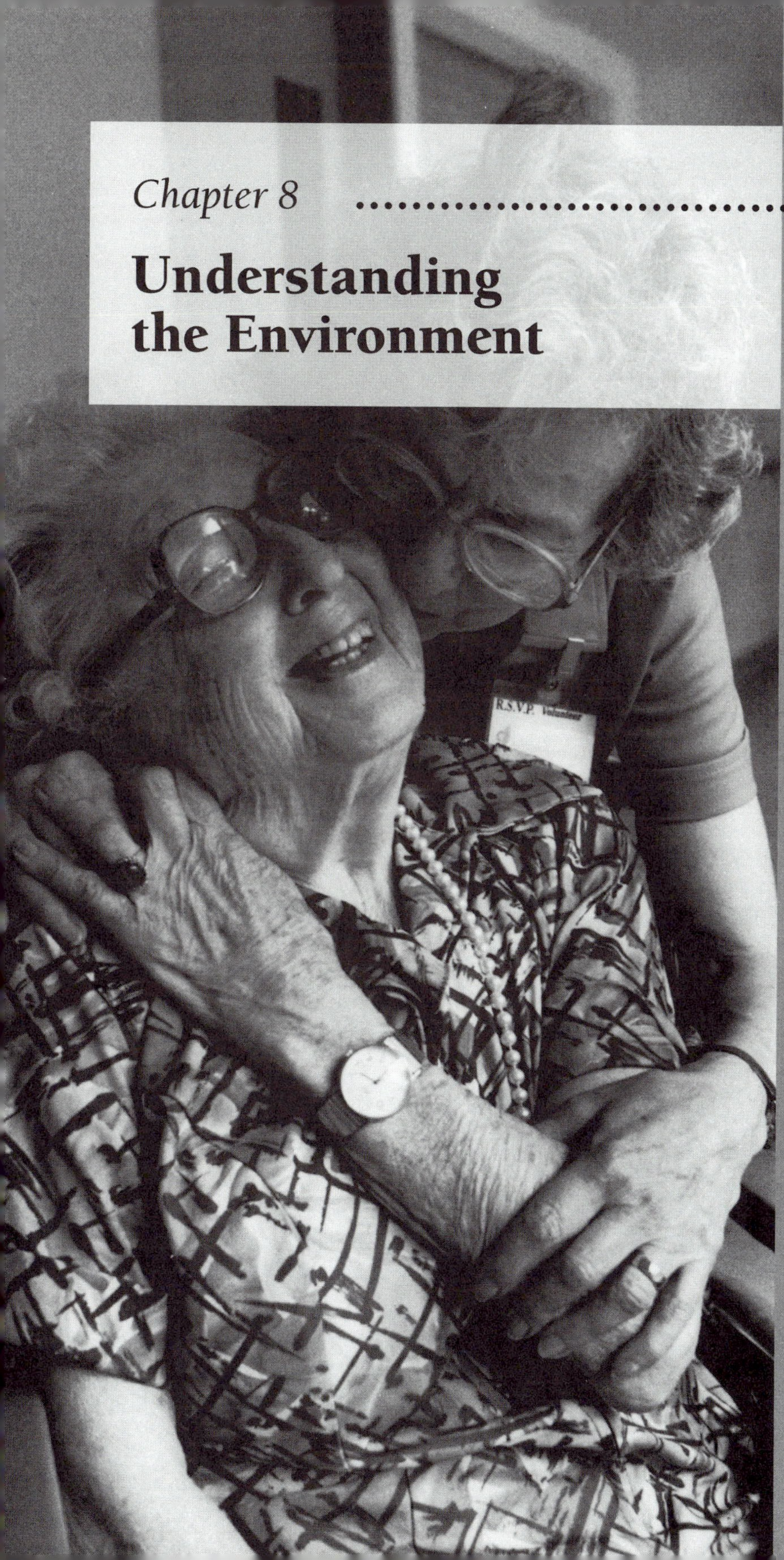

The Context

Understanding the environment in which human service activities occur is critical for the human service professional. The activities of the human service worker do not take place in a vacuum but are performed with clients in the context of their own environments. One important part of the problem-solving process is working with clients to consider problems in terms of their environments and developing useful strategies.

Working within the client's environment can be a challenge. Regardless of whether the worker is performing the role of planner or of broker, success depends on the helper's knowledge of community resources and client needs. This chapter provides the beginning human service professional with principles for understanding the client's environment and guidelines for understanding the system in which human services are delivered.

General Systems Theory

One helpful way to view the complicated environment of the client is through *systems theory,* the study of an organized whole. Systems theory is useful to the study of human services because it provides an organized way to describe the interaction between the individual and the environment. The application of systems theory is not restricted to individuals; it can provide a helpful perspective on any living system, including interactions among human service institutions and organizations.

Development of the theory is attributed to Ludwig Von Bertalanffy, a biologist who defined systems as elements that interact with each other (1968). The major focus of this theory is the interactions of elements in a system, including their relationships, their structures, and their interdependence. According to general systems theory, the following principles are important (Leiter & Webb, 1983):

1. Human beings are viewed as being in an environment that is an open system.
2. The human being functions as an individual and as a member of a community.
3. An individual must be viewed within the context of the immediate relationship groups (family) and within the context of the environment.
4. Human interaction is not a choice; individuals do not live in isolation.
5. General systems theory provides a representation of human social systems (groups, organizations, or communities) that are constantly interacting with one another.

When general systems theory is applied to human service systems, the system developed is very complex. It includes the individual client, the family or smaller group context of the client, and the larger environment. The individual worker and the environment of the worker must also be considered.

Understanding general systems theory can help you as a beginning human service professional in two ways. First, the theory allows you to think about individuals and organizations realistically. The definitions and models that follow present individuals, organizations, and actions in a flexible structure, which allows you to account for individuals and situations and the changes they may encounter. Second, the definitions and models presented help you notice patterns of interaction that can improve your understanding of clients' situations.

Melson (1980) considered the following terms to be basic to an understanding of general systems theory. Following the definitions are examples of how the terms may be used within the context of human service interaction and delivery.

Input—any energy (action or thought), materials (clothing, food, books), or individuals (worker, family member, neighbors) that exist in a particular system.

Transformation—the interaction between the inputs within the system.

Output—the product that results from the interaction of the inputs during the transformation.

An example of input, transformation, and output in the human services follows:

Harold is an 80-year-old male who has been hospitalized for a heart bypass but is now beginning his recovery at home. He continues to live alone and take care of himself. The social service personnel from the hospital have been working with his managed care organization for the past two weeks to plan Harold's transition from the hospital to his home. As they prepare for his discharge, they have developed a discharge plan that outlines the services he will need before he leaves the hospital and those he will need early in his home recovery. The plan calls for follow-up assessments later.

INPUT

The *input* for this case includes many actions and thoughts, both of Harold and of the hospital personnel involved in his care. Specific components of this input category are as follows:

- Harold explains his health-related goals.
- Medical and social service staff discuss Harold's needs.
- Financial arrangements are made with managed care to cover the costs of the services.
- Home health care is contracted for six weeks.
- Supplies, equipment, and medicine are purchased for Harold's home stay.
- Appropriate medical and social service contacts are scheduled with Harold.

TRANSFORMATION

The transformation occurs as Harold, the hospital personnel, and other referral services actually formulate and begin implementing the plan. This interaction is shaped within the context of Harold's needs and environment, the hospital setting, and the resources and constraints of the other social service agencies involved. Complications during the transformation may include the following:

- Harold does not want strangers in his home, and he argues against the use of the home health care "old ladies," as he calls them.
- Harold is depressed one day because he is not yet feeling better. Another day, he refuses to stay in bed because he feels "great."
- Harold's great grandniece Betsy, his only living relative, visits from a neighboring city. While she is there, she tells the hospital that Harold has no business leaving the hospital.
- Harold, the hospital social service worker, and the managed care case manager agree on home health care and then reassessment every two weeks.
- Before Harold is discharged, his surgeon gets sick. The surgeon's partner works with the discharge team.

OUTPUT

In the case of Harold, the outputs resulting from the transformation or interaction of the inputs may include these:

- Intense planning by the professional health care staff.
- A written plan of Harold's discharge.
- Interagency referrals to medical suppliers, druggists, and health care agencies, stating the types of services to be supplied and the dates.
- Meetings with Harold and the home health care staff.
- Planned assessments every two weeks and communication and review by the managed care case manager.
- Medical follow-ups after six weeks and three months.

Using the terms *input, transformation,* and *output* reminds the helper of the realities of the environment in which the case occurs. Using two other terms can reinforce this understanding of the context of the inputs and outputs: *interdependency* and *change.*

INTERDEPENDENCY

One of the characteristics of a system is that any change in one part affects another part. When individuals become involved in the human service system, both the world of the workers and the world of the clients have the potential for change. Such change occurs within the context of the environment. Because of this interdependence, completion of one task is dependent on other factors within the system (Von Bertalanffy, 1968). For example, the arrival of Harold's great grandniece Betsy has the potential to change the situation. She could insist that Harold is not competent to take care of himself or make decisions about his own care. The staff would then have to resolve the issue of competence. This decision could have a major impact on hospital planning, the review made by the managed care organization, and Harold's future living situation and recovery. This is only one of many inputs that could have changed the situation. For example, the availability of home health care services could have affected the planning. Although the hospital is not responsible for such services, its discharge planning is dependent on the delivery of high-quality home health care services.

CHANGE

When input interacts within a system, two types of responses can result: homeostasis or adaptation. In the state of homeostasis, inputs are introduced, but the system withstands change and maintains itself, retaining its original state. Sometimes inputs introduce factors that contribute to major change, and adaptation results. During adaptation, the system is changed from its original state. Change can take many forms: change of organizational structure, change in patterns of interaction, or change in patterns of interdependency.

In Harold's situation, the switch of doctors had the potential to effect great change. The new surgeon could have requested a new discharge plan requiring

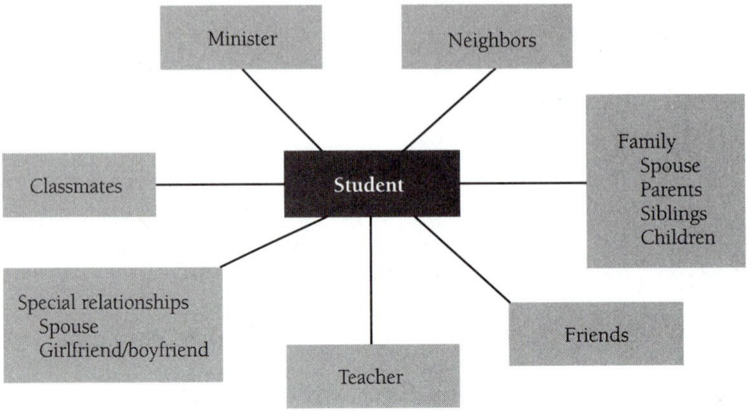

Figure 8-1 ✦ Life system model of a student

a more lengthy hospital stay and full-time nursing care for the next six weeks. This input would have drastically altered the discharge plan and Harold's own view of his recovery. The hospital staff, as well as Harold, would have had to adapt their previous ideas about recovery. As it was, the new doctor made few changes. Homeostasis (balance) was maintained.

Uses of General Systems Theory

General systems theory is a model human service professionals may use to study the organization of human service systems and the individual client. It is flexible enough to be helpful as the helper views both the world of agencies and organizations and the perspectives of individuals and families.

THE INDIVIDUAL CLIENT

General systems theory provides helpers with a model for understanding and providing assistance to individual clients and families. Systematic use of the concepts of input, transformation, and output can reduce the confusing complexities of working within both the human service system and the client environment. Figures 8-1, 8-2, and 8-3 provide a model for thinking about clients' situations. General systems theory and the philosophy of human services support the representations in each figure. The client, whether a student, a patient in a nursing home, or a victim of a violent crime, is the central focus. Environment is considered as it relates to the client.

Many factors affect the client, and the human service professionals must be aware of the important parts of the client's world. Such influences can be described using a *life system model,* a diagram that illustrates the influences on the client (B. Legg, personal communication, January 27, 1989). Using the life system view of the client is an efficient way to assess the client and the environment. This model helps the worker determine efficient ways to gather and think about pertinent information.

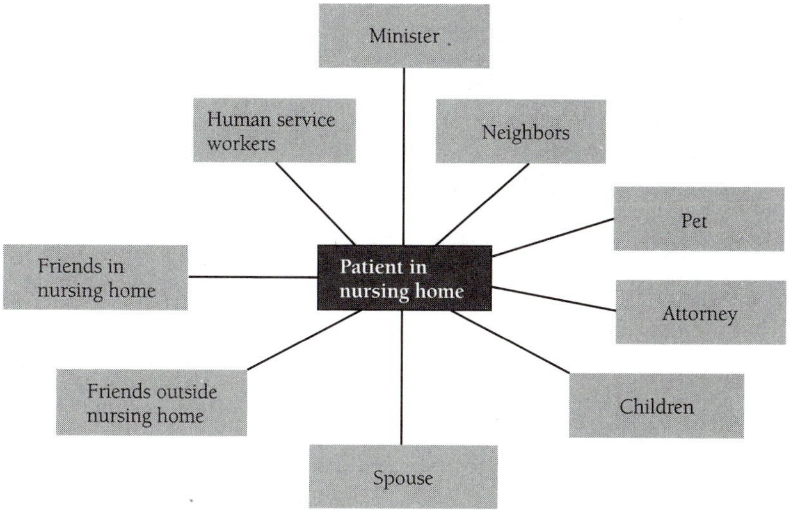

Figure 8-2 ✦ Life system model of a nursing home patient

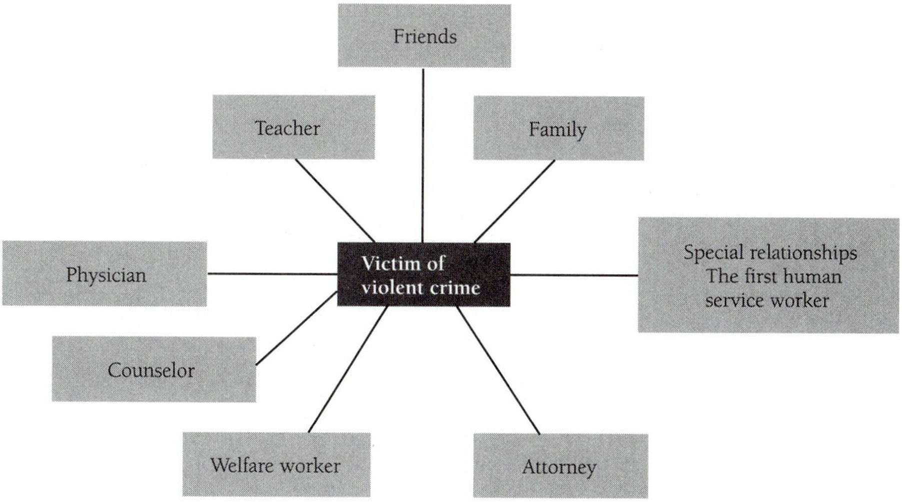

Figure 8-3 ✦ Life system model of a victim of violent crime

A model of a life system only *identifies* the influences in a person's life; it does not indicate their relative importance. For example, Figure 8-1 represents the life system of a student. It may be similar to yours. Note that it does not suggest which influences are most important; nor does it represent the internal characteristics of the client, such as knowledge, skills, and social and religious values.

The life system of a patient in a nursing home (see Figure 8-2) is more contained than that of a student but is equally complex. Environment is listed as a part of the system because the environment of the nursing home can be specifically defined and because it has a major impact on the client's life. The model includes people from the client's previous environment as well as significant others from the present nursing home environment.

How do human service professionals develop life system models for their own clients—ones that will be useful to the helping process? The helper first listens to the client talk about personal experiences so he or she can build the system model from the client's perspective. Using the following case, a firsthand account of a client's experience, we can practice developing a system model.

Victim of Violent Crime

I first became involved with human services in January 1996. As a victim of aggravated assault, attempted murder, and mayhem in a case of random violence, my situation was severe. As the result of the assault, I was blinded in my right eye and impaired in my left eye. The first person I saw was my physician, who gave me the prognosis and told me what medical treatment I would need, including surgery. The second person was a hospital administrator, who told me I had no major insurance that would cover my needs and the costs of surgery. The third person I talked to gave me hope. He was a case manager who worked with victims of violent crime. He talked with me for 2 hours about what legal processes were involved, how to apply for assistance, and whom to see in the different agencies. He told me to have faith in the system. And he told me that his job was to help link me to services that I need and then monitor my progress.

One day I was a healthy, employed college student, and the next day a nearly blind invalid. It seemed unfair, but I learned very quickly that I would need to swallow my pride and ask for help. It was not easy to do, but the people who worked with me truly cared. They were kind and empathetic, but most of all professional. All the professional men and women came together for me, but I did have difficulty working through the bureaucracy of managed care.

I needed to be declared indigent, because I could not work for nearly five months, until the final surgery. The costs of medicine and physician's visits were enormous. Medicare and rehabilitative services were needed; food stamps kept me fed; and counseling helped immensely. The final surgical procedure was the removal of the right eye and the insertion of a prosthetic, or artificial eye. It was a long five months. Without the professional help of my human service workers and the financial and emotional support given to our family, I am not sure I could have made it.

Today I am finishing my college degree, thanks to vocational rehabilitation and blind services. My major is human services. I want to give back to those who need a little help from one who knows what it means.

This victim of violent crime has a complex life system (see Figure 8-3) because of his involvement in the human service delivery system. His life system model resembles that of the patient in the nursing home, with many components coming from the personal sector of the system before involvement in the human service system. One obvious limitation of the model in this case is that it represents different inputs but does not show how they interact. For example, the victim states, "All the professional men and women came together for me," but the interaction and interdependence are not clear from the diagram.

Now it is your turn to practice building a life system model for a client. The following case describes a victim of child abuse during a critical year in her life. Read the case and identify the systems, institutions, organizations, and people mentioned in the client's story. Then draw the client's life system model.

VICTIM OF CHILD ABUSE

When the school made allegations of child abuse against my parents, they were shocked and appalled. They considered themselves hardworking, upstanding citizens who had opened their home as foster parents to help those less fortunate. They saw my behavior as a case of revenge from a resentful child trying to cause problems. After the allegations were made, I was placed under the observation of a child care worker who was investigating the charges made by the school.

Except through the poor and unwanted children who lived in our home, I knew very little about human services and was apprehensive about what I should say to this woman. From our first visit, several things she did caused even greater fear and anxiety. This woman, who was supposedly placed in my life to help make a bad situation better, seemed to always be preoccupied with irrelevant talk of what she was doing that evening. She constantly praised my parents on the commendable way they cared for the mentally retarded and other less fortunate children living in their home. It was obvious to me that I could not trust this woman, who made me doubt myself and my view of what was taking place in my life. I began to wonder if I really was jealous of the foster children, if I really was an "evil little brat" who constantly got in trouble to get attention. It was as if my bruises and missing teeth were self-inflicted.

As the tension and hatred between my parents, my sister, and me became almost unbearable, I tried to reach out to this strange woman, even though I needed to hide much of the truth for the sake of my sister and me. Amazingly enough, the incidents that we discussed would later be repeated back to us by our parents. As the threats and mental torment worsened, the only emotions I felt toward this woman were betrayal and distrust

Several months later, the school became legally involved once again, when one of my teachers found me alone and feeling quite desperate in the bathroom. After asking a lot of questions about the marks and bruises that covered my body, the teacher tucked me away in an office until she could take some action to prevent any future abuse. The child care worker was not available when the teacher called to express the urgency of the situation. When my parents arrived at the school, shouting and making violent threats, the school had to call the police to come and prevent my father from causing further trouble. A second call was placed to the worker, who was still unavailable, and my parents were escorted to the office as I was led outside to the waiting police car. I was quickly carried to a juvenile home, where I was to stay until a decision could be made by the proper authorities concerning my safety and welfare.

The previous child care worker was no longer in charge of my case because of the change in my situation. She was replaced by a man whose attitude and style were different and much more effective.

After collecting a lot of information, including interviews with people who knew about my situation, he was ready to go before a judge with the question of whether I should return to my home or be placed elsewhere. In spite of everything that had happened in the past, I figured that I had nothing to lose by telling this man the whole truth, even though I expected the same attitudes and responses as the previous worker had shown me. To my surprise, this man went before the judge and took my side. He presented all the information he had gathered, a good portion of which the previous worker had disbelieved or neglected to follow up on.

The system eventually proved my innocence. Instead of being labeled a child who continuously misbehaved and could be controlled only by severe discipline, I escaped my childhood prison. I now lead a reasonably normal life, but the scars of my childhood remain an obstacle that I encounter nearly every day. At least some of this turmoil might have been avoided by more timely and appropriate action from the people in human services.

In summary, by developing a life system model of a client, the human service professional can begin to understand the system or environment in which the client functions. Its advantage lies in its simplicity, for it allows the worker to describe the client's environment. Its obvious limitations are that it does not represent the chronology of events, distinguish the relative importance of system components, or describe interactions in the system.

Organizing Human Services

Scholars in the field of human services suggest that human service agencies are a part of an organization system (Austin, Kopp, & Smith, 1986; Lewis, Lewis, & Souflee, 1991). According to their research, human service professionals must understand the system better if they are to meet client needs effectively. Agencies are viewed as part of a human service system whose primary responsibility is to address the problem of meeting human needs. The three responsibilities of the human service system (discussed in Chapter 1) are social care, social control, and rehabilitation. Austin, Kopp, and Smith (1986) have defined a system as interacting parts that monitor the input and output of the system. This definition complements the central principle of general systems theory: The different parts of the system interact. Human service professionals serve a vital function, linking clients and services.

When human service professionals address the needs of clients, they focus on the needs of the whole person, recognizing that clients often have more than one problem and may require the services of several professionals and agencies. This multidisciplinary approach expands the role of the human service professional from that of the self-contained, one-on-one caregiver to the much more complex role of case manager and referral agent who connects the client with many agencies and services. To serve in this capacity, the helper must understand the human service system.

When thinking about the human service system, difficult but necessary questions concern the organization of the system. How are services defined? What interaction occurs? What interdependencies exist? How is change effected?

The human service system, which is an assembly of human service agencies and organizations, can be regarded in many ways. Each system has its own unique patterns and interactions. Instead of discussing organizational patterns you may encounter, we prefer to suggest ways to think about the human service system. You can then determine which model you find to be the most useful conceptualization of the system.

First, it may be helpful to think about the services that might be provided in any community by the human service system. Table 8-1 is not intended to be all-inclusive but rather a working list of services. It is used to demonstrate various ways of organizing services, depending on how one thinks about the services.

HUMAN NEEDS

In visualizing the services offered in the community in which you work, it may be helpful to organize them around the human needs they meet: physical, emotional, and social. These are the basic needs that individuals must meet to survive, to establish relationships with others, and to develop to their highest potential. The list of services provided in Table 8-2 are categorized by the type of human need they satisfy.

Advantages: One advantage of thinking about services in relation to human needs is the obvious connection between client problems and service delivery. Once the need is categorized as physical, social, or emotional, the worker has a ready list of possible alternatives for help.

Limitations: The use of only three categories makes broad distinctions between client needs. A client needing child care has a very different social need from the client incarcerated for a violent crime.

TABLE 8-1 ✦ HUMAN SERVICES DELIVERED IN THE COMMUNITY

Casework	Institutions
Child care	Law enforcement
Consulting	Libraries
Consumer protection	Mental health
Consumer affairs	Physical health
Corrections	Public health
Courts	Public welfare
Counseling	Recreation
Education	Rehabilitation
Employment/unemployment	Religion
Family development	Retirement plans
Financial counseling	Social Security
Fire prevention/fire fighting	Substance abuse treatment
Hotlines/crisis centers	Substitute care (short term)
Housing code enforcement	Therapy

SOURCE: Adapted from *Introduction to Social Welfare Institutions: Social Problems; Services, and Current Issue,* by C. Zastrow. Copyright © 1990 by Wadsworth, Inc. (1978 by Dorsey Press). Reprinted by permission of Wadsworth, Inc.

THE ROLE OF SERVICES

According to Zastrow (1990), human services are people-oriented, and the services that are provided to a family cluster or an individual may be grouped into the categories of protection, personal service, information and advice, and maintenance (see Figure 8-4). Organizing services in this way concentrates more on what the worker does than on what the client needs. It reflects a more general orientation to human service delivery, with a focus that spans populations. To use this model, the worker would determine whether the client, regardless of the problem, needs information, maintenance, service, or protection.

Advantages: This system is useful in many different settings and with different problems.
Limitations: It can be complex to use if the client has multiple problems and needs several types of services.

THE REFERRING PROBLEM

Another way to approach the complexities of the human service system and of clients and their problems is to begin by using the referring problem as the point of entry and the focus of referral. If the organization and structure of human services are viewed this way, the organizations are categorized according to the primary service they provide or the special population they serve. For example, if the referring problem is a crime, the corrections system is the

TABLE 8-2 ✦ SERVICES ACCORDING TO THE HUMAN NEEDS THEY FILL

Physical	*Emotional*	*Social*
Fire prevention/fire fighting	Counseling	Child care
Housing code enforcement	Financial counseling	Consulting
Physical health	Hotlines/crisis centers	Consumer affairs
Public health	Mental health	Corrections
Public welfare	Religion	Courts
Rehabilitation	Therapy	Education
Retirement plans		Employment/unemployment
Social Security		Family development
Substitute care (short term)		Law enforcement
		Libraries
		Recreation

organization to which the client is referred; if the problem is alcohol abuse, a provider of substance abuse treatment is the organization to receive the referral; if the patient is a suspected Alzheimer's patient, the patient is referred to a health care facility with a special treatment unit for that disease.

The following list of human services is organized by specific services. Below each referring problem are listed examples of agencies with the primary function of providing assistance in that area of care.

CHILD CARE

St. John's Baptist Church Child Center: Private day care sponsored by St. John's Baptist Church. Must have ability to pay.

Rainbow House: Sponsored child and family services for clients of this agency. Fee is determined by ability to pay.

CORRECTIONS

Project Lookout: Multifunded program serving adolescents 12–18. Clients are referred from juvenile court.

Trietre State House: State facility for institutionalized juvenile offenders. Clients are sentenced by the court.

COUNSELING/MENTAL HEALTH

Draper Mental Health Center: Private/public funding. Services available for battered women, sexually abused children, parents without partners, substance abusers, and mentally troubled adults. Fee is determined by ability to pay.

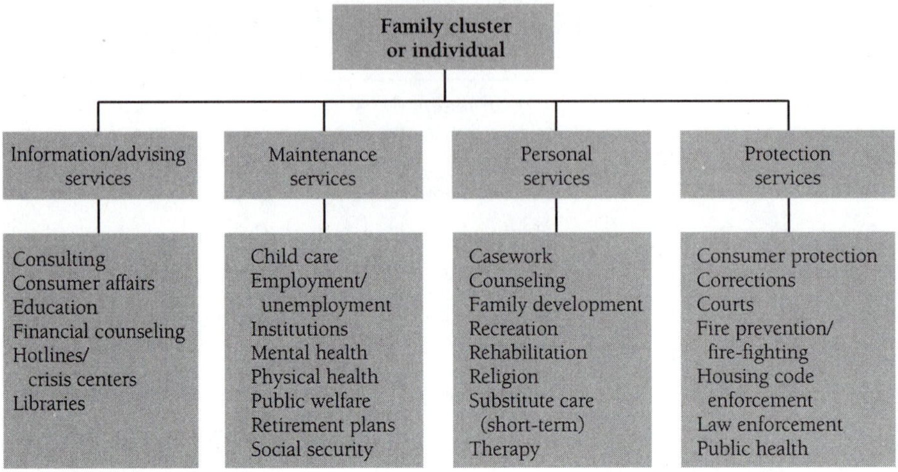

Figure 8-4 ✦ Sample network of human service systems that affect an individual

NOTE: This schema or network of human services is useful for analytical purposes and assumes that a service system may provide more than one form of service. The correctional system, which has a primary goal of protection, also includes elements of (1) personal service (casework, therapy), (2) information/advising services (consulting, crisis centers, education), and (3) maintenance services (institutions).

SOURCE: Adapted from *Introduction to Social Welfare Institutions: Social Problems, Services, and Current Issues,* by C. Zastrow. Copyright © 1990 Wadsworth, Inc. (1978 by the Dorsey Press). Reprinted by permission of Wadsworth, Inc.

County Mental Health Association: County- and state-funded support services for troubled children, adolescents, and adults. Fee is based on ability to pay.

Advantages: The referring problem leads to a specific source of help.
Limitations: The referring problem is often not the most immediate problem to be solved, and may be only one of many. Also, when the agency is listed according to the referring problem, the total services of the agency are left unexplained.

USING THE ORGANIZATION'S STRUCTURE

Another way of thinking about human services is to understand how services are organized within the area in which you work. The paragraphs that follow describe models that you may encounter when studying how services are organized and delivered.

Multiple delivery of similar services The multiple delivery model focuses on services needed by a specific population and provided by a variety of agencies within a geographic area. For example, the service of adoption is an important human service function: identifying potential adoptive children and adoptive parents and attempting to match the two client groups. In many communities, the service of adoption is performed by many different agencies: public agencies, private homes for unwed mothers, private child or family service centers, and church-related organizations.

Advantages: Clients have many choices of where to get the needed services. They can choose on such factors as location, eligibility for service, and cost.

Limitations: It is difficult for a referring worker to become familiar with the policies of service delivery of each agency.

Noninstitutional comprehensive service A collection of related services in one building and under one administration is representative of the noninstitutional comprehensive model. This set of services is grouped together to address the needs of the client with multiple problems. An example is a comprehensive rehabilitation center. In one place, the client who requires rehabilitation receives a comprehensive diagnosis, team treatment planning, and treatment, which includes counseling, educational training, vocational training, training in job and work values, skills coaching, job placement, and follow-up.

Advantages: Services are readily available for the client with multiple problems. There is potential for effective case management and good interdisciplinary work for the client.

Limitations: Clients are limited to one philosophy of service.

Single-service approach Single-service delivery is very restrictive. Only one service is offered, and the eligibility for service is strictly determined. An example of this approach is a food stamps office, where eligibility is determined and stamps are issued.

Advantages: Worker and client can easily identify who delivers the services and learn the criteria for the services available.

Limitations: The service offered may be only one of many that clients need. The multiproblem client may be frustrated because referrals to other agencies may be necessary.

Institutional Clients live in institutional settings. Institutions often provide comprehensive services because the clients are isolated and unable to receive services elsewhere. The offering of services depends on the type and the philosophy of the institution. For example, if a correctional institution for adults is committed only to social control and social care, the inmates will receive basic food, housing, clothing, medical care, and protection from violence. Special programs might include work experience, recreation and exercise, opportunities for reading, and religious growth. However, if the correctional institution is also committed to rehabilitation, opportunities for further development would be available in addition to those listed. These services might include high school or undergraduate education, vocational development, and other programs that emphasize the growth and development of people in the correctional program, focusing on their future positive contributions to society.

Advantages: Services are accessible to the client. Workers are able to plan for service delivery within a cooperative environment.

Limitations: Clients are restricted to the services that are available within the institution and some clients have limits on the ones they can use. Demand often exceeds the availability of services.

Community-based programs Programs based in the community serve populations who previously were institutionalized. The community-based program provides services for them in the "least restrictive environment." Clients continue to have mental health and other needs after deinstitutionalization, and these programs attempt to meet those needs through outpatient services. Persons with mental illness have been served primarily by community-based programs since the process of deinstitutionalization began in the 1950s. The services include housing, day care treatment, drug therapy, frequent assessment of client status, and supervision.

Clients with other needs also receive community-based support as the trend toward serving clients within their own environment continues to grow. These clients usually have multiple problems, and the community-based services are provided in an organized manner. An example of a community-based service for a population different from the traditionally served persons with mental illness is a needle-exchange program. In such a service, clean needles are dispensed to drug users from a mobile van that runs from neighborhood to neighborhood. Another relatively new community-based program supports parent educators who work with families in their homes, teaching parenting skills, good nutrition, and financial planning.

Advantages: Clients may live with more freedom and choices, increasing their opportunity for personal growth and development. Potentially, a broad range of services outside the institutional setting are accessible.

Limitations: Managing the client's case may be difficult. Many professionals must work together to integrate the variety of services the client needs and receives.

Service to a specific population Several populations are recognized as needy by our society, and services have been developed specifically to meet their needs. If an individual or a group of individuals can be categorized as part of a special group needing services, thinking about services to that group can help service providers focus on the group's particular needs. The following list of special populations and services available for them illustrates this way of organizing services.

Children: Services for children include adoption, foster care, day care, education for the disabled in special centers, health care, recreation in structured programs, care for the emotionally disturbed, counseling, and group therapy.

Substance abusers: Service for substance abusers includes assistance in overcoming alcohol and drug abuse, residential treatment, outpatient treatment, individual and group counseling, and establishment of self-help groups and group homes.

Elderly: Treatment for older people is as varied as the needs of the population. A primary focus is health care, which includes institutional care (skilled and unskilled) as well as services provided in public health clinics and community health centers, mobile health units, and home health care units. Other services include recreation, care in day care centers, transportation, provision of food or financial support, grief counseling, retirement counseling, and financial counseling and assistance.

Children, substance abusers, the elderly, those diagnosed as HIV-positive and AIDS patients are all examples of special populations. Other populations who receive special attention include veterans (especially Vietnam veterans), individuals with eating disorders, people with mental illness, and the homeless.

Advantages: Service providers have a rich understanding of the population and its needs. Services can be tailored to the target group.

Limitations: Services are too restricted to the population, neglecting the environment.

LEVELS OF ASSISTANCE

One final way of thinking about human service delivery is to determine how help is provided at several different levels: individual, family, agency, community or neighborhood, and society (Lewis, Lewis, & Souflee, 1991; Teare & McPheeters, 1970). A human service problem is approached in different ways, depending on the level of assistance to be provided. For example, for the problem of the homeless, an *individual client* perspective concentrates first on providing the basics to the homeless person and second on alleviating the homelessness of the individual as a long-term goal. The *family* focus for the short-term care of the homeless may include working with the extended family, establishing a family context for the individual, or determining the needs of adults to provide their children with housing, food, and education. Also, agencies develop networks, using the services currently available to address the needs of the homeless population and developing mechanisms to enable their clients to use the services more effectively.

The homeless are found in a *community* or *neighborhood.* Human service action at this level focuses on concerns beyond the individual, addressing the following questions: What are the effects of the homeless on the community?

How can the neighborhood provide relevant service to this population? How can the support of other institutions, such as government, schools, and churches, be enlisted to assess and solve this problem?

A societal focus is one of the broader approaches to the problem. It includes prevention, social care, and rehabilitation on a larger scale. The study of the problem at this level relies on assessing the economic, political, social, and cultural forces that affect society, as well as determining what interventions can successfully address the problems. The homeless are being studied by federal and state governments, which view the increasing number of homeless people as a serious national problem. For example, there have been presentations about the homeless before the Special Committee on Aging of the U.S. Senate.

Advantages: Using the levels-of-intervention model helps workers understand what types of impact they may have on a particular problem. When workers work only with the individual, they may not understand the broader context of the problem.

Limitations: The levels of focus often work at cross-purposes; proponents of the various levels do not view the problem as a common one.

Using the System

An important part of the human service professional's responsibility is to work within the larger context of the human service delivery system and the client's environment. This is not always an easy task. An understanding of the referral process and related issues will help the professional succeed within this larger context. Again, understanding general systems theory is helpful here, for referral relates directly to the interaction between the individual and the environment. The human service professional relates to the human service network during the referral process. Thus, the helper, in seeking services for a client, provides an input into the human service delivery system. The transformation occurs as the professional calls colleagues and other agencies to find the needed services, negotiates introductions and meeting times, and establishes the groundwork for the client to visit another agency. A successful referral, with the client receiving the services needed, could be one of the outputs. The referral process is described in this section.

Referral

One of the most important roles a human service professional performs is *brokering*, or referring a client to another agency or service. The actual referral involves a two-step process: first, assessing the client's problems and needs, and, second, providing the link between the client and the needed service. To understand the process of referral, the worker must know when to refer, how to refer, where to refer, and how to develop the referral. Successful brokering requires considerable time and skill. According to Crimando and Riggar (1996), effective referral is dependent on two factors: expectations and cooperation. The human service professional and the client need to understand the services that are provided by the agency or the worker who is receiving the referral. Cooperation is another key ingredient to an effective referral. Both helpers involved must keep the client's needs as the primary focus. If difficulties arise, they need to remember that the goal is to serve the client well.

To make a good referral, the helper must have information about a service or agency. This includes its history, possible legislation that affects it, its purpose or intent, and the specific client services it provides (Crimando & Riggar, 1996). In addition, to be considered a community resource, the agency must meet the following criteria (Crimando & Riggar, 1996):

Be able to provide the needed service
Be willing to provide these services on referral
Be accessible geographically
Have reasonable eligibility standards

In other words, if the services exist but are not readily available to your clients, they are not a good referral source.

WHEN TO REFER

A human service professional may send a client to another professional for several reasons. The referral may be client-initiated—that is, the client may request a referral. The client may realize that other services would be helpful, and he or she may suggest a specific referral. The client may request that the referral come from the worker, to give the client more credibility with the new service. In another case, the client may have come to the helper in the first place specifically to ask for help in working with other agencies.

Referral may be appropriate because the helper is not able to provide the assistance necessary to solve the client's problems. The client may present requests or have problems that the worker cannot solve, or the worker may discover that the client has a major problem that must be addressed before the others can be solved and that requires more specialized assistance than the worker can provide. Another reason for referral is that the client may be in serious psychological distress—suicidal or violent—and require intensive therapy or crisis intervention that the worker cannot provide in the human service setting. The human service professional may also decide to refer the client because he or she has had little success with that particular client and believes a new professional would be more effective.

HOW TO REFER

Once the helper has decided that the client needs to be referred, the complex process of referral begins. A key word in the referral process is *communication*. The following four-step process provides guidelines for linking the client with another service.

Home Health Source

Home health services are rapidly changing in the managed care environment and there are increasing demands for these services. They are one example of the emerging community-based care that is now preferred over institutional care as a method of service delivery. Home health care can be provided in homes now because of the advanced technology that allows high-quality care outside the hospital setting.

HISTORY/LEGISLATION

The roots of home health care services are in the late 1800s in New York City. The New York City Mission hired nurses to provide medical care and religious services and to teach health and sanitation to the poor. Later, the Metropolitan Life Insurance Company offered these services to their clients; and in the 1940s, Montefiore Hospital in New York City provided holistic home health care. Medicare mandated home health care, and Medicaid allows minimum home health care to be a part of state plans.

LICENSURE, CERTIFICATION, AND ACCREDITATION

Home health care is licensed by several organizations, such as the Joint Commission on Accreditation of Hospitals (JCAH) and the National League of Nursing (NLN).

PURPOSE/INTENT

"Home health care can be defined as all the services and products that maintain, restore, or promote physical, mental, and emotional health provided to clients in their homes. The purpose of home health care is to preserve the quality of life for the individual at home by increasing the client's level of independence and reducing the effects of existing disabilities through noninstitutional supportive services" (p. 23).

CLIENT SERVICES

High technology services
Client or family care services
Personal care
Standard health services
Advanced physician, dental, and pharmaceutical services
Hospice care

SOURCE: Adapted from "Home Health Services," by Beverly E. Holland, 1996, in W. Crimando and T. F. Riggar (Eds.), *Utilizing Community Resources: An Overview of Human Services*, pp. 21–28, Boca Raton, Florida: St. Lucie.

1. *Explain.* The client needs to understand why the referral is taking place. Even if the client initiates the referral, the client must understand that he or she is not just being passed on to the next human service professional. Referral is a thoughtful activity, initiated for the good of the client.
2. *Describe the services.* The client needs to be informed about the referral agency and its services. The more information the worker can give about the intake process, the services available, the fee structure, and the professionals in the agency, the more comfortable the client will be in making the initial contact.
3. *Know the contact.* Talk to the agency and get the name of the contact person, the telephone number, the address, and directions to the agency. Help the client make the appointment for the initial visit to the agency.
4. *Transmit information.* Send appropriate information about the client to the new service, always considering what that agency needs to know about the client. This will allow the agency to plan.

WHERE TO REFER

To determine where to refer the client, the human service professional must first identify the client's problems. Then the worker must find services to meet those needs. The worker may use services that are already known or may investigate other possibilities. Both formal and informal networks (described later) are useful in determining what services are available and appropriate to meet the client's needs.

EVALUATING THE REFERRAL

The referral process does not end once the referral has been made; it continues with systematic follow-up. The helper can call the agency to learn whether the client has kept the appointment and can call the client to get the client's evaluation of the service. The worker needs to know whether the service was effective and whether the help received matched the worker's assessment of the problem. Such follow-up can be very time-consuming for the helper but will be valuable not only for this client but for others in the future. It is especially good feedback for the professional and increases the client's faith in the system. The follow-up also reinforces the professional's care for and commitment to the client.

Making referrals is difficult for several reasons. Agencies are constantly changing, and maintaining an accurate picture of an agency, its current staff, and the services it provides is difficult. Sometimes services are not designed to meet the exact needs of the client, and the referring worker cannot guarantee treatment to the client. Each agency must independently assess the client's needs and the agency's ability to meet those needs. The service may not be provided because the client does not meet the eligibility criteria, because the services needed may not exist, or because there is a waiting list for assistance. The agency may not cooperate fully with the referring agency in the referral process or the follow-up. Also, many agencies are so understaffed that they simply do not have the staff to follow up.

BUILDING AN INFORMATION NETWORK

To make successful referrals, the human service professional must make effective use of all the human service agencies in a community. First, the helper must know what services are available. The beginning worker is at a particular disadvantage because of a lack of experience in the system, a lack of personal contacts with other professionals in the system, and a lack of knowledge about the many problems that clients may have. Therefore, the beginning worker must develop a systematic way of *building a file of information* about the human service network for referral purposes. The worker must first decide how to categorize the information to be gathered. We suggest that the beginning worker choose categories or divisions of services based on one of the models suggested earlier in this chapter. Whether services are being organized by the physical, social, and emotional needs of the clients, the specific populations served, or one of the other organizational frameworks mentioned, the categories will help the worker think about how services are delivered in the community.

The helper can then begin to collect information and record it using computer software, a card file, a file box, a loose-leaf notebook, or any other storage device that allows the helper to add or revise information easily. The summary information needed includes a description of the agency or service, the types of clients it serves, the payment required for the service, the phone number and address, and a contact person. The worker may collect information about community services from colleagues, clients, handbooks of agencies, newspapers, professional meetings, the phone book, and any community service directories that other agencies may have produced.

There is also more detailed information about each agency that is helpful to know. It includes the purpose of the agency, eligibility requirements for services, organizational patterns of staffing, and the nature of the agency funding. Prior to using an agency for referral it is important for a human service worker to know what services it provides, to whom they are provided (individuals or families), whether it uses case management services, and whether it has a good record as a client advocate. Other helpful information includes the qualifications of the staff, their caseload, and their experience with specific populations. The human service professional will have better knowledge of the agency if he or she has visited the facility to determine its accessibility and its psychological and physical environment. Also critical is knowing how the agency receives referrals, if there is a waiting list, how long a client must wait for services, and what follow-up procedure is used to inform the referring agency of the disposition of the referred client's case (Crimando & Riggar, 1996). All this requires a detailed understanding of the organization and represents quite a bit of information to gather. But once you have this information, updating it can be done with relative ease.

Understanding that creating the file is only one part of building a network, the worker should also begin to make personal contacts with other human service professionals. Then the worker should try to establish communication as a cooperative effort—sharing information with other agencies, following up on referrals, and providing feedback to other agencies that have made referrals. These efforts will begin to build the new helper's credibility as a serious professional interested in building and maintaining networks among agencies.

Network building takes time, but it makes the referral process more effective. The better the worker knows the services available, the more appropriate his or her referrals will be. A network is difficult to maintain. It is a never-ending project, no matter how long the human service professional has been serving the community, because agencies are constantly in flux.

Know the Formal and Informal Networks

According to *Webster's New World Dictionary of the American Language*, a *network* is "a fabric or structure of threads, cords, or wires that cross each other at regular intervals and are knotted or secured at the crossings" (1986, p. 1520). In human service settings, the fabric of the system is formed by the elaborate channels of communication among the agencies and the workers. The securing takes place when both parties confirm that they wish to communicate, engage in two-way communication, and establish channels of communication. Human service delivery is a complex system containing two networks of communication: the formal and the informal. Both must be mastered if human service professionals are to participate fully in the system (Booth & Owen, 1985).

The *formal* network is composed of organizations such as public and private human service agencies; self-help groups; schools; churches; businesses; and federal, state, and local government agencies. To understand this network, the worker must discover the answers to certain questions. What are the politics of these organizations? Who bears the major responsibilities within each? What are the formal ways to "hook up" the client to the services and resources available?

Beyond the formal network is a valuable *informal* network that is more difficult to recognize. It is not described in agency policy, formal reporting, or organizational diagrams. It is determined by an established history of agencies working together, personal friendships among workers, and political pressures, and it is maintained by mutual satisfaction and support. The informal network may also include informal helpers such as family and friends who provide needed support. Understanding this informal network is difficult, and accessing it takes time and effort.

There are three types of formal and informal networks: personal, professional, and organizational. Personal networks are made up of individuals, families, and groups of people that are part of the helper's family or part of his or her social support. Individuals in this context often know you very well and can also reach out to a variety of others who can help in the referral process. These can include people in church, social clubs, and exercise and other activity-based environments. Professional and organizational networks are made up of individuals with whom you work and includes colleagues, teachers, and supervisors (Carroll, 1986; Hagebak, 1982). Networking with these individuals can help reduce duplication and fragmentation of services and eliminate service gaps.

One example of formal and informal networks that human service professionals find in the client population is in the description of service needs and support networks of members of the Prairie Band Potawatomi elders (John, 1986). This elderly population, which lives in a Native American reservation community, has housing, transportation, employment, income, health, medical, social, and recreational needs. Both formal and informal networks play major roles in meeting those needs. The elderly depend on the professionals in the formal network for financial and medical support, but individuals within the informal network provide services in all the areas mentioned. Children most often assume the care of the elders, especially during times of illness, death, or divorce. Siblings and other family members also play a supporting role.

A human service worker wishing to help the elderly in this Native American population would need in-depth knowledge of the two networks. A special knowledge of the informal system allows the worker to build on the services that are already present rather than duplicate or attempt to replace them with formal services. The worker may learn about the special relationships between helpers in the informal and the formal networks by asking the following questions: What formal services are available? How do the informal and formal systems communicate? Who are the key individuals in both networks who provide services effectively or who assist the elderly in accessing the services?

The Gatekeeper Role

A role often performed by human service professionals is that of gatekeeper. In this position, the worker sees clients who have additional problems beyond those for which they have been referred. This is a pivotal role in the delivery of human services because of the importance of successfully identifying the client's problem and making an accurate referral. Problem solving without successful identification of the problem frustrates clients and workers alike. Moreover, clients are often discouraged by the complexities of their problems and of the human service system. They give up on the system before their needs can be matched to the correct service.

What makes gatekeeping so difficult is that few human service professionals are trained to work with all the types of clients they will encounter. Obviously, workers will have trouble identifying and referring problems that are unfamiliar. They will not know the right questions to ask in the interview, nor will they understand what symptoms and signs to look for. They will also be unaware of what services are available. Two examples will illustrate the problems that gatekeepers face.

There is currently a growing population of people with Alzheimer's disease and a similarly increasing number of family members who are committed to caring for these individuals in noninstitutional settings. Such care requires time, effort, and financial resources, but few family members understand what type of care is required and will be needed as the disease progresses. Family caregivers cannot identify what their needs are and have few formal or informal links to the human service system. Families do not utilize available services for several reasons: lack of awareness, lack of trust of strangers, and a perception of the care as still being a minor burden (Caserata, Lund, Wright, & Redburn, 1987; Walker, Pomeroy, McNeil, & Franklin, 1994). Workers who provide services to the elderly must understand the Alzheimer's patients' care needs. As gatekeepers, they can educate families to recognize the needs and can facilitate the "hookup" between clients and services.

Another area where gatekeeping has been less than effective is the referral of women who are suffering from alcohol abuse (Rhodes & Johnson, 1994). Again, the problem occurs because human service professionals who work with women are not familiar with the problem of alcohol abuse as it relates to women, including its incidence, symptoms, and treatment. For example, employee assistance programs (EAPs) in industry list a primary diagnosis for men as alcohol abuse and for women as personality problems. For men, poor work performance is attributed to drinking on the job, but for women, poor performance is attributed to the pressures of family life. Alcohol abuse is often obvious for males, who tend to drink during the day and on the job. The problem of women abusers is often less visible because they drink more at home than at work. Experts suggest that many gatekeepers do not detect a woman's alcohol abuse problem because they do not even suspect it. When they think of alcohol abuse, they are looking for male-related symptoms (Rhodes & Johnson, 1994; Turner, 1992). Also, referral for alcohol abuse is often more difficult for women than for men. Women are less free to accept institutionalization because of their family commitments. Treatment is also less likely to be effective because it is based on men's issues, not women's. Gatekeepers need not only to recognize alcoholism as a women's problem but also to know where women can be referred for effective treatment.

We prefer to think of the human service professional as a "gate opener" rather than a gatekeeper. In this role, part of the responsibility is to be aware of client needs and of personal limitations as a service provider.

Watching for Generalizations

The study of human problems and special populations helps workers understand clients in general terms. The training of the generalist in human services is based on a broad perspective of clients and problems. Although each person must be treated as an individual, helpers are encouraged to think about individuals and their problems using developmental models or theories of behavior and growth. In Chapter 4, we approached the understanding of clients from several of these perspectives.

Complementary to models of or theories about human growth and development is a consideration of the environment of the client. In many cases, this is the environment to which the client will return; both the client and the problem need to be evaluated in this environmental context. Because this context can be so critical to identifying the problem and delivering the appropriate services, the general ways in which workers perceive problems of populations or specific clients may be only a starting point for thinking about the problems. One of the most striking ways to illustrate this point is to look at problems of clients in rural and urban settings, for the experience of the elderly rural client is much different from that of his or her urban counterpart.

Research on the elderly in rural areas suggests that their lives are more difficult than those of the urban elderly. Their incomes are lower; housing is not as substantial; and many rural elderly lack the basics of good food, clothing, and shelter. They are often poor, in failing health, lonely, and geographically isolated from their children. They have less access to services because transportation is difficult. Moreover, the rural setting lacks the variety of services that urban settings have to offer. In spite of the bleak assessment of the lives of the rural elderly, research reports also indicate that they have higher levels of well-being than the urban elderly (Rowles, 1986). Once we look at the context of the rural setting, these conflicting reports are easier to understand.

For the rural elderly, food and shelter may not be a severe problem. Many of the elderly do not depend on the cash economy. They own their own homes and do not have to pay monthly rent. In addition, they grow their own food, freeze and can for the winter, and obtain goods and services on the barter economy (Atchley & Miller, 1979; Beall, Thompson, Godwin, & Donahue, 1981). In fact, the rural setting may be better suited for the elderly than urban settings.

Psychological health is promoted in several ways. There is less fear of crime and violence in rural areas; the daily lifestyle reflects previous decades, when people did not lock their homes and cars and were not afraid to be out at night. There is a slower pace to rural life. The rural population is more stable, and the elderly can use this familiarity to sustain their sense of reality (Bornstein, 1979; Lee & Lassey, 1980). Further reducing their sense of isolation and alienation are local newspapers, television, and bulletins that report nearby events and news of familiar people and places. Finally, a functional part of the rural informal network is the clustering of the older generation for support. Members of the younger generation provide assistance for everyday activities such as grocery shopping as well as for crises such as illness and death.

The elderly still have problems. Many services may not be available, and the elderly may not be able to get to the services that do exist. In addition, the winter months bring isolation and loneliness for this population. Churches often provide transportation and arrange many social events to counter isolation. Isolation and loneliness are difficult to overcome for those elderly who are new to the rural area, for making a place in the community is difficult. One serious problem encountered by the rural elderly is depression. This is also true of the aging population in general. According to the literature, depression of the rural elderly is associated with sleep problems, inadequate social support systems, and recent stressful life events (Ganguli, Gilby, Seaberg, & Belle, 1995).

Many human service professionals who work with mental health issues have begun to learn how to gain the trust of their clients. They have discovered that the most important variable is not their expertise but their ability to relate to their clients. The rural elderly are most likely to be slow to accept their need for services, especially in the mental health area. The elderly trust those helpers who know how to be low key, who bother to learn the local language and culture, and who keep their professional and personal lives separate (Vissing, Salloway, & Siress, 1994).

Physical health for the elderly in rural settings is viewed by many as an absence of illness. Rural women see social networks, endurance, and flexibility factors as related to health and believe that giving and productivity foster good health (DePoy & Butler, 1996). This population seeks medical treatment more often than those living in urban areas only if they know the helper who will provide the professional attention. They value the continuity of the professional/client relationship. Transportation does not seem to be a barrier, but cost of services is (Blazer, Landermann, Fillenbaum, & Horner, 1995).

Although a rural setting is often a positive environment for the elderly, several other populations are at risk within this isolated environment. One such population is rural elderly African Americans (Carlton, 1991; Heard, 1995; Ralston, 1993; Spence, 1993). One of the problems is accessibility. This population is underrepresented in number of visits to see physicians and number of days in the hospital (Heard, 1995). Ralston (1993) suggested that elderly blacks underuse services because they are not aware of the services, they are not part of the planning for services, they have no political voice, and they feel alienated in the human service delivery system.

Another population that has difficulty in rural areas is homosexual individuals—women, men, and families who live invisible lives in the rural setting because they are afraid of community reaction to their lifestyle (D'Augelli & Hart, 1987). Residents of rural areas often center their spiritual and social activities around the church, uphold traditional values, and have less tolerance for diversity than many urban residents. Most rural inhabitants do take responsibility for caring for members of the community, however, and many social service roles and tasks are performed by residents rather than by formal social service agencies. Even so, residents are often unable or unwilling to provide the services the homosexual population needs.

Homosexual individuals need to develop personal competence within a positive social setting. According to Danish, D'Augelli, and Ginsberg (1984), such development is facilitated by accurate information about life issues; personal, interpersonal, and social skills to meet life goals and needs; the ability to take risks to try new behaviors; and the creation of a social support system. The rural environment is not well suited to meeting any of these needs. Little information is available and there are few opportunities to socialize with others in the same situation or to develop a sense of community. Rural homosexuals often feel a sense of isolation and rejection that may lead to hopelessness and despair.

There is also evidence that helping professionals do not want to work with rural homosexual populations because of their fear of AIDS and their homophobia. D'Augelli (1989) found that rural nursing personnel showed an irrational fear of casual-contact transmission of AIDS. These nurses held negative views of gay men and lesbians, even though they had not had any or had had limited contact with this population. He also found the same unwillingness among volunteers working in rural areas: they feared AIDS transmission and were homophobic (Poullard & D'Augelli, 1989).

Developing Services in Response to Community Needs

In developing, maintaining, and reevaluating the delivery of human services, these services must be considered a response to community needs. The community has a dual role in the causation and resolution of client problems. On one hand, the community is a source of client problems. On the other hand, it provides many of the resources needed for resolving problems. Two issues are presented here: advocacy for nonexistent services and planning based on community needs.

Advocating the establishment of services that are nonexistent is one of the most difficult responsibilities of the human service professional. The advocate is one who speaks up for the rights of others and defends those who cannot defend themselves. When helpers discover that their clients have needs that cannot be met through the human service delivery system, they have a responsibility to work with others to develop alternative ways of meeting those needs. To do so requires skills that incorporate working with the individual, agencies, and legal and legislative bodies. Regardless of the type of advocacy, the process is much the same:

- Identify the needs of the individual or the population
- Identify how to meet the needs
- Work with a network of individuals or agencies that can help provide the services
- Identify the barriers that must be overcome
- Teach clients about the advocacy process and give them a role
- Negotiate to meet goals and objectives
- Develop a framework that continues the success of the advocacy process

Many professionals are successful in acting as advocates for their individual clients and can use their networking skills to find food where no food services exist, glasses and other special medical needs where resources are unavailable, and housing for those who temporarily need shelter. More difficult is the advocacy that involves developing a political voice for the larger issues that require community, state, or national attention. Ralph Nader lobbying for consumer protection, Maggie Kuhn championing the rights of the elderly, and Betty Ford heightening awareness of breast cancer are examples of individuals who are advocates in the community, state, and national arenas for issues of concern.

Planning human service delivery cannot always take place in the community, but professionals must be sensitive to potential problems. Workers and

INTERNATIONAL FOCUS

Kaumathua Housing: A Special Housing Scheme for Older Maori People

In New Zealand there is an effort to address the problems of the aging population. Their focus has been on developing community-based care with a special emphasis on providing quality services and empowering the elderly. Much attention has been given to developing services that make sense according to the culture of the elderly populations instead of developing a program nationwide that must fit everyone. Government policy has been to support care of the elderly with the family or religious, voluntary, and community groups. The housing needs of the aging Maori population have been addressed with the following program:

> The Maori population has historically been a youthful population characterized by high fertility and high mortality. During the 1920s and 1930s about half the Maori populations were children under fifteen years of age. Since 1971 there has been a marked decrease in fertility so that by 1986 under 40% of the Maori populations were in this age group. What has received less attention are the changes which are taking place in terms of ageing. In 1986 Maori comprised 4% of those over sixty years of age and only just over 2% of those aged over sixty-five years, compared with 12.4% of the total population being Maori . . . beneath these figures however is a pattern of rapid increase in the numbers of Maori surviving into old age. Between 1986 and 1991 the number of Maori aged sixty to seventy-four increased by over a fifth and between 1981, 1986, and 1991 the number aged seventy-five and over increased by over 50% in each census period . . .
>
> The building of blocks of housing for older Maori people began in the late 1960s through a Special Maori Housing Fund administered by the Department of Maori and Island Affairs. The siting of this housing was focused around the *marae* (meeting house). This allowed some elderly Maori to remain in their home communities and be close to the focus of communal life on the *marae*. Another group for whom the scheme was attractive were those who had moved into urban areas and now wished to spend their old age back in their original tribal communities. Legislation was passed to allow Maori land to be gifted to the Crown for this kind of housing and to allow Maori trusts and incorporations to play a part in such development. The programme became formally referred to as "kaumathua housing." (pp. 179–180)

SOURCE: From "New Zealand and Community Care for Older People: A Demographic Window of Opportunity," by S. Uttley, 1995, in T. Scharf and G. C. Wengar, *International Perspectives on Community Care for Older People* (pp. 171–189), Brookfield, Vermont: Avebury.

The Council on the Ageing (Western Australia) Incorporated

ACTIVITY

The Council on the Ageing of Western Australia (COTA) was established in 1959, out of concerns for the ageing population in this state, and the associated needs and problems of seniors. The Council is a "peak" advocacy body, addressing issues confronting seniors living in the community. The COTA seeks to protect and promote the well-being of all older people through the improvement of policy and programs for seniors, through information, advice, and referral, along with general community education about all aspects of ageing. COTA is connected to the National Council on the Ageing based in Melbourne, which seeks to provide "the voice of older Australians" to the federal government in Canberra. The Council in Western Australia is staffed almost entirely by volunteer effort, though it has sometimes received a measure of governmental funding over the years.

HISTORY

In almost forty years since its inception the Council has pioneered many initiatives, some of which have been subsequently mimicked by more formal governmental programs. In 1961, for example, the Council established a volunteer-based "Golden Age Visiting Service" to address the needs of frail and lonely older people, a program which is mirrored in recent federal and state activities. In the same year the Council invented "Old People's Week," which was the forerunner of the modern "Seniors' Week" promoting positive images of ageing, and organized by the State government now for over a decade. In 1974 the Council established the "Residential Aged Care Association," now relabelled as Aged Care Australia, which looks after the interests of those frail or sick seniors living in residential care facilities. In the same year the Council launched its "Guide to Services for Older People in WA," which in its many revised editions has been an invaluable resource for seniors and for those working with seniors in this state. In 1992 the Council conducted extensive consultations with Aboriginal and Ethnic elders in outback and metropolitan regions, and integrated this feedback into recommendations for the State Strategy on Ageing, which was designed to address seniors' issues into the twenty-first century. In the same year the Council also initiated and sponsored the now independently incorporated

agencies from outside the community need to make a special effort to understand the culture of the community and the available resources. They must try to get to know the local professionals and identify the natural or informal helpers (Daley & Poole, 1985).

According to Moroney (1976), four types of needs should be considered when services are being developed. The first is the *normative* need—what professionals and experts in the human services field have determined is

Intergenerational Activity Network, which seeks to promote exchange, empathy, and understanding between the generations.

MISSION

Across the western world during the eighties and nineties, the Welfare State has been in retreat, and Western Australia has not been immune from this trend. The non-government organizations have had increasing tasks but less resources, and in the case of the Council it is now, as it was in the beginning, almost entirely supported through voluntary effort. Nevertheless, the Council looks forward to serving seniors in the future. At its recent AGM, President Bettine Heathcote spoke of "hope," "optimism," and "progress," and noted two recent programs in evidence. First, the "Be Wise with Medicines" seminars seek to educate seniors and the community about polypharmacy and its associated dangers, and constitutes a most worthwhile project in the "community education" tradition. Second, the establishment of the "Seniors Computer Centre" trains older citizens in the ways of computers and connects them with the modern world of the "information superhighway," in this way empowering older people to participate more completely in our rapidly changing technological society.

SUMMARY

Thus in terms of its helping agenda on behalf of seniors, its history of pioneering social programs later adopted by government, and its struggle to complete its mission for its clients while doing more with less, the Council on the Ageing of Western Australia provides a useful insight into the voluntary and informal human service sector within this country.

REFERENCES

Heathcote, B. (1996). President's Report, to the AGM of the Council on the Ageing (WA) Incorporated, held on Monday, 14 October, at the Auditorium Wesley Centre, Perth.

Hooper, J. (1990). The History of WACOTA: The origins and development of the WA Council on the Ageing 1959–1988. Perth: Murdoch University.

SOURCE: Prepared by: David Wiles, Ph.D., Lecturer in Human Services and Gerontology, Edith Cowan University (Joondalup, Perth), Department of Human Services, 5 December 1996.

necessary for effective service delivery. Professionals usually make this determination after study of and experience with the problem. The second kind is the *perceived* or *expressed* need—what the community itself defines as the services that would best serve it. The expressed need of the *individuals* seeking the services is also important to consider; they may have opinions very different from those of the experts or the community at large. *Relative* need—the difference between what the community could use and what it already has

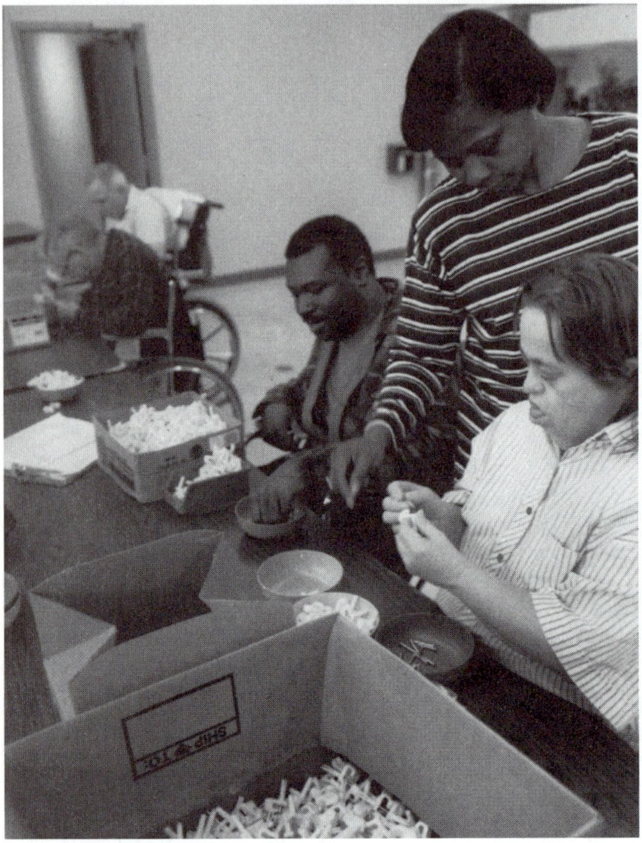

Sheltered workships provide clients with meaningful employment.

available—is also important to consider. Often, in planning service delivery, some services are already available. How the new services fit into the network of the existing services is an important question for planners to answer when building an effective service network.

It is important to consider all four types of needs so that planning can occur within the context of the environment. One principle to follow in developing services was proposed by Kreitner (1983): The development of services should follow the guidelines of Maslow's hierarchy, with services to meet basic needs developed first. If basic service needs go unmet, other services will not succeed. Following Maslow's hierarchy, physical needs must receive attention first, before planning for safety and security needs takes place. The needs assessment for the elderly described in Table 8-3 is based on Maslow's hierarchy.

A critical component in developing services is knowing what the needs are and knowing the characteristics of the populations in need. The following case study illustrates the importance of being able to identify the problems and develop programs that address those specific problems when planning for services (Butterfield, 1996).

TABLE 8-3 ✦ COMMUNITY SERVICE IDENTIFICATION USING THE IDENTIFICATION OF NEEDS

WIDOWS AGED 85+ LIVING ALONE IN WEST KINGSTON

Type of need	*Services typically designed to meet need*	*Services available in this community*
Self-actualization needs	Education programs Volunteer opportunities	Available at Kingston Senior Center
Esteem needs	Support groups Psychosocial counseling Mental Health centers	Two support groups Mental Health center has limited services
Social needs	Recreational and social Groups Senior centers Home visitors	One senior center
Safety and security needs	Emergency response system Adult family homes Congregate care facilities Senior housing Continuing care retirement Communities Wellness clinics Telephone contact	No emergency system Three unlicensed homes One congregate facility No senior housing No retirement community Public health department has wellness clinic Church runs telephone reassurance program
Survival needs	Home delivered meals Senior discounts Mobile meals Transportation Homemaker Home health Personal care Medical care	Limited delivered meals program Twenty mobile meals slots No bus system, one senior van available One licensed homemaker program No home health provider Two licensed personal care agencies One community hospital and one nursing home

SOURCE: From *Social Work Macro Practice*, by F. E. Netting, P. M. Kettner, & S. L. McMurtry, p. 98.

In 1996, the city of Boston recorded a substantial drop in homicide rates. Researchers believe that this progress in reducing deaths by violence is attributed to a new cooperative arrangement between the juvenile court and the criminal justice system, two systems that do not usually work together. Two critical needs were identified prior to the program's implementation with the discovery that three-quarters of juvenile killers and victims had been involved with gangs. These were repeat offenders with established criminal records. Specifically, 75% of killers and victims had been to court at least once. Half these youths had been on probation before and one-third of them had been previously incarcerated. In addition, firearms dealers were selling guns to these juveniles. The central concepts that support the new program were these: letting probation officers ride in patrol cars, and reducing the number of firearms sold to youth (Butterfield, 1996).

The first program allowed the probation officer to arrest youths who had broken parole by violating their 8 P.M. curfew. The beginning of the experiment paired Bill Stewart, a probation officer, with city detective Robert Fratalia. The first night they worked together they received a call that a boy had been shot. When they arrived at the scene, Mr. Stewart discovered that the victim was on his caseload, he also saw 35 other youths who were on probation and violating curfew.

The benefits to the probation system are numerous with this new partnership. Many probation officers see their work as worthless, for there is a revolving door in the criminal justice system; it allows many of their clients to go free and later commit other crimes. They also have difficulty enforcing the rules of probation because they do not carry guns themselves and cannot safely arrest their clients for breaking parole or curfew. The police also benefit from this new arrangement. They are armed and have the power to arrest, but they do not know all the youths on probation so they cannot identify those who are breaking curfew. Because these youths are on probation, they can be incarcerated without a new trial and parole officers do not need probable cause to talk with them or to visit them in their homes. Since this program was implemented, the number of youths arrested for breaking curfew has tripled and compliance with conditions of probation has risen from 15% to 70% (Butterfield, 1996).

The second program focused on reducing arms sales. Several strategies were used. City officials made clear that they have zero tolerance for guns, and they called in gang members to talk to them about the tougher policies. These meetings included representatives from the United States District Attorney's office; the county District Attorney's office; the Federal Bureau of Alcohol, Tobacco and Firearms; and the state Department of Probation and Division of Youth Services. Also attending were school police and city employees who work with gangs. One major arrest was made of 23 gang members who refused to heed the warnings.

Boston has not had a single juvenile death since July 1995. This statistic speaks to the success of providing services based on identified needs and target population. It is also a good example of human service professionals working together to develop services in response to community needs (Butterfield, 1996).

Suppose you are a human service professional planning for services to reduce youth-related violence in your city or rural area. What needs must be considered? How would you discover what those needs are? What problems might you anticipate in implementing new programs in the community? What actions might you take to ensure successful planning and implementation?

In answering these questions, you may realize how difficult planning is. Your responses should consider a variety of viewpoints and take into consideration how the services fit within the context of the current environment.

✧ Things to Remember

1. The activities of the human service professional do not occur in a vacuum but are performed with clients within the context of their own environments.
2. Systems theory focuses on the interaction of elements in a system, including their relationships, their structures, and their interdependence.
3. One of the characteristics of a system is that any change in one part affects another part.
4. The worker must be aware of the many influences on the client, which can be represented in a life system model.
5. Scholars in the field of human services suggest that human service agencies are a part of an organization system.
6. The level at which assistance is to be provided (individual, family, agency, community or neighborhood, or society) determines how the human service problem is approached and how the services are delivered.
7. One of the most important roles of a human service professional is brokering, or referring a client to another agency or service.
8. The referral process involves the worker, the client, and the other agency to which the client is referred.
9. In referral, the beginning human service professional is at a disadvantage because of a lack of experience in the system, a lack of personal contacts with workers in the system, and a lack of knowledge about the many problems that clients may have.
10. The beginning professional must develop a systematic way of building a file of information about the human service network for referral purposes.
11. Human service delivery is a complex system containing two networks of communication: the formal and the informal.
12. When workers are unfamiliar with problems, they do not know the right questions to ask in the interview, nor do they understand what symptoms and signs to look for. They are also unaware of what services are available.
13. The context in which client problems occur is important and may present a starting point from which workers can begin to think about the problem.

14. In developing, maintaining, and reevaluating the delivery of human services, it is important to consider human services as a response to community needs.

Additional Readings: Focus on Organizations

Deal, T. E., & Jenkins, W. A. (1994). *Managing the hidden organization*. New York: Warner Books.
With actual case histories and diagnostic tests, the authors offer specific strategies to help managers achieve their most important goal for the coming decade: connecting workers to the core missions of a company.

Homan, M. S. (1994). *Promoting community change: Making it happen in the real world*. Pacific Grove, CA: Brooks/Cole.
The author illustrates how you personally can become an effective change agent by discussing topics such as raising money, building power, negotiating, working with irritating people, working with the media, and motivating other people.

Keidel, R. W. (1995). *Seeing organizational patterns: A new theory and language of organizational design*. San Francisco: Berrett-Koehler.
The author explains that most organizational issues are a balance of three variables: individual autonomy, hierarchical control, and spontaneous cooperation. By learning to frame issues as trade-offs among these design variables, one becomes able to see the underlying patterns.

Chapter 9

Professional Concerns

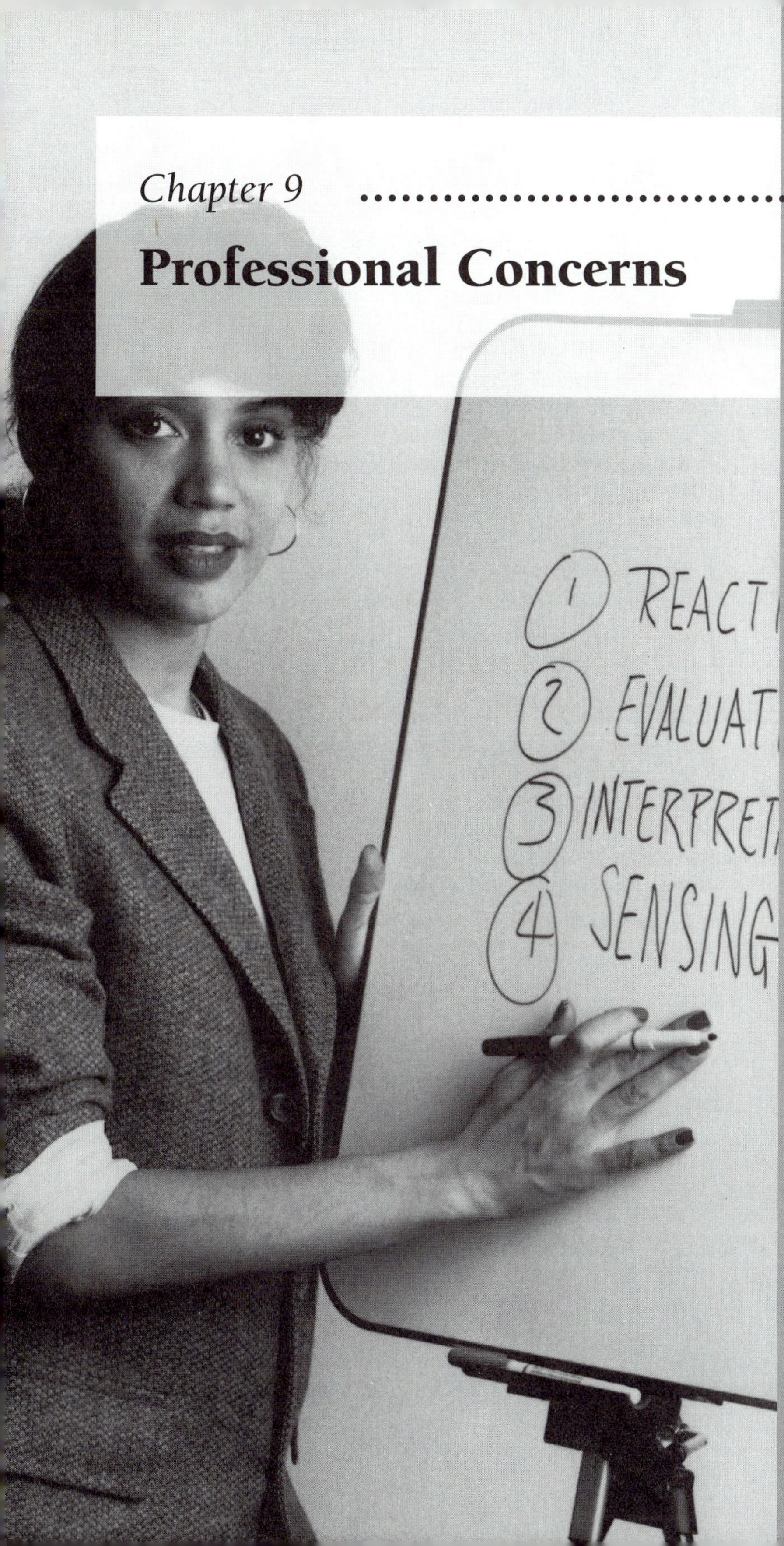

This final chapter focuses on the professional concerns of the human service worker. As we discuss ethical considerations and professional issues, we ask you to shift your orientation from that of a beginning worker to that of a more seasoned professional. The reason for this shift is twofold. First, after your intense study of human services, you are no longer an outsider looking in. Your knowledge of the history of human services, the work of the professional, and the nature of clients and settings allows you to imagine yourself in the role of the worker. Second, the professional concerns discussed in this chapter are experienced not only by the beginning professional but by all helpers, regardless of the length of their service or the populations they serve.

The professional concerns highlighted in this chapter are divided into two areas: ethical considerations and professional development. As pointed out in Chapter 1, both are important facets of the human service profession. This chapter discusses the ethical standards of professional behavior and the dilemmas encountered in a complex working environment. The discussion of these issues centers around professional development, because the professional growth of the human service worker does not end with getting a job. Although a substantial part of professional development does begin with that first job, developing as a professional is a lifelong process.

Ethical Considerations

As you deliver human services, situations will arise in which you may be unsure about the appropriate action to take. A third party requests information about a client; you observe a colleague joking about a client in the break room at work; a client requests information about obtaining an abortion, but your agency opposes providing this type of information. These situations represent ethical dilemmas for the human service professional. Even though education and training in human services emphasize the values of confidentiality, acceptance, individualism, self-determination, and tolerance, situations will inevitably occur in which simply possessing these values will not be enough to determine the right course of action.

In the past decade, increased public awareness of professional behavior, coupled with the passage of federal and state legislation controlling the helping professions, has underscored the importance of ethical concerns in service delivery. Stadler (1986) cites the Family Educational Rights and Privacy Act of 1974, state legislation requiring reporting of child abuse, and *Tarasoff* v. *Regents of the University of California,* which imposed a duty to warn potential victims, as examples of government action that directly affects the ethics of service provision. The human service professional must obey the law and must also be cognizant of the implications of the law.

In this section, we explore codes of ethics or statements of standards of behavior as guides for professional behavior, as well as some major areas of ethical concern for the human service professional. Then we describe an ethical decision-making model that can be applied to dilemmas for which there is no relevant guideline. Vignettes are used to illustrate the range of dilemmas that may arise.

Codes of Ethics

Professionals have responded to the dilemmas of service provision by developing *codes of ethics* or *statements of ethical standards of behavior* for the members of their profession. VanHoose (1986) suggested that codes of ethics or ethical standards reflect professional concerns and define the guiding principles of professional activities. As an aid to ethical decision making in dilemmas arising in service delivery, such standards or codes help clarify the professional's responsibilities to clients, to the agency, and to society. Typically, a code of ethics includes items that state the goals or aims of the profession, protect the client, provide guidance to professional behavior, and contribute to a professional identity for the worker. A complete understanding of a code of ethics or ethical standards requires knowledge of the code's strengths and purposes as well as its limitations.

PURPOSES AND LIMITATIONS

The primary functions of a code of ethics or ethical standards are to establish guidelines for professional behavior and to assist members of the profession in establishing a professional identity (Mabe & Rollin, 1986). Other purposes include protecting members from practices that may result in public condemnation, providing for self-regulating measures, protecting clients from incompetent helpers, and protecting helpers from malpractice lawsuits (VanHoose & Paradise, 1979).

Ethical codes do have limitations; they cannot cover every situation. They do, however, present a framework for ethical behavior, although their exact interpretation will depend on the situation to which they are being applied. As a result of this vagueness, codes may have a limited range, and some codes of ethics will likely conflict with others regarding some standard of behavior. Such conflicts pose problems for professionals who are members of more than one professional organization.

Parallel standard-setting entities may also issue ethical standards that conflict. For example, a code may not include a statement relating to the duty to warn, but the California Supreme Court has ruled in *Tarasoff* v. *Regents of the University of California* that there is a duty to warn potential victims of danger (Mabe & Rollin, 1986). Members bound by a code of ethics must be alert to the possibility that other forums may reach conclusions that differ from their code. Of course, this is especially critical when the other forum is a court of law or a legislative body.

Some other limitations of codes of ethics are beyond the scope of this text. However, human service professionals must be aware that such limitations do exist. The professional must develop ethical reasoning skills to help resolve ethical dilemmas that may arise. A first step in this process is differentiating ethical dilemmas from situations in which the guidelines are clear. For resolving problem situations for which there are no specific guidelines, an ethical decision-making model is presented later in this chapter.

ETHICS AND THE PROFESSION

A code of ethics is binding only on the members of the group or organization that adopts it. Several organizations in human services have issued codes of behavior expected of their membership—organizations such as the American Counseling Association, the National Council for Social Work Education, and others in the fields of corrections, mental health, gerontology, and education. Most codes of ethics stipulate that the worker's first responsibility is to enhance and protect the client's welfare. Codes also give guidance about the helper's responsibilities to employers, to colleagues in the profession and other fields, and to society in general.

Ethical codes adopted by a professional association are usually based on the premise that a profession polices itself. Members of helping professions are assumed to be responsible, sensitive persons who are accountable for their behavior and the behavior of their colleagues. Self-regulation involves two types of discipline: informal and formal. Informal discipline is seen in the subtle and not-so-subtle pressure colleagues exert on one another in the form of consultations, client referrals, and informal and formal discussions. Formal discipline occurs when professional associations publicly criticize or censure their members—in extreme cases, barring them from membership.

CODES OF ETHICS AND THE LAW

The law is generally supportive of, or at least neutral toward, ethical codes and standards. It is supportive in that it enforces minimum standards for practitioners through licensing requirements and generally protects the confidentiality of statements and records provided by clients during service provision. It is neutral in that it allows each profession to police itself and govern the helper's relations with clients and fellow professionals. The law intervenes and overrides professional codes of ethics only when necessary to protect the public health, safety, and welfare. One instance of legal intervention occurs when the profession's standards of confidentiality (deemed necessary to ensure effective treatment) call for the suppression of information that government authorities require to be disclosed to prevent harm to others.

The California Supreme Court's ruling in the case of *Tarasoff* v. *Regents of the University of California* (1976) legally supported a "duty to warn" possible victims of clients once counselors have this information. The court stated that

> when a therapist determines, or pursuant to the standards of his profession should determine, that his patient presents a serious danger of violence to another, he incurs an obligation to use reasonable care to protect the intended victim against such danger. The discharge of this duty may require the therapist to take one or more steps, depending on the nature of the case. Thus, it may call for him or her to warn the intended victim or others likely to apprise the victim of the danger, to notify the police, or to take whatever other steps are reasonably necessary under the circumstances. (p. 340)

Competence and Responsibility

Before any involvement with clients, helpers must concern themselves with two areas: their *competence* as professionals and their *responsibility* to the individuals, groups, or organizations with whom they are affiliated or whom they serve as clients. Ethical concerns of competence and responsibility pervade all areas of professional practice.

Competence is a difficult concept to define from an ethical standpoint. One way to define it is by identifying the standards for practice within the

Ethical Standards for Psychologists American Psychological Association

PRINCIPLE TWO: COMPETENCE

Psychologists strive to maintain high standards of competence in their work. They recognize the boundaries of their particular competencies and the limitations of their expertise. They provide only those services and use only those techniques for which they are qualified by education, training, or experience. Psychologists are cognizant of the fact that the competencies required in serving, teaching, and/or studying groups of people vary with the distinctive characteristics of those groups. In those areas in which recognized professional standards do not yet exist, psychologists exercise careful judgment and take appropriate precautions to protect the welfare of those with whom they work. They maintain knowledge of relevant scientific and professional information related to the services they render, and they recognize the need for ongoing education. Psychologists make appropriate use of scientific, professional, technical, and administrative resources.

profession. Most codes of ethics in helping professions include statements about academic training, practical training or supervised experience, and areas of specialization in which the helper is most knowledgeable or competent. During their training, human service professionals must acquire knowledge about the helping process, professional ethics, the limits of professional practice, and the pertinent legislation that governs practice.

In addition to the competence acquired through preparation to be a professional, the human service worker in practice also has an obligation to ensure that available services meet acceptable standards. He or she has a further obligation to improve services and skills through activities such as involvement in ongoing research and study, participation in peer consultation, and review of the current professional literature. All these activities contribute to the competence of the helper.

The second concept that pervades all phases of service delivery is *responsibility.* Rinas and Clyne-Jackson (1988) defined it as "an obligation to promote and safeguard the dignity, well-being, and growth of clients, colleagues, the . . . profession itself, and society as a whole" (p. 3). The idea that helpers have obligations to others in addition to the client may present dilemmas for the helper in cases of conflict. It is important for the helper to understand the nature of the conflict and be able to explain to the client how this may limit the client-helper relationship.

Ethical Standards for School Counselors
American School Counselor Association

F. RESPONSIBILITIES TO THE PROFESSION

The school counselor:

1. Conducts herself/himself in such a manner as to bring credit to self and the profession.
2. Conducts appropriate research and reports findings in a manner consistent with acceptable educational and psychological research practices. When using client data for research, statistical or program planning purposes, the counselor ensures protection of the identity of the individual(s).
3. Actively participates in local, state, and national associations which foster the development and improvement of school counseling.
4. Adheres to ethical standards of the profession, other official policy statements pertaining to counseling, and relevant statutes established by federal, state, and local governments.
5. Clearly distinguishes between statements and actions made as a private individual and as a representative of the school counseling profession.
6. Contributes to the development of the profession through the sharing of skills, ideas, and expertise with colleagues.

SOURCE: Reprinted from *The ASCA Counselor,* 29(4), April 1992, pp. 13–16.

To fulfill their commitment to be responsible, helpers must know the ethical and legal procedures that are pertinent to their service delivery functions. These include the profession's code of ethics, its standards of behavior, and the consequences of failure to conform to codes and standards.

In many instances, ethical standards of competence and responsibility are compatible. For example, human service professionals are obligated to provide high-quality service to their clients. Discharging this obligation relies to a certain extent on the competence of the worker, as the worker is expected to provide only those services he or she is trained and qualified to deliver. If the client has needs beyond the competence of the worker, the worker has a duty, according to codes and standards of professional behavior, to locate alternative services from a co-worker or another agency. In this situation, the competence of the human service professional is reflected in an awareness of available services and knowledge of how those services relate to the client's problems.

The responsibility of the helper extends beyond client contact. The helper is also concerned with having sufficient time to work with a client and the resources necessary for effective practice. Should these not be present, the helper is responsible for locating or developing resources such as grants for additional funding or increased staff for specialized caseloads. The overriding concern, of course, is the obligation and commitment to provide good-quality services to whoever needs those services.

The vignettes that follow illustrate some of the dilemmas that a helper might face while working with human service clients. The primary issues in these vignettes are competence and responsibility.

Case 1

Carmen is a night counselor for a cerebral palsy group home. She works five nights a week, arriving at 4 P.M. *and staying until 7* A.M. *the next day. Right now the group home is in the process of hiring three new staff members: a van driver, an evening visiting nurse, and a day teacher/counselor. Until these professionals are hired, much of the responsibility falls to Carmen. She does not mind doing all that she can for the group home and the clients, but she feels that she is not qualified to do some of the things asked of her.*

Case 2

George has a job as a caseworker for a mental health outpatient service. He provides individual and group counseling for adult clients. One of his clients, Kim, is having trouble relating to her husband, her son, and her father. George suggests to Kim that she practice various forms of sexual intimacy with him as a part of her therapy to improve her relationships with men.

Case 3

Dim Su is a social service worker in a health care facility for the elderly. He is in a dilemma because several of his clients are requesting that he provide them with cigarettes even though smoking has been discouraged by the doctor. Dim Su's colleague, Betty, laughs when he tells her of his dilemma. She tells him that there is no dilemma. She has provided cigarettes for patients for the past three years.

Case 4

Jim, the sports program director for the Millerville Home for Boys, walks by a group of new workers who are discussing their recent orientation session. They mention the newest rule that prohibits workers from transporting a client in a private car. Jim had heard about the new rule, but so far he has ignored it, hoping to plead ignorance if someone were to challenge his behavior. Many of the relationships he forms with the children are established during one-on-one private outings to the mall, movies, and out to dinner. He hates to give them up.

CASE 5

Bradley's job as coordinator of the hospice program in a local hospital is very demanding. His hours are 8 to 5, Monday through Friday, but the needs of the clients do not follow these regular hours. He is operating the program with little help: one half-time secretary to answer the phone and one hospice nurse. He often works 15 to 18 hours a day. He feels committed to his work but is often so tired that he is afraid he cannot be effective.

CASE 6

Susan Deerpath is a traveling health department worker in a rural area. She is the only worker serving clients in 12 counties. Once every two weeks, she meets with other health department officials from the district, but for the most part she has limited contact with other professionals. She read her last professional magazine two years ago, and she has attended only one inservice meeting in the past five years.

CASE 7

Luis works for an outpatient AIDS clinic whose major goals include prevention and therapeutic counseling. Luis feels that meeting the demands of his clients is the most important service he provides, and he has difficulty ignoring the clients. Consequently, he is booked solid each day, seeing individual AIDS victims and their families. The director thinks he should spend more time on preventive efforts to promote the agency's other main goal.

CASE 8

Enrique is an intake worker for a local community development corporation. He screens individuals for eligibility for housing, seeing more than 70 clients a week. A majority of them qualify for the services, but only two to five housing units become available each week. There are few alternatives for the other clients. Enrique worries about the welfare of these clients, who remain on a waiting list for as long as six months. The dilemma occurs because his job responsibilities do not include referral.

In each of these situations, the worker faces a dilemma regarding worker competence and responsibility for which there is no easy solution. *Competence* is a personal issue that demands professional self-assessment and then commitment to professional development. *Responsibility* involves the interpersonal relationships the worker has with individual clients or groups and human service agencies. The common ground between responsibility and competence is the helper's primary commitment to serving the client.

Confidentiality

Confidentiality is the helper's assurance that information the client divulges will remain between the two of them. If information is to be shared, it will be shared only with those designated by the client. These two statements regarding the concept of confidentiality provide only general guidelines for the helper. In some situations, laws require confidentiality to be breached: Parents have the legal right to information about their offspring in most circumstances; courts may require the disclosure of information that would otherwise be confidential; and helpers have a duty to alert authorities if they suspect child abuse (Rinas & Clyne-Jackson, 1988). The concept is a complex one. This section provides an introduction to confidentiality and gives examples of the complex situations workers may encounter in human service practice.

Wilson (1978) suggested that there are two kinds of confidentiality. One is *absolute confidentiality,* meaning that information learned or observed by the worker is *never* shared in any form. It is never discussed with a supervisor, recorded in the client's file, or entered in the computer. The beginning human service professional rarely encounters this type of confidentiality. Some private practitioners have a right of *privileged communication* that may be considered absolute confidentiality. (Human service workers are seldom granted this degree of confidentiality.) Such practitioners may legally refuse to release certain information in response to a subpoena. The term *legally* is used because privileged communication is a right granted to a group of professionals by state law-making bodies. Situations in which helpers are ethically or legally obligated to breach confidentiality include the following:

1. When the client requests it
2. When the client brings charges against the counselor
3. When the counselor believes the client poses a clear and imminent danger to others and that revealing confidential information may avert danger (Herlihy & Sheeley, 1987)

The second type of confidentiality is *relative confidentiality*—the informal sharing of information that occurs in an agency or organizational setting among co-workers or treatment team members and supervisors. The client's permission is not required for this type of exchange to take place. Typically, agency policy will also guide this sharing by determining who has access to confidential information. The Federal Privacy Act of 1974, which governs confidentiality in federally funded and administered programs such as the Department of Veterans Affairs and the Social Security Administration, states that clients have access to their records and establishes procedures for this to occur. It also supports the concept of relative confidentiality by providing for the sharing of information among those workers within the agency who need the information in the performance of their duties.

In summary, absolute confidentiality rarely exists for the beginning human service professional, but relative confidentiality is a concept that deserves the worker's attention. Agency guidelines, the profession's code of ethics, and the laws of the state in which one practices are important considerations in the delivery of services. A worker should be familiar with all three as guides to dilemmas that may arise. The following vignettes provide examples of confidentiality dilemmas that you may face as a beginning worker.

CASE 1

Sue Lee works for the Department of Human Services in Child Protective Services and visits families once a week to review the status of the home environment. Yesterday she received a subpoena and will be required to testify in court that the father in one of the families in her caseload was not at home the last two times she visited. He is charged with armed robbery and states in his defense that he was at home during the time of the crime. That time coincides with her visit.

CASE 2

Joe Cullinane works in a small agency that provides educational services to children with developmental disabilities. He promises clients that his records are confidential and is very careful not to divulge the names of the clients or the nature of their problems. The mother of one of his young clients reports to him that "someone at her church" had heard that her child was receiving his services. If it was not Joe who breached confidentiality, it might be the secretary who answers the phones or the typist who keeps the records.

CASE 3

Faye Goldstein is a counselor/recreation specialist working in an after-school recreation facility. One of her favorite teenagers has just told her "in confidence" that she is pregnant. Should she keep this confidential?

CASE 4

Freda Tehaar is a group therapist for a grief group at the local mental health center. She has explained to the group the importance of confidentiality. One of the members asks, "How can I place my trust in a bunch of strangers?"

CASE 5

David Root is a recovering alcoholic and has not had a drink in the last two years. He understands and practices confidentiality in his human service work, but he cannot help but wonder how well he would do in this regard if he were to go on a drinking binge.

Code of Professional Ethics for Rehabilitation Counselors: Confidentiality

CANON 6—CONFIDENTIALITY

Rehabilitation counselors shall respect the confidentiality of information obtained from clients in the course of their work.

Rules of Professional Conduct

R6.1 Rehabilitation counselors will inform clients at the onset of the counseling relationship of the limits of confidentiality.

R6.2 Rehabilitation counselors will take reasonable personal action, or inform responsible authorities, or inform those persons at risk, when the conditions or actions of clients indicate that there is clear and imminent danger to clients or others after advising clients that this must be done. Consultation with other professionals may be used where appropriate. The assumption of responsibility for clients must be taken only after careful deliberation and clients must be involved in the resumption of responsibility as quickly as possible.

R6.3 Rehabilitation counselors will not forward to another person, agency, or potential employer, any confidential information without the written permission of clients or their legal guardians.

R6.4 Rehabilitation counselors will ensure that there are defined policies and practices in other agencies cooperatively serving rehabilitation clients which effectively protect information confidentiality.

R6.5 Rehabilitation counselors will safeguard the maintenance, storage, and disposal of the records of clients so that unauthorized persons shall not have access to these records. All non-professional persons who must have access to these records will be thoroughly briefed concerning the confidential standards to be observed.

R6.6 Rehabilitation counselors, in the preparation of written and oral reports, will present only germane data and will make every effort to avoid undue invasion of privacy.

R6.7 Rehabilitation counselors will obtain written permission from clients or their legal guardians prior to taping or otherwise recording counseling sessions. Even with guardians' written consent, rehabilitation counselors will not record sessions against the expressed wishes of clients.

R6.8 Rehabilitation counselors will persist in claiming the privileged status of confidential information obtained from clients, where communications are privileged by statute for rehabilitation counselors.

R6.9 Rehabilitation counselors will provide prospective employers with only job relevant information about clients and will secure the permission of clients or their legal guardians for the release of any information which might be considered confidential.

SOURCE: Material from "Code of Professional Ethics for Rehabilitation Counselors." Reprinted by permission of the Commission on Rehabilitation Counselor Certification.

Case 6

Cynthia Loomis works in a high-stress hospice program. Working with the dying patient and family and friends is emotionally draining, and she often "takes her work home." To help her relieve the stress, can she tell her friends and family anything about her work without breaching her promise of confidentiality?

Case 7

Jefferson Smith works with adults on probation and has just heard one of his clients tell how she abuses her six-month-old child. Does he report this information? To whom does he report it?

Case 8

Raphael Sanchez is a vocational rehabilitation counselor working with a Vietnam veteran. His client has been very depressed during the last month, and during his last individual conference with Raphael, he talked of "ending all the agony." Raphael wonders what he should do and whom he should tell.

These are just a few examples of the many conflicts that can arise over the issue of confidentiality. Many of the troublesome dilemmas result from the constant tension between worker responsibilities, agency policies, and client needs. Absolute and relative confidentiality are difficult principles to follow. The preceding cases illustrate the problems helpers may encounter as they translate their values into action in the workplace. An equally complex issue human service professionals encounter concerns clients' rights.

Clients' Rights

Clients are first and foremost citizens of a democratic society; as such, they have certain rights and privileges. In a helping situation, the client's trust in the helper is important for the development of the helping relationship. In exchange for the trust of the client, the helper is ethically obligated to protect the rights of the client. Two examples of clients' rights are the right to privacy and informed consent.

Clients have the right to share whatever information they wish with a helper. They also have the right to withhold information they do not want to share. The helper is ethically bound to respect clients' *right to privacy* by not pressuring them to reveal things they do not wish to reveal.

Informed consent is another example of the rights of clients involved in the helping process. It is the client's right to know about the qualifications of the helper, treatment procedures, costs of services, confidentiality, and access to records. The concept of informed consent extends beyond simply telling the client about such matters. The client must comprehend this information and consent voluntarily. In some cases, the helper must educate the client about his or her rights with regard to consent.

Informed consent is a particularly critical aspect of client rights with respect to decision making. In the helping process, the client is an active participant who has a voice in what is happening. In the absence of informed consent, the client's right to self-determination is compromised. The helper has an ethical obligation to make sure that clients receive and understand the appropriate information.

One way the client can become informed about the helper is for the helper to write and to share with the client a *professional disclosure statement.* This should include information about the worker and the worker's credentials, which will allow the client to make an informed assessment of the worker's competence. According to Gill (1982, p. 444), the American Counseling Association recommended that the following be included:

> The counselor's name, business address and telephone number, philosophy of counseling, formal education and training, competency areas, continuing education, fee schedule, and the name and address and telephone number of the state government agency regulating the practice of counseling.

Another approach to the professional disclosure statement discussed by Gill (1982) involves workers asking themselves several questions as they develop a professional disclosure statement. Gill's questions have been adapted as follows for the beginning human service worker developing a professional disclosure statement:

1. What is your purpose in helping?
2. What should your clients expect as a result of a helping relationship with you?
3. What are the usual methods, strategies, and techniques that you use?
4. Under what circumstances should your clients expect referral to another helper or agency?

Developing a personal professional disclosure statement has several benefits. As the helper shares the statement with the client, it promotes the development of a helping relationship. Not only does it signal to the client that this relationship is different from informal helping relationships, but it also acquaints the client with the person in whom the client will soon place his or her trust. While working out the statement, the helper has an opportunity to think about and put into words exactly who he or she is as a human service professional. It also allows the worker to define himself or herself as a professional and links the individual to the common knowledge, skills, and values of the profession.

The following sample professional disclosure statement was written by a vocational evaluator, Carmen Rodriguez, introduced in Chapter 6.

American Counseling Association Code of Ethics and Standards of Practice: Clients' Rights

A.3. CLIENT RIGHTS

a. *Disclosure to Clients.* When counseling is initiated, and throughout the counseling process as necessary, counselors inform clients of the purposes, goals, techniques, procedures, limitations, potential risks and benefits of services to be performed, and other pertinent information. Counselors take steps to ensure that clients understand the implications of diagnosis, the intended use of tests and reports, fees, and billing arrangements. Clients have the right to expect confidentiality and to be provided with an explanation of its limitations, including supervision and/or treatment team professionals; to obtain clear information about their case records; to participate in the ongoing counseling plans; and to refuse any recommended services and be advised of the consequences of such refusal. (See E.5.a. and G.2.)

b. *Freedom of Choice.* Counselors offer clients the freedom to choose whether to enter into a counseling relationship and to determine which professional(s) will provide counseling.

c. *Inability to Give Consent.* When counseling minors or persons unable to give voluntary informed consent, counselors act in these clients' best interests. (See B.3.)

SOURCE: Material from "American Counseling Association Code of Ethics and Standards of Practice." Reprinted by permission of the American Counseling Association.

My name is Carmen Rodriguez, and I am involved in vocational rehabilitation of the handicapped. My purpose is to help my clients understand who they are and what they can do to make their lives more satisfying. Specifically, I evaluate clients to determine what knowledge, skills, and abilities they possess and explain to them what potential work opportunities are available for them.

Once a client meets the eligibility requirements established by the agency, there is no charge for my services. I have worked for this agency for four years as a vocational evaluator. I received training in college for this work and frequently attend workshops to update my knowledge.

Evaluations can take from two weeks to six weeks. This may depend on the client, the disability, and what we want to know. I often refer my client to other team members in my agency and to other professionals in the community. The clients I see usually have such complex problems that I cannot address them all by myself, so I work with a team. Because my agency uses this team approach, I may share information about clients with co-workers within the agency but not with outsiders or other clients.

Now that you have read Carmen's statement, can you write one of your own? It may be easier to write such a statement if you imagine that you work in a specific agency with a well-defined population.

Protection is another of the helper's obligations to clients. Clients have the right to expect the helper to protect them from harm (Rinas & Clyne-Jackson, 1988). It is the helper's responsibility to be sensitive to situations in which the client risks economic or physical harm, and, if possible, to prevent harm from occurring. If there is a clear and imminent danger to a third party, the helper has a duty to take action to protect the individual at risk. Determining when a situation warrants action may be difficult for the human service professional; when questionable occasions arise, consultation with.colleagues or supervisors will be helpful in deciding on a course of action.

The following cases provide examples of dilemmas that a human service worker may encounter in relation to clients' rights. Several of the cases present ethical situations in which the human service worker is confronted with a difficult decision about what action to take. In other cases, the dilemma is one over which the worker has little or no control.

CASE 1

Susan Yew and her client, Mr. Rodriguez, have agreed on what referral information should be sent to a local educational reading clinic. The clinic, however, wants more information. Specifically, they want to know whether Mr. Rodriguez is a veteran, but he feels they will treat him "special" if they know that he fought in Vietnam. Susan has agreed that the file to be sent should include a short note explaining why he does not want to answer that particular question.

CASE 2

Once a week, the staff members at the battered women's shelter discuss the cases in which they are involved. One client, age 56, told the worker "in confidence" that she had had an abortion when she was 13. She asked the worker not to tell the other staff members.

CASE 3

The local mental health institution has a new professional worker: the patient advocate, who has been hired by the mental health association to protect the rights of the clients in the institution. The patient advocate explains to each patient his or her rights when he or she enters the institution, but many patients forget or are unable to comprehend how they might use the services of the advocate. Sometimes Ron, a social worker on a treatment team serving the men's locked ward, sees clients' rights being abused, but to recommend that a client see the advocate might cause trouble for the treatment team to which Ron belongs.

CASE 4

Youvella is a patient in a health care facility. She wants to see her medical records before they are examined by the team of specialists who will decide what protocol to prescribe for the treatment of her cancer-ridden pancreas. Although Youvella is entitled to review these records, the nurse questions the wisdom of this decision because of Youvella's emotional instability. The nurse requests assistance from the hospital social service worker in this dilemma.

CASE 5

Emile is a human service student working with rehabilitation services. For the next two weeks, he will be administering vocational aptitude tests to new clients. He is unsure whether he should tell his clients that he is a student. He wants them to trust him and have confidence in him, as they would if he were a seasoned worker.

CASE 6

The adoption agency is reviewing the files of a young couple considering adoption. Unfortunately, the adoption counselor has received some damaging information from the couple's landlord of ten years ago that will make it impossible for the agency to consider them suitable as parents. The counselor really likes this couple and believes that they would make wonderful parents, but she also knows that the information cannot be withheld. The adoption counselor must tell the couple of the agency's decision not to consider them "fit" to adopt and must tell them of the negative recommendation.

CASE 7

The Annas are involved in marital therapy; the stated purpose of the counseling is to "save the marriage." They receive individual counseling once a week, and once a month they participate in counseling sessions together. Ms. Anna has recently told the counselor of her desire to harm Mr. Anna. The counselor wonders how to handle this information, since it was given in confidence and also may jeopardize the goal of saving the marriage.

In clients' rights issues, the worker's judgment and the agency's judgment are often not the only considerations. Legal rulings must also be taken into account. Sometimes legal pronouncements, ethical standards, and personal commitments conflict, presenting a difficult dilemma for the worker. The worker then must decide what action is most ethical.

Ethical Standards of Human Service Professionals

During 1990 and 1991, both the National Organization for Human Service Education (NOHSE) and the Council for Standards in Human Service Education (CSHSE) recognized the need for the development of a separate and distinct ethical code for human service professionals. Previously, students and graduates were guided by the codes of ethics or ethical standards of various other professions, some of which have been excerpted in this chapter. These codes did not reflect the unique history or philosophy of the human service profession.

In 1990, the governing boards of NOHSE and CSHSE expressed the desire to enhance the professional identity of human service professionals; this resulted in the appointment of a committee by NOHSE to develop a code of ethics. Developing a code of ethics or ethical standards for a profession is a lengthy process. In this case, there was a review of the code of ethics of related professions: the American Counseling Association (ACA), the National Association of Social Workers (NASW), and the American Psychological Association (APA). An examination of literature on ethical guidelines followed. These steps led to written ethical guidelines that were eventually approved by the boards of two human service organizations and their memberships in 1995.

As you read these ethical standards, you will note that they address the topics discussed at the beginning of this chapter. The Preamble introduces the goals or aims of the profession. The ethical standards then divide professional responsibilities in six areas: to clients, to the community and society, to colleagues, to the profession, to employers, and to self.

These ethical standards as well as those in other helping professions provide guidelines only. They do not provide answers to all ethical dilemmas. The ethical decision making that follows the ethical standards is helpful when these situations arise.

Ethical Decision Making

Clearly, no code of ethics or statement of standards can provide a course of action for every situation that might arise in the practice of human services. What does the human service professional do in situations for which there are no guidelines or guidelines that conflict? In such *ethical dilemmas,* the helper "experiences conflict in determining an appropriate standard of conduct regarding obligations to two or more constituencies" (Hayman & Covert, 1986, p. 318). The areas of confidentiality, role conflict, and counselor competence frequently present ethical dilemmas. Rather than attempt to provide possible solutions to every situation that comes to mind, this subsection will introduce a model for ethical decision making that can be applied to many dilemmas to determine a course of action.

The key question in the decision-making model is "What is the best action under the circumstances and with the individuals involved?" In asking this question, the helper must assume an attitude of *moral responsibleness.* This should be distinguished from the kind of responsibility discussed earlier. That responsibility is imposed by some higher authority, such as the profession or the

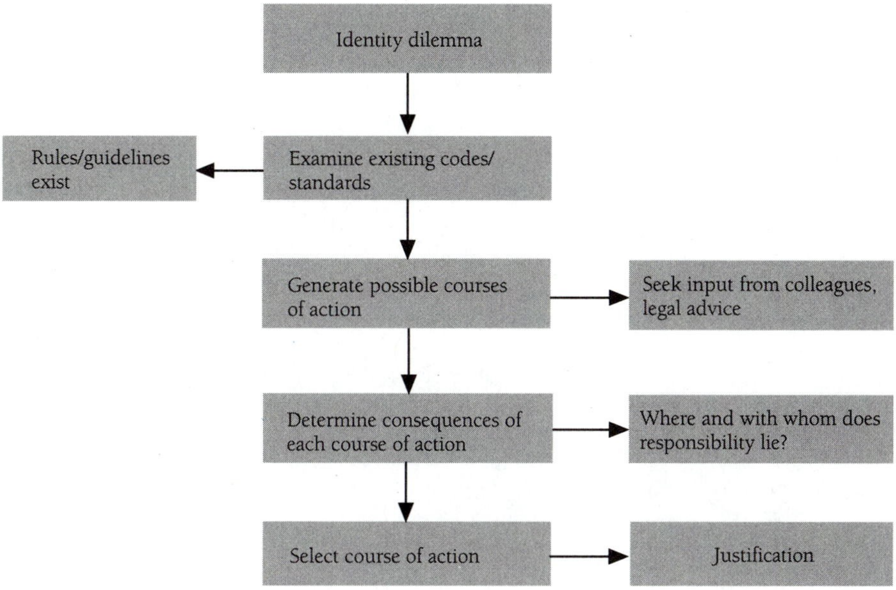

Figure 9-1 ✦ Ethical decision-making model

government; it may be interpreted as one's duty. Moral responsibleness, on the other hand, comes from within the individual, who assumes that there is a course of action that is morally right (Tennyson & Strom, 1986). A commitment to rational thinking and a knowledge of moral principles are necessary components of moral reasoning.

The ethical decision-making model proposed by VanHoose and Paradise (1979) consists of five steps. The first is identification of the problem or dilemma. Second is an examination of existing rules or guiding principles that may be applied to resolve the dilemma. If none are found, the worker proceeds to a third step: generating possible courses of action. The fourth step is consideration of the consequences of each proposed course of action, and the final step is selection of the best course of action.

We have discussed dilemmas that involve competency and responsibility, confidentiality, and clients' rights and have presented short cases to illustrate problems that might arise in actual practice. The following questions may be useful as you consider how you would respond to each case. These questions correspond to the ethical decision-making model proposed by VanHoose and Paradise (1979) and illustrated in Figure 9-1.

1. State the dilemma clearly. There may be more than one; if so, please think of all that you can.
2. What options are available to you?
3. What are the disadvantages and advantages of choosing each option?
4. What action do you choose?
5. What factor most influenced your decision?

Ethical Standards of Human Service Professionals

PREAMBLE

Human services is a profession developing in response to and in anticipation of the direction of human needs and human problems in the late twentieth century. Characterized particularly by an appreciation of human beings in all their diversity, human services offers assistance to its clients within the context of their community and environment. Human service professionals, regardless of whether they are students, faculty or practitioners, promote and encourage the unique values and characteristics of human services. In so doing human service professionals uphold the integrity and ethics of the profession, partake in constructive criticism of the profession, promote client and community well-being, and enhance their own professional growth.

The ethical guidelines presented are a set of standards of conduct which the human service professional considers in ethical and professional decision making. It is hoped that these guidelines will be of assistance when the human service professional is challenged by difficult ethical dilemmas. Although ethical codes are not legal documents, they may be used to assist in the adjudication of issues related to ethical human service behavior.

Human service professionals function in many ways and carry out many roles. They enter into professional-client relationships with individuals, families, groups and communities who are all referred to as "clients" in these standards. Among their roles are caregiver, case manager, broker, teacher/educator, behavior changer, consultant, outreach professional, mobilizer, advocate, community planner, community change organizer, evaluator and administrator (SREB, 1967). The following standards are written with these multifaceted roles in mind.

THE HUMAN SERVICE PROFESSIONAL'S RESPONSIBILITY TO CLIENTS

STATEMENT 1 Human service professionals negotiate with clients the purpose, goals, and nature of the helping relationship prior to its onset, as well as inform clients of the limitations of the proposed relationship.

STATEMENT 2 Human service professionals respect the integrity and welfare of the client at all times. Each client is treated with respect, acceptance and dignity.

STATEMENT 3 Human service professionals protect the client's right to privacy and confidentiality except when such confidentiality would cause harm to the client or others, when agency guidelines state otherwise, or under other stated conditions (e.g., local, state, or federal laws). Professionals inform clients of the limits of confidentiality prior to the onset of the helping relationship.

STATEMENT 4 If it is suspected that danger or harm may occur to the client or to others as a result of a client's behavior, the human service professional acts in an appropriate and professional manner to protect the safety of those individuals. This may involve seeking consultation, supervision, and/or breaking the confidentiality of the relationship.

STATEMENT 5 Human service professionals protect the integrity, safety, and security of client records. All written client information that is shared with other professionals, except in the course of professional supervision, must have the client's prior written consent.

STATEMENT 6 Human service professionals are aware that in their relationships with clients power and status are unequal. Therefore they recognize that dual or multiple relationships may increase the risk of harm to, or exploitation of, clients, and may impair their professional judgment. However, in some communities and situations it may not be feasible to avoid social or other nonprofessional contact with clients. Human service professionals support the trust implicit in the helping relationship by avoiding dual relationships that may impair professional judgment, increase risk of harm to clients or lead to exploitation.

STATEMENT 7 Sexual relationships with current clients are not considered to be in the best interest of the client and are prohibited. Sexual relationships with previous clients are considered dual relationships and are addressed in Statement 6 (above).

STATEMENT 8 The client's right to self-determination is protected by human service professionals. They recognize the client's right to receive or refuse services.

STATEMENT 9 Human service professionals recognize and build on client strengths.

THE HUMAN SERVICE PROFESSIONAL'S RESPONSIBILITY TO THE COMMUNITY AND SOCIETY

STATEMENT 10 Human service professionals are aware of local, state, and federal laws. They advocate for change in regulations and statutes when such legislation conflicts with ethical guidelines and/or client rights. Where laws are harmful to individuals, groups, or communities, human service professionals consider the conflict between the values of obeying the law and the values of serving people and may decide to initiate social action.

STATEMENT 11 Human service professionals keep informed about current social issues as they affect the client and the community. They share that information with clients, groups and community as part of their work.

STATEMENT 12 Human service professionals understand the complex interaction between individuals, their families, the communities in which they live, and society.

STATEMENT 13 Human service professionals act as advocates in addressing unmet client and community needs. Human service professionals provide a mechanism for identifying unmet client needs, calling attention to these needs, and assisting in planning and mobilizing to advocate for those needs at the local community level.

STATEMENT 14 Human service professionals represent their qualifications to the public accurately.

STATEMENT 15 Human service professionals describe the effectiveness of programs, treatments, and/or techniques accurately.

(continued)

(continued)

STATEMENT 16 Human service professionals advocate for the rights of all members of society, particularly those who are members of minorities and groups at which discriminatory practices have historically been directed.

STATEMENT 17 Human service professionals provide services without discrimination or preference based on age, ethnicity, culture, race, disability, gender, religion, sexual orientation or socioeconomic status.

STATEMENT 18 Human service professionals are knowledgeable about the cultures and communities within which they practice. They are aware of multiculturalism in society and its impact on the community as well as individuals within the community. They respect individuals and groups, their cultures and beliefs.

STATEMENT 19 Human service professionals are aware of their own cultural backgrounds, beliefs, and values, recognizing the potential for impact on their relationships with others.

STATEMENT 20 Human service professionals are aware of sociopolitical issues that differentially affect clients from diverse backgrounds.

STATEMENT 21 Human service professionals seek the training, experience, education and supervision necessary to ensure their effectiveness in working with culturally diverse client populations.

THE HUMAN SERVICE PROFESSIONAL'S RESPONSIBILITY TO COLLEAGUES

STATEMENT 22 Human service professionals avoid duplicating another professional's helping relationship with a client. They consult with other professionals who are assisting the client in a different type of relationship when it is in the best interest of the client to do so.

STATEMENT 23 When a human service professional has a conflict with a colleague, he or she first seeks out the colleague in an attempt to manage the problem. If necessary, the professional then seeks the assistance of supervisors, consultants or other professionals in efforts to manage the problem.

STATEMENT 24 Human service professionals respond appropriately to unethical behavior of colleagues. Usually this means initially talking directly with the colleague and, if no resolution is forthcoming, reporting the colleague's behavior to supervisory or administrative staff and/or to the professional organization(s) to which the colleague belongs.

STATEMENT 25 All consultations between human service professionals are kept confidential unless to do so would result in harm to clients or communities.

THE HUMAN SERVICE PROFESSIONAL'S RESPONSIBILITY TO THE PROFESSION

STATEMENT 26 Human service professionals know the limit and scope of their professional knowledge and offer services only within their knowledge and skill base.

STATEMENT 27 Human service professionals seek appropriate consultation and supervision to assist in decision-making when there are legal, ethical or other dilemmas.

STATEMENT 28 Human service professionals act with integrity, honesty, genuineness, and objectivity.

STATEMENT 29 Human service professionals promote cooperation among related disciplines (e.g., psychology, counseling, social work, nursing, family and consumer sciences, medicine, education) to foster professional growth and interests within the various fields.

STATEMENT 30 Human service professionals promote the continuing development of their profession. They encourage membership in professional associations, support research endeavors, foster educational advancement, advocate for appropriate legislative actions, and participate in other related professional activities.

STATEMENT 31 Human service professionals continually seek out new and effective approaches to enhance their professional abilities.

THE HUMAN SERVICE PROFESSIONAL'S RESPONSIBILITY TO EMPLOYERS

STATEMENT 32 Human service professionals adhere to commitments made to their employers.

STATEMENT 33 Human service professionals participate in efforts to establish and maintain employment conditions which are conducive to high quality client services. They assist in evaluating the effectiveness of the agency through reliable and valid assessment measures.

STATEMENT 34 When a conflict arises between fulfilling the responsibilities to the employer and the responsibility to the client, human service professionals advise both of the conflict and work conjointly with all involved to manage the conflict.

THE HUMAN SERVICE PROFESSIONAL'S RESPONSIBILITY TO SELF

STATEMENT 35 Human service professionals strive to personify those characteristics typically associated with the profession (e.g., accountability, respect for others, genuineness, empathy, pragmatism).

STATEMENT 36 Human service professionals foster self-awareness and personal growth in themselves. They recognize that when professionals are aware of their own values, attitudes, cultural background, and personal needs, the process of helping others is less likely to be negatively impacted by those factors.

STATEMENT 37 Human service professionals recognize a commitment to lifelong learning and continually upgrade knowledge and skills to service the population better.[1]

[1] Southern Regional Education Board. (1967). *Roles and Functions for Mental Health Workers: A Report of a Symposium.* Atlanta, GA: Community Mental Health Worker Project.

SOURCE: Ethical Standards of Human Service Professionals (1996). *Human Service Education, 16,* 11–17.

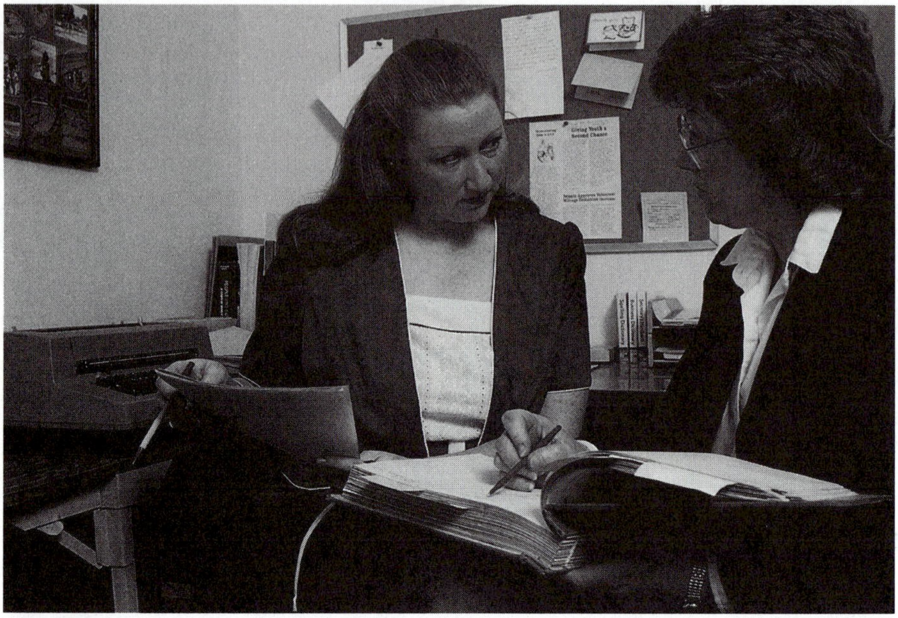

When deciding among possible courses of action, human service professionals may find it helpful to solicit input from a co-worker.

Another place to use the ethical decision-making model is with dilemmas that are unique to a specific setting, for it provides a purposeful way of thinking about them. Human services in a correctional setting provides examples of such ethical conflicts. The dilemmas correctional workers face illustrate the conflict between human service workers' responsibilities to the client, to the agency, and to society. As an officer of the court, the corrections worker has the primary role of ensuring that clients do not break the law or injure others. This role places the professional in the position of judge, evaluator, and reporter, making establishing and maintaining helping relationships difficult. The following two dilemmas arise from a conflict between this primary role of the corrections worker and the human service worker's overriding concern for the welfare of the client (Page, 1979).

One dilemma may arise when the courts mandate counseling sessions for public offenders. The fact that counseling is imposed will probably impede the helping relationship. The second dilemma, which further complicates the relationship, occurs when the worker explains what confidentiality means in the corrections setting. If a client has violated an institution's rules or any state or federal law and tells the worker of the violations, the professional is expected to report this information to the appropriate authorities. Many clients never develop the trust needed for a good helping relationship, refusing to share problems with the worker. Other clients may be reluctant to disclose real problems they are experiencing, as the worker is often in a position to provide information and make recommendations about clients. Thus, clients may tell the helper only good news, in hopes of securing a positive recommendation.

In situations like these, the professional should begin by identifying exactly what the conflict is. After reviewing ethical guidelines, the helper then considers possible courses of action and the consequences of each. It may be helpful at this point to ask co-workers for input and clarification as the professional explores what each course of action will mean to the client, to the agency, and to the helper. At some point, the helper will have to select a course of action. This ethical decision-making model provides only a structure for thinking about a dilemma; selecting a course of action may still be very difficult. Apply what you have learned about ethical decision making to the following case.

The Ethical Dilemma of Counselor B

Background

Counselor B is working as a youth services counselor for the Child Welfare Board of an urban city. She has been asked by the court to see ten-year-old Nancy L. to determine if she should be returned to the custody of her mother. Nancy L. has been living with foster parents for the past two years.

The foster parents, Mr. and Mrs. S., have become quite attached to Nancy and have initiated legal proceedings to adopt her. Shortly after they informed the Child Welfare Board of their intentions, Nancy's natural mother, Mrs. L., hired a lawyer to regain custody of her daughter.

Nancy had been sent to live with her foster parents after her mother was convicted of prostitution. After serving six months, Mrs. L. was paroled and began working in a department store. She has recently married a former boyfriend. They have been married for almost a year and would like to have Nancy live with them.

For several weeks, Counselor B has been seeing all parties involved in the situation. The following background information has been obtained: Nancy has a loving relationship with her foster parents and does not want to be separated from them, even though she believes them to be very strict parents. During the first year that Nancy lived with them, her mother made no attempts to contact her or to see her. The foster parents believe that it was only after the mother learned of the impending adoption that she began to take an interest in her daughter. Counselor B has also learned through a former neighbor of Nancy's mother that the man Mrs. L. has married was also involved in the prostitution activities that caused her arrest. However, in talking with Mrs. L. and her husband, it was determined that both seem sincere in their desire to have Nancy in their home. Mrs. L. and her husband feel that Mrs. L. has paid for her past actions and that she has a right to have custody of her daughter. Mrs. L. states that prison was a very difficult adjustment for her and that it took some time for her to "get back on her feet." This is why she did not attempt to contact her daughter earlier. Mrs. L.'s husband claims he has a good job that will support Nancy and her mother and that Mrs. L. will be able to stay at home and devote her attentions to Nancy. Although he had some minor scrapes with the law as a juvenile, and although the police suspect him of continued involvement in prostitution, he has no police record.

The court would like the counselor's recommendation, as to whether Nancy should be returned to the custody of her natural mother, as soon as possible.

THE PROBLEM

Should the counselor recommend that Nancy be returned to her mother, overriding Nancy's wishes to remain with her foster parents? While Nancy's natural mother appears to be making a constructive change in her life, there is some suspicion as to whether this is really the case. Counselor B has just learned from the Child Welfare Agency that several unsubstantiated complaints have been filed against Mr. and Mrs. S., the foster parents, for the apparent harsh discipline they have exercised on previous children in their care.

THE DILEMMA

Should a mother be deprived of her child? Should Counselor B act on her suspicions about Nancy's mother and stepfather? Does Mrs. L. deserve to be punished again for past actions? What would you recommend? Why? To help you decide what Counselor B should do, answer the following questions:

1. *Exactly who is Counselor B's client?*
2. *What are the counselor's responsibilities to Nancy?*
3. *What are the counselor's responsibilities to Nancy's natural mother?*
4. *What impact do the wishes of ten-year-old Nancy have on Counselor B's recommendations?*
5. *What are the counselor's responsibilities to the court?*
6. *What are the counselor's responsibilities to society (i.e., the welfare of this child and others like her)?*
7. *Generate possible alternative courses of action stating why they were chosen.*
8. *What are the possible and probable consequences of the actions that Counselor B could take?*
9. *As Counselor B, what would you do and why? Which ethical standards support your decision?*

SOURCE: From *Ethics in Counseling and Psychotherapy: Perspectives in Issues and Decision Making*, by William H. VanHoose and Louis V. Paradise (1979). New York, NY: Sulzburger & Graham, pp. 65–68.

Professional Issues

Among the professional issues that all human service professionals face, three are most relevant to the beginning worker: how to advance as a worker, the emotional stress of the job, and professional development.

Advancement in the profession is a concern for most human service professionals. Knowledge of the history of the profession and the ways it is regulated is important for understanding advancement. Basic to this discussion is the assumption that human services is a career. Chapter 1 (definitions of human services) and Chapter 2 (history of the profession) explain in detail the rationale supporting this assumption.

The word *ladder* within the term *career ladder* connotes a possibility of climbing higher. In professional terms, this means advancing as a professional by getting a "better" job, with more responsibility, prestige, recognition, and a higher salary. The career ladder for human services is not as well defined as in some other professions, but nevertheless it does exist.

Another issue to be covered in this section involves the stresses and strains experienced by workers in helping professions. Such tensions are likely to result in workers' becoming "encapsulated"—retreating from the engagement of helping and becoming rigid, insensitive, uncaring professionals. Another result of the pressures of the job may be burnout, a syndrome that can result in poor work performance or a decision to leave the profession.

One key to resolving such professional issues is a commitment to professional development. We recommend such a commitment as a means of keeping the worker engaged and well supported in the delivery of services.

The History of the Career Ladder in Human Services

As noted in Chapter 2, the community mental health movement and the War on Poverty during the 1960s and 1970s created an increased demand for human service professionals. The challenge of this time was to train the human service professionals needed by the burgeoning social programs as quickly and cost effectively as possible. Two factors were critical. First, traditional staffing patterns could not meet the demand. Up to this time, professionals with advanced degrees, such as social workers, psychologists, and vocational rehabilitation counselors, had provided most of the human services. The increased demand forced social services to expand to include other types of workers. According to Vidaver (1973), the new workers, commonly called human service workers, included four categories. First, *nonprofessionals,* who had no professional training, were hired to perform jobs involving low-level responsibilities. Second, *indigenous community workers* were hired to work with people from their own communities. Often, such workers had previously been clients. Hiring these workers gave jobs to a needy population and provided workers to whom the clients could relate. The third category was comprised of people who switched to human services after working in related fields. For these individuals, human services offered a midlife career change that allowed them to work with people and contribute to the betterment of society. The fourth category consisted of specially trained *entry-level workers* who were formally educated at the associate or baccalaureate level. Some of this training was specific to the type of client to be served (as in the cases of mental health and criminal justice workers), but much of the training focused on generic education for human service work.

PROFESSIONALS OR PARAPROFESSIONALS?

During this time, only those individuals holding advanced degrees were viewed as professionals, and the four groups described by Vidaver (1973) were considered nonprofessionals or paraprofessionals. The use of the word *paraprofessional* implied that these workers were only substitutes or were pretending to be professional but were not really capable of doing professional work. This usage reflected a concern that these workers could not provide effective human services and questions about how clients would receive such workers. Because of the questions about the performance of "non" or "para" professionals, supervision of these workers became a critical issue. The reluctance of professionals to accept the new workers also stemmed from the fear that professionals would lose control of the education and training for the profession, which would then become diluted by the paraprofessionals.

During the 1960s and 1970s, the prevailing attitude was that one was either a professional or not, and being a professional was determined by one's education rather than the responsibilities and roles one performed on the job. The assumption was that advanced, formal training instilled an understanding of social behavior and an important knowledge base, without which a worker could not perform in a professional manner. In summary, education was the key; only an advanced degree entitled an individual to be regarded as a professional in human services.

The concept of the paraprofessional is now outdated. The categorization used by Okun (1997)—professional helpers, entry-level professionals, and nonprofessionals—reflects the new view of the professional. One of the most important changes is that an advanced degree is no longer necessary for professional status. The expanded definition of *professional* has resulted from the success enjoyed by those formerly labeled paraprofessionals—their positive impact on the human service system. Not only have these workers been able to assume the roles and perform the responsibilities asked of them, but they have performed them with a commitment and efficiency that was not anticipated. These workers also did not require as much supervision as was assumed necessary. Moreover, clients often did not distinguish between the paraprofessionals and the professionals but treated both with the same respect.

In summary, the traditional two levels of workers (professionals who held advanced degrees and paraprofessionals) have now become three. The replacement of the word *paraprofessional* with *nonprofessional* was supported by

Schulman (1982), because the term *paraprofessional* implies an inferior status. In reality, these workers are assisting the professionals, working with them to achieve a common goal for the client. The career path for the nonprofessional is determined by his or her level of education and training. The worker's experience is not discounted, but to become eligible for most entry-level positions, a nonprofessional would need more education.

Entry-level professionals, a completely new level of workers, are those who have associate or baccalaureate degrees and who assume major responsibilities in working with clients. This category includes workers with a wide range of different types of training and job descriptions. The jobs of these workers are often defined and advertised in terms of the degrees held (such as the A.A., B.A., B.S., or B.S.W.) but not the major field of study. Therefore, this group may include graduates of human service programs, students who graduate with a related major such as psychology or sociology, those who have an unrelated major such as business or physics, and people who have degrees and previous work experience that may be related (such as education) or unrelated (such as sales). In an attempt to achieve a more diverse work force, human service agencies seeking to fill entry-level positions recruit more members of minority groups and students who are older than the average graduate. Two-year programs play a critical role in this recruitment. The associate degree, under-valued in the 1960s and 1970s, has become a distinct educational goal for people who wish to enter the field of human services. The degree not only provides education and training in the human services but also gives graduates easy access to four-year programs of higher education.

These entry-level professionals have a flexible career path within the profession. They are able to make lateral career moves (for example, from working with the elderly to working with community mental health) because their skills are considered transferable. Still, in certain career paths, an advanced degree remains critical to professional advancement.

REGULATING THE PROFESSION

Another issue directly related to advancement in the profession is the way in which human services regulates its professional workers. Basically, there are three ways that professions can be regulated: registry, certification, and licensure. *Registry* is the least restrictive of the regulatory measures. Individuals who have met certain criteria (often, education or experience in the field) can apply to be placed in a registry—a list of individuals who claim to be qualified for professional work. This is useful for workers who need professional status and for employers who need some documentation of the expertise of their workers. *Certification,* a more restrictive form of regulation, purports to guarantee the competence of individual workers. Actual certification is based on performance on a test or other procedures designed to demonstrate knowledge and skills. Usually what is certified is a certain level of qualifications or competence, and workers voluntarily participate in certification procedures. Once certified, they have documents that attest to their qualifications.

The third and most restrictive way of regulating professionals is *licensure.* Usually a state or federally mandated procedure, licensure guarantees minimum competency in a particular field or area of expertise through comprehensive testing, certification of educational experience, performance in the field, and testimonies to moral and ethical character and practice. The system of licensing was originally developed to meet several goals. It was feared that unsuspecting clients would fall prey to untrained and unethical individuals claiming the title of a professional. Licensure became a way of protecting vulnerable clients. It also gives the licensed workers some influence over the profession by regulating who becomes recognized as a professional and by providing input into the educational process.

Competence—defining it and determining who has it—becomes an issue in regulating a human service profession. Certification and licensure are attempts to ensure that individuals have the abilities necessary for professional work. These include the knowledge, skills, values, and personal characteristics suitable for work in that profession as well as the ability to apply these in the work environment. Middleman (1984) wrote, "Competence is inferred from performance according to specific measures and may be taken to mean some aggregate of knowledge, judgment, experience, style, self-image, and skill, that is applied when and where needed to accomplish the impinging task" (p. 149). His point is that testing for competence is more than just testing for knowledge. Middleman suggested four levels of assessment: knowledge and understanding, qualities and attitudes, practice, and work management and relationships.

Although human services is a relatively new profession, it has some experience with professional regulation. The National Commission for Human Service Workers (NCHSW), established under the direction of the Southern Regional Education Board, focused on establishing registration and certification procedures for the new human service profession. Because human services represented a variety of professional settings and roles, the NCHSW decided to develop regulations that would organize the complex human service system. The vision of the commission was that the regulation would provide visibility for human services, expand traditional thinking about competence to include experience as well as education, and assist in providing quality services to clients. The certification system was to be a complex one that required applicants to be tested for professional knowledge and application, to compile a portfolio documenting successful work experience, to provide evidence of academic achievement, and to submit references to document strong ethical standards. Unfortunately, the registration and certification procedures established by the commission failed, and the National Commission for Human Service Workers no longer exists. Although there is no national regulation of human service workers, opportunities do exist for human service workers to become registered, certified, or recognized as professionals at the national, state, and local levels.

Pitfalls for the New Professional

Becoming a human service professional is an exciting time of new experiences, challenges, and personal and professional development. Unfortunately, the excitement of the first job can fade, and new workers may not grow as professionals during this time of transition. They can become disenchanted, experience disequilibrium, and behave in ways that are less than professional. Two pitfalls may limit professional development: encapsulation and burnout.

ENCAPSULATED WORKERS

New workers faced with the difficulties of developing as professionals may become static in their work. They may feel so threatened and frightened by the difficult tasks they are asked to perform that they quit learning and growing—thus becoming *encapsulated*. Encapsulated workers relate to clients in characteristic ways (Wrenn, 1962). First, they become rigid and inflexible, believing that there are enduring truths that must be upheld. Such truths can take many forms, such as "The system's rules are always right and just" or "Individuals who are unemployed do not deserve to be helped." If human service workers are not static but dynamic, their personal and professional experiences modify their ideas about clients and the human service system. They grow, learning about the system and how it operates as well as learning about the self. To cling to the "truths" workers have at the beginning of their professional careers limits what they can learn from their experiences.

Another characteristic of encapsulated human service professionals is their retention of the beliefs of the traditional culture. The history of human services (discussed in Chapter 2) is evidence that beliefs about people and their needs change. Often in history, cultural beliefs have limited the assistance available for those in need. From the 1930s until the late 1970s, the poor were considered worthy of help and support. By the 1980s, the trend had reversed itself; once again, helping the poor became less valued by the culture. Thoughtful workers in the 1990s must wrestle with issues such as "What are the rights of the poor?" and "What is the role of human services in helping people who cannot help themselves?" To become encapsulated means to accept the values of the times unquestioningly, no matter what pain those values may cause clients.

Encapsulated workers not only assume the traditions of the culture but ask clients to do so as well. Such workers may listen carefully and with great concern to clients and then ask them to conform to the social norms. However, many people who seek help are not part of the traditional culture. To ask them to give up their own beliefs, lifestyles, and culture is to violate the values of human services. To demand that clients conform to the traditional culture is hardly a sign of tolerance and concern for individual clients and respect for their self-determination.

Encapsulated workers depend only on their own personal experiences and frames of reference, which limits their understanding of clients. There are many different types of clients and client situations, and it is difficult for workers to be familiar with all of them. As a result, workers should constantly read, discuss, and observe clients so as to broaden the base from which they understand clients' experiences. Workers who do not expand their knowledge remain limited in the types of clients they can serve.

One way to address the problem of encapsulation is through a commitment to lifelong learning. Part of learning is making changes in behaviors and attitudes; change and growth can be very exciting parts of the learning process, though difficult at times. Part of the change process is *unlearning*, which can counteract the encapsulated workers' tendencies to cling to truths and to accept the values of the traditional culture. To avoid or counteract encapsulation, workers must constantly try to develop professionally by revising and updating the knowledge, skills, and values of the profession.

BURNOUT

Another result of the stress and strain new professionals experience is *burnout*. This condition results from negative changes in attitudes and behavior that are precipitated by job strain (Cherniss, 1980). Beginning human service professionals are certainly subject to pressure that leads to burnout. Loss of idealism and disappointment in client motivations may result in a loss of commitment to both job and clients. New professionals who experience burnout may also be reacting to a less-than-perfect work setting—one that is too demanding, too frustrating, or too boring.

Some symptoms of burnout are a change in attitudes about work, lower expectations of performance, severe emotional detachment from work, reduced psychological involvement with clients, and an intense concern with self. As workers burn out, they are likely to perceive work more negatively, resulting in sick days, tardiness, and clock watching. The syndrome also affects how workers perceive clients. They may call them names behind their backs, become angry with them, or feel that they are irresponsible and ungrateful for the help that is given them.

There are also some physical symptoms of burnout, such as chronic fatigue, frequent colds, serious illness, stomach trouble, lower back pain, and perhaps even substance abuse. Burnout may also affect the person's relationships with others outside of work, and the worker may be unable to take up new hobbies or to concentrate on anything for long periods of time.

Burnout is not temporary strain, but rather a pattern of being and thinking that cannot easily be interrupted unless specific efforts are made to alleviate it. Especially for new workers, it is not just "poor adjustment" that can be corrected with increased time on the job. Recovery from burnout is a long process that necessitates many changes in the life and work of the workers affected.

Changing one's career orientation, encouraging institutional change, increasing the intrinsic rewards of work, and improving the quality of life outside work are all ways workers can counteract burnout. To develop a different career orientation, workers adopt a more realistic view of what a career means to them, both personally and professionally. This also means realistically assessing what workers can expect to do for clients, what they can expect from the organization, and how much fulfillment they should expect from their jobs. Part of this assessment is deciding what job activities are rewarding and then concentrating on those aspects. Because extrinsic rewards are not always available, workers must often depend on intrinsic rewards. They can learn to measure their performance by their own professional standards and begin to identify and articulate what they do well, rather than glossing over their successes in light of perceived failures.

The issues of realistic expectations and intrinsic rewards are also directly related to improving the quality of life outside of work. When work is an individual's major or only focus, it must fill psychological and social needs, such as the need to be close to others, to belong, to be creative, and to relax. Rarely can any one activity, even work in the human services, satisfy all these needs. Some can be met through well-chosen activities outside of work.

The human service organization can counteract burnout in other ways. Bureaucracies may not know how to protect their workers; professionals may have to provide the leadership to promote these changes. One effective strategy is to establish a work structure that helps workers avoid boredom by varying work, responsibility, and routine. When individuals work in predictable patterns day after day, they get tired and begin to function like machines rather than human beings. A slight change in responsibility, timing, or setting may prevent boredom. Another strategy is to implement ways of recognizing and rewarding workers' efforts. Such extrinsic rewards as certificates of merit, small promotions, asking workers' opinions, raises, changes of job title, and support for education or professional development can all provide workers with formal recognition for jobs well done. Another approach is to provide a mechanism for workers to give feedback and effect even small changes in agency role, procedure, or policy. This provides workers with evidence that they can make a difference and that the bureaucracy is not indifferent to those who are working on the front line.

Another effective response to burnout is a focus on wellness—considering the well-being of individuals from the perspectives of their social, psychological, nutritional, safety, physical, and creative needs. The wellness movement is committed to educating individuals to take responsibility for their own lives, promoting a fuller, more satisfying lifestyle. The ultimate goal of the wellness movement is to promote the growth and development of individuals and to encourage them to strive for self-actualization, the highest stage of development in Maslow's hierarchy.

Professional Development

The issue of professional development relates directly to professional mobility and the pitfalls new workers encounter. Critical to improving one's professional standing is a commitment to developing new knowledge and skills. This is one goal of professional development that can also help counteract encapsulation and burnout.

One characteristic of professionals, regardless of their area of expertise, is their commitment to professional development. Human service professionals are strongly supportive of continuing education and lifelong learning. Both formal and informal approaches to continuing education are important to professional growth. Returning to school for an advanced degree—whether it be an associate, baccalaureate, master's, doctorate, or specialist degree—is a legitimate way to continue professional education in the human services. Such formal education will also open alternative career paths and allow workers to increase their qualifications and competence. The possibilities of formal education are many and include earning A.A. or A.S. degrees in human services or a more specialized program such as child care or mental health technology; earning B.A. or B.S. degrees in human services, social work, liberal arts, or education; or earning master's or doctoral degrees in social work, public health, rehabilitation, child and family studies, or business or law. Such degrees give workers additional expertise and flexibility for future career moves and also enhance their performance in their current positions.

Inservice training is also an excellent way to develop new expertise. Many workshops and conferences are available within an organization, or within the working radius of the professional, to broaden his or her understanding of client needs and the changing times. Other education opportunities may focus on developing one or two specific skills in greater depth.

Commitment to the profession is also a part of professional development. When human service workers become active in an organization or become active members of the community, they expand their professional associations and their professional awareness. Any time they study political issues or become deeply involved in ethical situations that are difficult to comprehend, they are expanding their professional understanding. Even the continuous updating of their knowledge of the community, its workers, and its resources is an informal development process. Finally, working with students through guest lecturing in human service classes, assisting students with special projects, and supervising students in their field experiences are excellent ways to continue learning. The commitment to helping others learn involves growth on the part of the instructor as well.

Conclusion

This chapter on professional concerns concludes your introduction to the field of human services. The material on professional ethics and ethical dilemmas should help you reflect on professional issues in light of your new understanding of human services. Professional development represents a lifelong commitment to study and reflection. Whether it involves resolving ethical dilemmas or focuses on meeting the challenges of demanding clients, professional development supports the worker.

Let us return to Carmen Rodriguez and read her views of the professional issues we have just presented. In her work as a vocational evaluator for a state agency, Carmen has many professional concerns. As you read about her concerns, consider her responsibilities to clients, to the state agency that employs her, and to society in general. Identify any assets or plans that will assist Carmen in moving ahead in her profession.

When I first started this job as a vocational evaluator four years ago, one of the first things the agency did was to send me to the state office for inservice training. This really served as my orientation to the agency and its goals and services. It also helped me to realize how very important it is to attend meetings and conferences because they provide you with the latest information about legislation, new agency guidelines, and state-of-the-art ways of working with clients.

The agency I work for supports professional development by sponsoring workshops and providing financial support and leave time to attend other conferences. It organizes an annual conference in May for all its employees. I have attended for the past three years and found that it's a great way to meet other vocational evaluators from across the state. Sometimes, some business even takes place. For example, last year I was approached by two workers from another area who were referring a client to my facility. They wanted me to be on the lookout for the client and to help him adjust to the facility. It's really good business practice to know someone at a facility, because with a personal contact, referrals do tend to be smoother.

Another way the agency promotes networking is by requiring follow-up studies of clients. My workplace is a statewide facility—clients are referred to us from all over the state. For one week each summer, each worker at our facility is responsible for traveling to one section of the state to meet with workers and to follow up on the clients we have served during the past year. This is also a good way to meet other state employees, to hear their concerns about the agency and their work, and to promote the work of our facility. I must admit it's also nice to get away from the usual work setting.

I am quite excited about two other recent developments. One is that I hope to pursue my master's degree part-time while continuing to work here at the agency—which has agreed to pay part of my tuition; that will certainly be a big help. As you may know, I want to develop my counseling skills to work with clients as individuals or in groups in a more specialized way. Second, two months from now my facility will begin accepting clients who are deaf. In preparation to serve this new client group, all workers will attend a sign language class at the facility, three times a week. I am really excited about learning this new skill. I don't know whether I've ever been around a deaf person before, and I don't know anything about deafness. It should be an interesting experience and will certainly increase my skills. I may even think about becoming an interpreter.

Besides opportunities for professional development, other professional concerns arise periodically. Often there are no quick answers, and in these situations I've found my co-workers to be very helpful. For example, we deal with a lot of confidential information about our clients, and it's sometimes very confusing trying to determine who has access to the files. Of course, all the workers within the agency do, because they need the information to provide services to the client. But other agencies frequently request information. I always check with my co-workers and supervisor before I release anything.

I had something very interesting happen to me after I was on the job two months. One of the first things I learned was that client information was confidential. What was discussed between the client and the worker was also confidential. I did try to summarize important conversations or interview information in the client's case file for future reference. Was I surprised when my records on a client were subpoenaed one day! The agency's attorney came to the facility to pick up the records to take them to court. I learned how important it is to document carefully and objectively, but I still haven't resolved for myself what kinds of information should be documented. I mean, if I tell the client that our conversations are confidential, and then that information is taken to court, they really aren't confidential. The agency's stand on this is that all pertinent information relating to the client should be documented and that this comes before worker-client confidentiality. I haven't quite resolved that dilemma yet.

Another difficult time for me is when I work with a client in planning services for the future. One of the first things that the planning form calls for is a documented disability that is a handicap to employment. It is important that the client understand the disability, the limitations it involves, and how those limitations relate to the plan. It's a little like the notion of informed consent. Clients must understand what is going on and by their signatures indicate that they are aware of the vocational plan that has been developed. It's really a good idea to have client input. But do you have any idea how difficult it is to explain to someone what "mentally retarded" means or why you can't recommend a college program?

Professional development activities, such as attending conferences and participating in inservice training, have helped me think about the dilemmas in my work. I haven't resolved them all, but talking with other workers, reading professional journals, and participating in professional organizations are important ways to grow as a professional.

✧ Things to Remember

1. In the course of delivering human services, the human service professional may encounter numerous ethical dilemmas; for some of these, the worker may be unsure of the appropriate action to take.
2. Professionals have responded to the dilemmas of service provision by developing codes of ethics or statements of ethical standards of behavior for the members of their profession. Items are included that state the

goals or aims of the profession, protect the client, provide guidance as to professional behavior, and contribute to a professional identity for the worker.

3. Most codes of ethics indicate that the helper's first responsibility is to enhance and protect the client's welfare.
4. Two areas with which helpers concern themselves are their *competence* as professionals and their *responsibility* to the individuals, groups, or organizations with whom they are affiliated or whom they serve as clients.
5. *Confidentiality* is the worker's assurance to the client that information divulged by the client will remain between the two of them.
6. Two examples of clients' rights are the *right to privacy* and *informed consent.*
7. The word *ladder* within the term *career ladder* connotes the ability to climb higher; in professional terms, this means advancing as a professional by getting a "better" job, with more responsibility, prestige, recognition, and a higher salary. The career ladder for human services is not as well defined as in some other professions, but it does exist.
8. Basically, there are three ways that professions can be regulated: registry, certification, and licensure.
9. Two possible pitfalls limit professional development: encapsulation and burnout.

Additional Readings: Focus on Professionalism

Bollas, C., & Sundelson, D. (1995). *The new informants: The betrayal of confidentiality in psychoanalysis and psychotherapy.* Northvale, NJ: Aronson.

The authors survey, analyze, and attack the trend away from secrecy, which they attribute partly to the let-it-all-hang-out standard of contemporary culture.

Dickenson, D. T. (1995). *Law and the health and human services.* New York: Free Press.

This book focuses specifically on the law as it applies to the broad field of health and human services and on the legal issues that challenge its many professionals.

Johnson, D. W. (1993). *Reaching out: Interpersonal effectiveness and self-actualization* (5th ed.). Boston: Allyn & Bacon.

Reaching Out outlines the theory and experience necessary to develop effective interpersonal skills such as building relationships, resolving interpersonal conflicts, and increasing communication skills.

Rinas, J., & Clyne-Jackson, S. (1988). *Professional conduct and legal concerns in mental health practice.* Norwalk, CT: Appleton & Lange.

The authors describe in detail the current status of ethical and legal issues such as responsibility, competency, client rights, and third-party interactions. The issues are illustrated in terms of treatment, assessment, and research.

References

A world in need. (1996, June 24). *U.S. News & World Report, 120,* 20.

Afifi, A., & Breslow, L. (1994). The maturing paradigm of public health. *Annual Review of Public Health, 15,* 223–235.

Aguilera, D. C., & Messick, J. M. (1993). *Crisis intervention: Theory and methodology* (7th ed.). St. Louis: C. V. Mosby.

Albee, G. W. (1961a). *Action for mental health.* New York: Basic Books.

Albee, G. W. (1961b). *Mental health manpower trends.* New York: Basic Books.

Alley, S., & Blanton, J. (1976). A study of paraprofessionals in mental health. *Community Mental Health Journal, 12*(2), 151–160.

Atchley, R. C., & Miller, S. J. (1979). Housing and households of the rural aged. In T. O. Byerts, S. C. Howell, & L. A. Pastalan (Eds.), *Environmental context of aging: Life-styles, environmental quality and living arrangements* (pp. 62–79). New York: Garland STPM Press.

Auletta, K. (1982). *The underclass.* New York: Random House.

Austin, C. (1983). Case management: A systems perspective. *Families in Society: The Journal of Contemporary Human Services, 79*(9), 451–459.

Austin, D. M. (1993). The political economy of human services. *Policy and Politics, 11*(3), 343–359.

Austin, M. J., Kopp, J., & Smith, P. L. (1986). *Delivering human services* (2nd ed.). New York: Longman.

Austin, M. J., Skelding, A. H., & Smith, P. L. (1977). *Delivering human services: An introductory programmed text.* New York: Harper & Row.

Axelson, J. A. (1985). *Counseling and development in a multicultural society.* Pacific Grove, CA: Brooks/Cole.

Barber, B. (1965). Some problems in the sociology of the professions. In K. Lynn (Ed.), *The professions in America* (pp. 15–34). Boston: Houghton Mifflin.

Barker, B. (1996). *The management of information.* Presentation conducted at the Managed Care Institute: Futurecare preparing for managed care and children's services, Nashville, Tennessee.

Barr, C. W. (1996a, August 28). World activists meet to combat child sex trade. *The Christian Science Monitor,* pp. 9–11.

Barr, C. W. (1996b, September 16). Getting adults to think in new ways. *The Christian Science Monitor,* pp. 9–11.

Baruth, L. G., & Huber, C. H. (1984). *An introduction to marital theory and therapy.* Pacific Grove, CA: Brooks/Cole.

Bassoff, E. (1987). Mothering adolescent daughters: A psychodynamic perspective. *Journal of Counseling and Development, 65*(9), 471–474.

Beall, G. T., Thompson, M. M., Godwin, F., & Donahue, W. T. (1981). *Housing older persons in rural America: A handbook on congregate housing.* Washington, DC: International Center for Social Gerontology.

Beckman, L., & Mays, V. (1985). Educating community gatekeepers about alcohol abuse in women: Changing attitudes, knowledge, and referral practice. *Journal of Drug Education, 15*(4), 289–309.

Beers, C. W. (1945). A *mind that found itself.* Garden City, NY: Doubleday, Doran & Co.

Bennett, L. W. (1995). Substance abuse and the domestic assault of women. *Social Work, 40*(6), 760–771.

Berglas, S. (1985). Why did this happen to me? *Psychology Today, 17*(2), 44–48.

Blake, W. M., & Darling, C. A. (1994). The dilemmas of the African American male. *Journal of Black Studies, 24*(4), 402–415.

Blankertz, L. E., & Cnaan, R. A. (1995). Assessing the impact of two residential programs for dually diagnosed homeless individuals. *Social Service Review, 68*(4), 536–560.

Blazer, D., Landermann, L. R., Fillenbaum, G., & Horner, R. (1995). Health services access and use among older adults in North Carolina: Urban vs. rural residents. *American Journal of Public Health, 85*(10), 1384–1390.

Bliss, W. (1908). *The new encyclopedia of social reform.* New York: Funk & Wagnalls.

Booth, N., & Owen, E. (1985). The relevance of formal and informal networks for community development. *Research in Rural Sociology and Development, 2,* 159–172.

Bornstein, M. H. (1979). The pace of life: Revisited. *International Journal of Psychology, 14,* 83–90.

Bosworth, K. (1994). [On-line]. Computer games and simulations as tools to reach and engage adolescents in health promotion activities. *Computers in Human Services, 11*(1/2). Abstract from http\\www.uta.edu\cuss\vol11.htm

Bowler, M. (1974). *The Nixon guaranteed income proposal: Substance and process in policy change.* Cambridge, MA: Ballinger.

Boy, A., & Pine, G. (1968). *The counselor in the schools: A reconceptualization.* Boston: Houghton Mifflin.

Brammer, L. M. (1977). Who can be a helper? *Personnel and Guidance Journal, 56*(6), 303–308.

Brammer, L. M. (1978). Informal helping systems in selected subcultures. *Personnel and Guidance Journal, 56*(8), 476–479.

Brammer, L. M. (1995). *The helping relationship* (6th ed.). Englewood Cliffs, NJ: Prentice Hall.

Brill, N. (1995). *Working with people* (5th ed.). White Plains, NY: Longman.

Brisman, J. (1996). Learning to listen: Therapeutic encounters and negotiations in the early stage of treatment. *Eating Disorders: The Journal of Treatment and Prevention,* 2(1), 68–73.

Brown, D., & Srebalus, D. J. (1995). *An introduction to the counseling profession* (2nd ed.). Englewood Cliffs, NJ: Prentice Hall.

Brown, T. (1991, June 3). Want to be a real team? *Industry Week,* p. 17.

Brown, T. (1992, March 2). Why teams go bust. *Industry Week,* p. 20.

Bruch, H. (1983). *Eating disorders: Obesity, anorexia nervosa, and the person within.* New York: Basic Books.

Budman, S. H., & Gurman, A. S. (1988). *Theory and practice of brief therapy.* New York: Guilford.

Butterfield, F. (1996, November 21). In Boston, nothing is something. *The New York Times,* p. A8.

Cahill, J. M. (1994). [On-line]. HEALTHWORKS: Interactive AIDS education mldeogrames. *Computers in Human Services, 11*(1/2). Abstract from http\\www.uta.edu\cuss\vol11.htm

Cahill, M. (1993). Computer technology and human services in the 90s: Advancing theory and practice: Teleshopping and social services in the United Kingdom. In M. Leiderman, C. Guzetta, L. Struminger, & M. Monnickdam (Eds.), *Technology in people services: Research, theory, and application* (pp. 231–245). New York: Haworth.

Campbell, J. C., Harris, M. J., & Lee, R. K. (1995, Summer). Violence research: An overview. Special issue: Nursing's response to our culture of violence. *Scholarly Inquiry for Nursing Practice, 9*(2), 105–126.

Caplan, G. (1964). *Principles of preventive psychiatry.* New York: Basic Books.

Career Track. (1991). *How to build and lead your team.* Boulder, CO: Author.

Carlton, L. I. (1991). Some consideration of the rural elderly black's underuse of social services. *Journal of Gerontological Social Work, 16*(1/2), 3–17.

Carroll, R. A. (1986). Resource exhange: A catalyst for networking in rehabilitation. *American Rehabilitation, 12*(4), 18–19.

Carter, J. (1979). *Message from the President of the United States transmitting a draft of proposed legislation to improve the provisions of mental health services and otherwise promote mental health throughout the United States; and for other purposes* (House Document No. 96–125). Washington, DC: U.S. Government Printing Office.

Caserata, M., Lund, D., Wright, S., & Redburn, D. (1987). Caregivers to dementia patients: The utilization of community services. *Gerontologist, 27*(2), 209–214.

Cherniss, C. (1980). *Professional burnout in human service organizations.* New York: Praeger.

Chilman, C. S. (1995). Programs and policies for working poor families: Major trends and some research issues. *Social Service Review, 69*(3), 516–524.

Cimmino, P. (1996). Basic concepts and definitions of human services. In H. S. Harris & D. C. Maloney (Eds.), *Human services: Contemporary issues and trends* (pp. 3–27). Boston, MA: Allyn & Bacon.

Clear, T. R., & Cole, G. F. (1990). *American corrections* (2nd ed.). Pacific Grove, CA: Brooks/Cole.

Cogan, D. B., & Wood, A. C. (1987). A survey of the introductory course in mental health and human services. *Human Service Education, 8*(2), 1–8.

Cohen, R., & Lavach, C. (1995). Strengthening partnerships between families and service providers. In P. Adams & K. Nelson (Eds.), *Reinventing human services: Community and family-centered practice* (pp. 262–277). New York: Aldine DeGruyter.

Collier, R. (1965). *The general next to God: The story of William Booth and the Salvation Army.* New York: Dutton.

Combs, A. W. (1969). *Florida studies in the helping professions.* Gainesville: University of Florida Press.

Committee Study of the Future of Public Health Institute of Medicine. (1988). *The future of public health.* Washington, DC: National Academy Press.

Conlin, M. M. (1995, November). Silent suffering: A case study of elder abuse and neglect. *Journal of the American Geriatrics Society, 43*(11), 1303–1308.

Cooney, C., & Howard, R. (1995, September). Abuse of patients with dementia by carers—out of sight but not out of mind. *International Journal of Geriatric Psychiatry, 10*(9), 735–741.

Cormier, M. (1979). From the Council president. *Bulletin: Council for Standards in Human Service Education, 1*(1), p. 1.

Council for Standards in Human Service Education (CSHSE). (1985). *Handbook* (2nd ed.). Atlanta: Author.

Craig, S. S., & Hennessy, J. J. (1989). Personality differences and expectations about counseling. *Journal of Counseling Psychology, 36*(4), 401–407.

Cranston, A. (1986, September). Psychology in the Veterans Administration. *American Psychologist, 41*(9), 990–995.

Crimando, W., & Riggar, T. F. (1996). *Utilizing community resources: An overview of human services.* Delray Beach, FL: St. Lucia.

Crossette, B. (1995, December 11). UNICEF sees children as major victims of war. *The New York Times,* p. A7.

Crossette, B. (1996, June 11). New tally of world tragedy: Women who die giving life. *The New York Times,* pp. A1, A7.

Daley, J. M., & Poole, D. L. (1985). Community development insights for planning public social service innovations. *Research in Rural Sociology and Development, 2,* 143–157.

Danish, S. J., D'Augelli, A. R., & Ginsberg, M. R. (1984). Life development intervention: The promotion of mental health through the development of competence. In S. D. Brown & R. W. Lent (Eds.), *Handbook of counseling psychology* (pp. 520–544). New York: Wiley.

Daum, K. (1996, September 17). Sexually exploited children in Canada: The law is not on their side. *The Christian Science Monitor,* p. 19.

D'Augelli, A. R. (1989). AIDS fears and homophobia among rural nursing personnel. *AIDS Education and Prevention, 1*(4), 277–284.

D'Augelli, A., & Hart, M. (1987). Gay women, men, and families in rural settings: Toward the development of helping communities. *American Journal of Community Psychology, 15*(l), 79–93.

Department of Veterans Affairs. (1996). *VA fact sheet.* Washington, DC: Office of Public Affairs News Service.

DePoy, E., & Butler, S. S. (1996). Health: Elderly rural women's conceptions. *Journal of Woman and Social Work, 11*(2), 207–220.

Desjarlais, R., Eisenberg, L., Good, B., & Kleinman, A. (1995). *World mental health: Problems and priorities in low-income counties.* New York: Oxford University Press.

DeVita, C. J. (1989). *America in the twenty-first century: A demographic overview.* Washington, DC: Population Reference Bureau.

DeWitt, Elmer P. (1994, July 25). Battle for the soul INTERNET. *Time,* pp. 50–56.

Dunn, G. (1987). Allegheny Community College mental health graduate data summary report. (Available from Gary Dunn, Willowbrook Road, Cumberland, MD 21502-2596).

Eckstein, E. (1995). CASA's kids. *Spirit.* Dallas, TX: American Airlines Magazine Publications.

Egan, G. (1994). *The skilled helper: A problem-management approach to helping* (5th ed.). Pacific Grove, CA: Brooks/Cole.

Ehrenreich, J. (1985). *The altruistic imagination.* Ithaca, NY. Cornell University Press.

Ellis, S. J., & Noyes, K. H. (1978). *By the people: A history of Americans as volunteers.* Philadelphia: Energize.

Emlet, C. A., & Hall, A. M. (1991). Integrating the community into geriatric case management: Public health interventions. *The Gerontologist, 31*(4), 556–560.

English, J. T., Kritzler, Z. A., & Scherl, D. J. (1984). Historical trends in the financing of psychiatric services. *Psychiatric Annals, 14*(5), 321–331.

Epstein, C. (1981). *Introduction to human services.* Englewood Cliffs, NJ: Prentice Hall.

Eriksen, K. (1981). *Human services today.* Reston, VA: Reston Publishing.

Erikson, E. (1963). *Childhood and society.* New York: Norton.

Ethical standards of human service professionals. (1996). *Human Service Education, 16,* 11–17.

Fast, J. (1970). *Body language.* New York: M. Evans.

Fernandes, N. (1995, October 15). Bombay street kids become entrepreneurs. *Seattle Times,* p. A4.

Figueira-McDonough, J. (1995, March). Community and the underclass: Exploring new practice directions. *Social Service Review, 69*(1), 57–85.

Fischer, P. J., Shapiro, S., Breakey, W. R., Anthony, J. C., & Kramer, M. (1986). Mental health and social characteristics of the homeless: A survey of mission users. *American Journal of Public Health, 76*(5), 419–524.

For a healthy nation. (1988). Washington, DC: U.S. Department of Health and Human Services, Public Health Services.

Fordham, G. (1993, October). Sustaining local involvement. *Community Development Journal, 28*(4), 299–304.

Foster, S. (1995, December). Rising to the challenge. *Counseling Today,* pp. 14, 16, 27.

Franklin, R. M. (1995, September). Emotion and the physician-patient relationship. *Motivation and Emotion, 19*(3), 163–173.

French, M. (1986). Pitt Community College graduate placement data. (Available from Margaret French, Pitt Community College).

Frenk, J. (1993). The new public health. *Annual Review of Public Health,* 14, 469–490.

Frey, D. (1984). The counselor's role in the treatment of anorexia nervosa and bulimia. *Journal of Counseling and Development, 63,* 248–249.

Friedman, D. (1996, March 25). Ahead: A very different nation. *U.S. News & World Report,* 120, p. 16.

Friedrich, 0. (1976). *Going crazy: An inquiry into madness in our time.* New York: Avon Books.

Fullerton, S. (1996). Theories as tools and resources for helping. In H. S. Harris & D. C. Maloney (Eds.), *Human services: Contemporary issues and trends* (pp. 113–120). Boston, MA: Allyn & Bacon.

Fujimura, L. E., Weis, D. M., & Cochran, J. R. (1985). Suicide: Dynamics and implications for counseling. *Journal of Counseling and Development, 63,* 612–615.

Ganguli, M., Gilby, J., Seaberg, E., & Belle, S. (1995). Depressive symptoms and associated factors in a rural elderly population. *American Journal of Geriatric Psychiatry, 3*(2), 144–160.

Gardner, M. (1996, March 21). Tide shifts on how to protect abused children. *The Christian Science Monitor,* p. 12.

Gariti, P., Alterman, A. I., Holub-Beyer, E., & Volpicelli, J. R. (1995, May–June). Effects of an appointment reminder call on patient show rates. *Journal of Substance Abuse Treatment, 12*(3), 207–212.

Gelles, R. J. (1981). The myth of battered husbands and new facts about family violence. In J. B. Williamson, L. Evans, & A. Munley (Eds.), *Social problems: The contemporary debates* (pp. 246–260). Boston: Little, Brown.

Gelman, D. (1988, March 7). Black and white in America. *Newsweek,* pp. 18–23.

Gill, S. (1982). Professional disclosure and consumer protection in counseling. *Personnel and Guidance Journal, 60*(7), 443–446.

Ginsberg, L. (1987). Economic, political, and social context. In L. H. Ginsberg (Ed.), *Encyclopedia of social work* (18th ed., pp. xxxiii–xli). Silver Spring, MD: National Association of Social Workers.

Golden, T. (1996, August 1). People on welfare, too, find a lot to criticize. *The New York Times,* p. A9.

Goodman, M., Brown, J., & Dietz, P. (1992). *Managing managed care.* Washington, DC: American Psychiatric Press.

Gould, P. L. (1992). Adult developmental brief computer-assisted therapy. In J. L. Feldman & R. J. Fitzpatrick (Eds.), *Managed mental healthcare* (pp. 347–358). Washington, DC: American Psychiatric Press.

Granello, M. S. (1995, March/April). Creating links: Electronically. *The Advocate, 18*(7), p. 6.

Gray, J. I. (1994). [On-line]. Problem solving in case management (PIC): A computer assisted instruction simulation. *Computers in Human Services, 11*(1/2). Abstract from http\\www.uta.edu\cuss\vol11.htm

Grebel, H. W. (1993). Information technology in the care of the mentally handicapped: An educational approach. In M. Leiderman, C. Guzetta, L. Struminger, & M. Monnickendam (Eds.), *Technology in people services: Research, theory, and application* (pp. 329–335). New York: Haworth.

Grier, P. (1996, March 6). New Census Bureau portrait of the American landscape. *The Christian Science Monitor,* p. 3.

Gross, A., & McMullen, P. (1982). The help seeking process. In V. Derlega & J. Grzelak (Eds.), *Cooperation and helping behavior* (pp. 306–324). New York: Academic Press.

Gruber, M. (Ed.). (1981). *Management systems in the human services.* Philadelphia: Temple University Press.

Haber, R., & Runyon, R. P. (1983). *Fundamentals of psychology.* Reading, MA: Addison-Wesley.

Hacker, A. (1995). *Two nations: Black and white, separate, hostile, unequal.* New York: Ballantine Books.

Hagebak, B. R. (1982). *Getting local agencies to cooperate.* Baltimore: University Park Press.

Hamlin, P. (1985). *Experiences in mental institutions: Case studies.* Unpublished manuscript.

Harris, H. S., & Maloney, D. C. (Eds.). (1996). *Human services: Contemporary issues and trends.* Boston: Allyn & Bacon.

Harris, P. R., & Moran, R. T. (1996). *Managing cultural differences* (4th ed.). Houston: Gulf.

Harrison, P. (1980). *Inside the Third World. The anatomy of poverty.* Brighton, U.K.: Harvester Press.

Hayman, P. M., & Covert, J. A. (1986). Ethical dilemmas in college counseling centers. *Journal of Counseling and Development, 64*(5), 318–320.

Hayman, P. M., Sommers-Flanagan, R., & Parsons, J. P. (1987). Aftermath of violence: Posttraumatic stress disorder among Vietnam veterans. *Journal of Counseling and Development, 65,* 363–366.

Hazard, T. G. (1844, April 10). Astonishing tenacity of life. *Providence Journal,* pp. 252–253.

Hazzard, W. R. (1995, November). Elder abuse: Definitions and implications for medical education. *Academic Medicine, 70*(11), 979–981.

Healthy people 2000: Midcourse review and 1995 revisions. (1995). Washington, DC: U.S. Department of Health and Human Services, Public Health Service.

Heard, B. C. (1995). *Patterns of health care utilization among rural elderly population of East Texas.* University of Texas at Arlington, *1*(3), Number 1251.

Hecht, D. (1996, July 25). Senegal's kid workers unite, demand rights. *The Christian Science Monitor,* p. 6.

Henton, J., Cate, R., & Emery, B. (1984). The dependent elderly: Targets for abuse. In W. H. Quinn & G. A. Hughson (Eds.), *Independent aging* (pp. 149–162). Rockville, MD: Aspen.

Herlihy, B., & Sheeley, V. L. (1987). Privileged communication in selected helping professions: A comparison among statutes. *Journal of Counseling and Development, 65*(9), 479–483.

Higginbotham, H. N. (1979). Culture and mental health services. In A. J. Marsella, R.G. Tharp, & T. Ciborowski (Eds.), *Perspectives on cross cultural psychology* (pp. 307–332). New York: Academic Press.

Highlights of the new law. (1996, August 23). *USA Today,* p. 3A.

Holland, B. E. (1996). Home health services. In W. Crimando & T. F. Riggar (Eds.), *Utilizing community resources: An overview of human services* (pp. 21–28). Delray, Florida: St. Lucie.

Holmes, S. (1996, March 14). Census sees a profound shift in ethnic U.S. *The New York Times,* p. A8.

Hornblower, Margot. (1996, June 3). It takes a school: A new approach to elementary education starts at birth and doesn't stop when the bell rings. *Time,* p. 37.

Husain, I. (1996, July 1). Global experience is bringing better antipoverty programs. *The Christian Science Monitor,* p. 19.

Hutchins, D. E., & Cole Vaught, C. (1997). *Helping relationships and strategies* (3rd ed.). Pacific Grove, CA: Brooks/Cole.

Iglehart, J. K. (1996). Health policy report: Politics and public health. *Health Policy Report, 334,* 203–207.

International Study Project. (1972). *Abraham H. Maslow: A memorial volume.* Pacific Grove, CA: Brooks/Cole.

Ivey, A. E. (1994). *Intentional interviewing and counseling.* Pacific Grove, CA: Brooks/Cole.

James, V. (1981, April). Mental health worker news: A forum for the mental health forum. *Bulletin: Council for Standards in Human Service Education,* p. 4.

Joe, T. (1984, March). Forgotten Americans: The "working poor." *USA Today,* pp. 85–86.

John, R. (1986). Aging in a Native American community: Service needs and support networks among Prairie Band Potawatomi elders. *Dissertation Abstracts International, 47*(6), 23–32A.

Johnson, D. (1996, July 31). One mother's ordeal with life on welfare. *The New York Times,* p. A7.

Johnson, D. E., & Vestermark, M. J. (1970). *Barriers and hazards in counseling.* Boston: Houghton Mifflin.

Johnson, D. W. (1993). *Reaching out: Interpersonal effectiveness and self-actualization* (5th ed.). Boston: Allyn & Bacon.

Johnson, L. B. (1964). President's Michigan speech on "The Great Society." *Congressional Quarterly, 20,* 874.

Joint Center for Political and Economic Studies. (1994). *Young black males in jeopardy: Risk factors and intervention strategies.* (SRI MAIN NO: 1996 R5685-19). Washington, DC: Author.

Jones, L., & Wattenberg, E. (1991). Working, still poor: A loan program's role in the lives of low-income single parents. *Social Work, 36*(2), 146–153.

Kantor, D. (1960). *Inducing preferences for mental health careers.* New York: National Association of Social Workers.

Kennedy, J. F. (1964a). Remarks intended for delivery to the Texas Democratic State Committee in the Municipal Auditorium in Austin, November 22, 1963. *Public papers of the presidents of the United States: John F. Kennedy* (January 1–November 22, 1963) (p. 897). Washington, DC: U.S. Government Printing Office.

Kennedy, J. F. (1964b). Remarks on proposed measures to combat mental illness and mental retardation. *Public papers of the presidents of the United States: John F. Kennedy* (January 1–November 22, 1963) (pp. 50–51). Washington, DC: U.S. Government Printing Office.

Kenny, D. T. (1995, September). Determinants of patient satisfaction with the medical consultation. *Psychology and Health, 10*(5), 427–437.

Kessler, K. (1989). Managed psychiatric care will continue to boom. *Clinical Psychiatry News, 17*(9), 6–7.

Kiesler, C. (1991). Homelessness and public priorities. *American Psychologist, 46*(11), 1245–1248.

Kondrates, A. (1991). Ending homelessness: Policy changes. *American Psychologist, 46*(11), 1126–1136.

Kreitner, R. (1983). *Management* (2nd ed.). Boston: Houghton Mifflin.

Kristof, N. D. (1996, April 14). Asian childhoods sacrificed to prosperity's best. *The New York Times,* pp. 1, 6.

Lawson, R., & Anderson, P. (1996). Community-based schools: Collaboration between human services and schools as radical educational reform. In H. S. Harris & D. C. Maloney (Eds.), *Human Services: Contemporary issues and trends* (pp. 161–172). Boston: Allyn & Bacon.

Lederer, E. M. (1996, June 2). 20,000 minds to tackle urbanization problem. *The Atlanta Journal/The Atlanta Constitution,* p. A12.

Lee, G. R., & Lassey, M. L. (1980). Rural-urban differences among the elderly: Economic, social and subjective factors. *Journal of Social Issues, 36,* 62ff.

Leiter, M. P., & Webb, M. (1983). *Developing human service network.* New York: Irvington.

Lenihan, G. O., & Sanders, C. D. (1984). Guidelines for group therapy with eating disorder victims. *Journal of Counseling and Development, 63,* 252–254.

Levinson, D. (1978). *The seasons of a man's life.* New York: Ballantine.

Lewis, J. A., Lewis, M. D., & Soufflée, F. (1991). *Management of human service programs.* Pacific Grove, CA: Brooks/Cole.

Littrell, J. M. (1996). *Resolution-focused counseling in action.* Presentation at the American Counseling Association Professional Development Seminar, Nashville, Tennessee.

Long, L., Paradise, L. V. & Long, T. J. (1981). *Questioning: Skills for the helping process.* Pacific Grove, CA: Brooks/Cole.

Lowry, R. J. (1973). *A. H. Maslow: An intellectual portrait.* Belmont, CA: Wadsworth.

Lyon, W., & Duke, B. J. (1981). *Introduction to human services.* Reston, VA: Reston Publishing.

Mabe, A. R., & Rollin, S. A. (1986). The role of a code of ethical standards in counseling. *Journal of Counseling and Development, 64*(5), 294–297.

Macht, J. (1990). A historical perspective. In S. Fullerton & D. Osher (Eds.), *History of the Human Services Movement,* 7, 90–22.

Maluccio, A. (1979). *Learning from clients.* New York: Free Press.

Mandell, B. R., & Schram, B. (1995). *Human services: Introduction and interventions* (3rd ed.). New York: Wiley.

Marino, T. W. (1966, January). Counselors in cyberspace debate whether client discussions are ethical. *Counseling Today,* p. 18.

Marshall, H. (1937). *The forgotten Samaritan.* Chapel Hill: University of North Carolina Press.

Martz, D. M., Handley, K. B., & Eisler, R. M. (1995). The relationship between feminine gender role stress, body image, and eating disorders. *Psychology of Women Quarterly, 19*(4), 493–508.

Masi, D. (1982). *Human services in industry.* Lexington, MA: Lexington Books.

Maslow, A. (1971). *The farther reaches of human nature.* New York: Viking Press.

Massey, D. S. (1994, December). America's apartheid and the urban underclass. *Social Service Review, 68*(4), 472–487.

Mayer, J. E., & Timms, N. (1969). Clash in perspective between worker and client. *Social Casework, 50*(1), 32–40.

McBride, S. M. (1992). Rehabilitation case managers: Ahead of their time. *Holistic Nursing Practice, 6*(2), 67–75.

McChesney, K. Y. (1995). A review of the empirical literature on contemporary urban homeless families. *Social Service Review, 69*(3), 429–460.

McClam, T. (1992). *Results of follow-up study of graduates: 1992.* Unpublished manuscript. University of Tennessee, Program in Human Services, Knoxville, Tennessee.

McClam, T. (1996). *Results of follow-up study of graduates: 1996.* Unpublished manuscript. University of Tennessee, Program in Human Services, Knoxville, Tennessee.

McClam, T., & Woodside, M. (1994). *Problem solving in the helping professions.* Pacific Grove, CA: Brooks/Cole.

McGinnis, J. M., & Foege, W. H. (1993). Actual causes of death in the United States. *Journal of the American Medical Association, 270,* 2207–2212.

Mehr, J. (1995). *Human services: Concepts and intervention strategies* (6th ed.). Boston: Allyn & Bacon.

Melson, G. F. (1980). *Family and environment: An ecosystem perspective.* Minneapolis: Burgess.

Merritt, J., & Neugeboren, B. (1990). Factors affecting agency capacity for interorganizational coordination. *Administration in Social Work, 15*(4), 73–85.

Middleman, R. R. (1984, March–April). How competent is social work's approach to the assessment of competence? *Social Work, 29*(2), 146–153.

Mills, L. (1996, May). Empowering battered women transnational: The case for postmodern interventions. *Social Work, 41*(3), 261–268.

Moorhouse, W. (1983). *Careers in training and development.* (Available from William Moorhouse, Human Resources Development Area, Oakland University, Rochester, MI 48063).

Moroney, R. (1976). Needs assessment for human services. In W. F. Anderson, B. J. Frieden, & M. J. Murphy (Eds.), *Managing human services.* Washington, DC: International City Management Association.

Morse, G. A., Calsyn, R. J., Allen, G., & Kenny, D. A. (1994, October). Helping homeless mentally ill people: What variables mediate and moderate program effects? *American Journal of Community Psychology,* 22(5), 661–268.

Mortenson, T. G. (Ed.). (1996). *Postsecondary education opportunity.* (SRI MAIN NO: 1996 B6300-1). Iowa City, IA: Postsecondary Education Opportunity.

Myers, J. E., & Shelton, B. (1987). Abuse and older persons: Issues and implications for counselors. *Journal of Counseling and Development, 65,* 376–380.

National Center for Children in Poverty. (1994). *Young children in poverty: A statistical update.* New York: Columbia University School of Public Health.

National Commission for Human Service Workers. (1982). *Registration and certification of human service workers.* Atlanta: Author.

National Institute of Mental Health (NIMH). (1971). *Mental illness and its treatment.* Social issues resources series (Vol. 1, Article #3) (DHEW Publication No. [HSM] 72-9030). Washington, DC: Author.

National Institute of Mental Health. (1985). *You are not alone: Facts about mental health and mental illness* (DHHS Publication No. ADM 85-1178). Washington, DC: U.S. Government Printing Office.

Netting, F. E., Kettner, P. M., & McMurtry, S. L. (1993). *Social work macro practice.* New York: Longman.

Neugebauer, R. (1979). Medieval and early modern theories of mental illness. *Archives of General Psychiatry, 36,* 477–483.

Neugeboren, B. (1991). *Organization, policy, and practice in the human services.* New York: Longman.

Neukrug, E. (1995). *Theory, practice, and trends in human services: An overview of an emerging profession.* Pacific Grove, CA: Brooks/Cole.

New interactive multimedia system for computerized cognitive therapy. (1995, June). *Counseling Today,* 37(12), 44.

Nifong, C. (1996, July 1). Work, or else: Welfare moms strive to meet the ultimatum. *The Christian Science Monitor, 1,* pp. 10–11.

Nifong, C. (1997, January 16). Welfare mom lays plans, with an eye on the clock. *The Christian Science Monitor, 1,* pp. 10–11.

Nooe, R. (1996). *Homeless in Knoxville/Knox County: A ten year examination 1968–1996.* Knoxville, TN: Knoxville Coalition for the Homeless.

Nord, M., & Luloff, A. E. (1995). Homeless children and their families in New Hampshire: A rural perspective. *Social Service Review, 69*(3), 461–478.

Oalcley, C. (1994). [on-line]. SMACK: A computer driven game for at-risk teens. *Computers in Human Services, 11*(1/2). Abstract from http\\www.uta.edu\cuss\vol11.htm

Occupational outlook handbook. (1992–1993). Bulletin 2400. Washington, DC: U.S. Department of Labor, Bureau of Labor Statistics.

Occupational outlook handbook. (1996). Washington, DC: U.S. Department of Labor, Bureau of Labor Statistics.

Okun, B. F. (1997). *Effective helping: Interviewing and counseling techniques* (5th ed.). Pacific Grove, CA: Brooks/Cole.

One-stop shopping for infants and pregnant women. (1992). *Public Welfare, 50*(1), 26–34.

Page, R. C. (1979). Major ethical issues in public offender counseling. *Counseling and Values, 24,* 33–40.

Parham, T. A., & McDavis, R. J. (1987). Black men, an endangered species: Who's really pulling the trigger? *Journal of Counseling and Development, 66,* 24–27.

Parker, G. (1991). Team players and teamwork. *Small Business Reports, 16,* 64–71.

Pattison, E. M. (1984). Cultural level interventions in the arena of alcoholism. *Alcoholism, 8*(2), 160–164.

Pendleton, S. (1992, August 19). Homelessness defies both parties. *Christian Science Monitor, 2,* p. 19.

Perlman, H. H. (1979). *Relationship: The heart of helping people.* Chicago: University of Chicago Press.

Perlman, R. (1975). *Consumers and social services.* New York: Wiley.

Pichot, P. (1985). Remedicalisation of psychiatry. *Psychiatrial Fennica, 16,* 9–17.

Pilisuk, M. (1980, April). The future of human services without funding. *American Journal of Orthopsychiatry, 50*(2), 200–204.

Pinkstaff, E. (1985). An experience in narrative writing to improve public health practice by students. *Journal of Nursing Education, 24*(1), 25–28.

Pins, A. M. (1963). *Who chooses social work, when and why.* New York: Council on Social Work Education.

Pohlman, M. (1986). Technology, corporate mobility and a decline in urban services. *Journal of Sociology and Social Welfare, 13*(1), 171–196.

Ponterotto, J. G. (1985). A counselor's guide to psychopharmacology. *Journal of Counseling and Development, 64,* 109–115.

Poor nations have many of year's 100 million new people. (1995, December 28). *The Knoxville News-Sentinel,* p. A1.

Poullard, J. D., & D'Augelli, A. R. (1989). AIDS fears and homophobia among volunteers in an AIDS prevention program. *Journal of Rural Community Psychology, 10*(1), 29–39.

Powell, G. (1991, April 17). Lessons: Teach the children well. *Knoxville Journal,* p. W4.

Ralston, P. A. (1993). Health promotion for rural black elderly: A comprehensive review. *Journal of Gerontological Social Work, 20*(1/2), 53–78.

Rapoport, L. (1962). The state of crisis: Some theoretical considerations. *Social Service Review, 36*(2), 211–217.

Raths, L. E., Harmin, M., & Simon, S. B. (1978). *Values and teaching: Working with values in the classroom.* Columbus, OH: Merrill.

Ray, J. R., & Warden, M. K. (1995). *Technology, computers, and the special needs learner.* Albany, NY: Delmar.

Reinhard, S. (1986). Financing long-term health care of the elderly: Dismantling the medical model. *Public Health Nursing, 3*(1), 3–22.

Resnick, H. (1994). [On-line]. Electronic technology and rehabilitation: A computerized simulation game for youthful offenders. *Computers in Hu-*

man Services, 11(1/2). Abstract from http\\www.uta.edu\cuss\vol11.htm

Rhodes, R., & Johnson, A. D. (1994). Women and alcoholism: A psychosocial approach. *AFFILIA Journal of Woman and Social Work, 20*(1/2), 53–78.

Richmond, M. (1917). *Social diagnosis.* New York: Russell Sage Foundation.

Riessman, F. (1979). Self-help. In S. Alley, J. Blanton, & R. Feldman (Eds.), *Paraprofessionals in mental health: Theory and practice* (pp. 319–328). New York: Human Sciences Press.

Rinas, J., & Clyne-Jackson, S. (1988). *Professional conduct and legal concerns in mental health practice.* Norwalk, CT: Appleton & Lange.

Ritchie, M. H. (1986). Counseling the involuntary client. *Journal of Counseling and Development, 64*(8), 516–518.

Rivlin, L. G. (1986). A new look at the homeless. *Social Policy, 16*(4), 3–10.

Rogers, C. (1958). The characteristics of a helping relationship. *Personnel and Guidance Journal, 37*(1), 6–16.

Roth, J. A. (1994). *Public Welfare, 52*(4), 33–43.

Rowles, G. D. (1986). The rural elderly and the church. *Journal of Religion and Aging, 2*(1–2), 79–98.

Sack, D. (1995, November, 25). Volunteering made easier for busy young workers. *The New York Times,* pp. A1, 9.

Sallee, M. (1986, October 2). *Teen pregnancy.* Address to the Annual Meeting of Planned Parenthood of East Tennessee.

The Samaritans. (1985). *Principles and practices.* Slough, U.K.: Author.

Schafer, K. (1996). *Managed care and children's services.* Presentation conducted at the Managed Care Institute: Futurecare preparing for managed care and children's services in Tennessee, Nashville.

Schneider-Braus, K. (1992). Managing a mental health department in a staff model HMO. In J. L. Feldman & R. T. Fitzpatrick (Eds.), *Managed mental health care* (pp. 125–141). Washington, DC: American Psychiatric Press.

Schmolling, P., Jr., Youkeles, M., & Burger, W. R. (1997). *Human services in contemporary America* (4th ed.). Pacific Grove, CA: Brooks/Cole.

Schoech, D., & Arangio, T. (1979, March). Computers in the human services. *Social Work, 24*(2), 96–102.

Schulman, E. (1982). *Intervention in human services.* St. Louis: C. V. Mosby.

Sciolino, E. (1996, November 12). A painful road from Vietnam to forgiveness. *The New York Times,* pp. A1, 8.

Scott, C., & Jaffe, D. (1991). *Empowerment: A practical guide for success.* Menlo Park, CA: Crisp Publications.

Sheehy, G. (1995). *New passages: Mapping your life across time.* New York: Ballantine.

Sherraden, M. W. (1984). Working over the "underclass." *Social Work, 29*(4), 391–392.

Shirreffs, J. H. (1982). *Community health: Contemporary perspectives.* Englewood Cliffs, NJ: Prentice Hall.

Shisslak, C. M., Crago, M., & Estes, L. S. (1995). The spectrum of eating disturbances. *International Journal of Eating Disorders, 18*(3), 209–219.

Sielski, L. M. (1979). Understanding body language. *Personnel and Guidance Journal,* 57(5), 238–242.

Sijuwada, P. O. (1995). Cross-cultural perspectives on elder abuse as a family dilemma. *Social Behavior and Personality, 23*(3), 247–251.

Smith, C. (1996, September). The link between childhood maltreatment and teenage pregnancy. *Social Work Research, 20*(3), 131–141.

Smith, L. D. (1977). Crisis intervention theory and practice. *Community Mental Health Review,* 2(1), 1, 5–13.

Smothers, R. (1996, July 1). As Olympics approach, homeless are not feeling at home. *The New York Times,* p. A11.

Snyder, W. T. (1996, February). *Opportunities for partnering between profes-*

sional societies and universities. Paper presented at the meeting of WATTEC, Knoxville, Tennessee.

Southern Regional Education Board. (1969). *Roles and functions for different levels of mental health workers.* Atlanta: Author.

Southern Regional Education Board. (1979). *Staff roles for mental health personnel: A history and a rationale.* Atlanta: Author.

Spence, S. A. (1993). Rural elderly African Americans and service delivery: A study of health and social service needs and service accessibility. *Journal of Gerontological Social Work, 20* (3/4), 187–202.

Spicuzza, F., & Spicuzza, B. (1979). A human services model of helping: Theory and practice. *Journal of Humanics, 7*(1), 3–18.

Stadler, H. (1986). Preface to the special issue. *Journal of Counseling and Development, 64*(5), 291–292.

Steinmetz, S. K. (1982). Battered parents. In J. B. Williamson, L. Evans, & A. Munley (Eds.), *Social problems: The contemporary debates* (pp. 257–260). Boston: Little, Brown.

Stevens, A. (1985, January 13). Caring about the working poor. *New York Times Book Review,* p. 7.

Sullivan, W., Wolk, J., & Hartman, D. (1992). Case management in alcohol and drug treatment: Improving client outcome. *Families in Society: The Journal of Contemporary Human Services, 73*(9), 195–204.

Swisher, R. (1991). The underclass debate. *Journal of Planning, 6,* 93–99.

Talmon, M. (1990). *Single-session therapy: Maximizing the effect of the first (and often only) therapeutic encounter.* San Francisco: Jossey-Bass.

Tarasoff v. *Regents of the University of California.* (1976). *Pacific Reporter,* 2nd Series, 551, 340.

Taylor, C. (1985). *Carl Rogers and client-centered therapy.* Unpublished manuscript. Knoxville, Tennessee.

Taylor, M., Bradley, V., & Warren, R. (1996). *The community support skill standards.* Washington, DC: Human Service Research Institute.

Teague, D. (1970). *Background information.* Boulder, CO: WICHE Project for Manpower Utilization. Unpublished manuscript.

Teare, R. J., & McPheeters, H. L. (1970). *Manpower utilization in social welfare.* Social and Rehabilitation Service Grant. Atlanta: Southern Regional Education Board.

Tennyson, W. W., & Strom, S. M. (1986). Beyond professional standards: Developing responsibleness. *Journal of Counseling and Development, 64*(5), 298–302.

Tims, M. (1961). *Jane Addams of Hull House: 1860–1935: A centenary study.* London: Allen & Unwin.

Toczek-McPeake, A., & Matthews, M. (1995, September–October). Quality management: A survey of client and career satisfaction with speech pathology and physiotherapy services in a rehabilitation setting. *Journal of Cognitive Rehabilitation, 13(5), 12–18.*

Trattner, W. I. (1994). *From poor law to welfare state: A history of social welfare in America* (5th ed.). New York: Free Press.

Truesdale, L. (1987). Sample list of employers. (Available from Linda Truesdale, Midlands Technical College, P.O. Box 2408, Columbia, SC 29202)

20 Hot Job Tracks: Career Guide 1996. (1995, October 30). *U.S. News & World Report, 119*(17), pp. 104, 108.

20 Hot Job Tracks: Career Guide 1997. (1996, October 28). *U.S. News & World Report, 121*(17), p. 95.

Turner, S. (1992). Alcoholism and depression in women. *AFFILIA Journal of Women and Social Work, 7*(3), 8–22.

Tyson, A. S. (1995, December 6). Keeping it together—barely. *The Christian Science Monitor,* pp. 10–11.

United Nations world population chart. (1992). New York: Population Division, Department of Economic and Social Development, United Nations.

U.S. Census Bureau. (1996). *Population projections of the United States by age, sex, race and Hispanic origin: 1995 to 2050.* Washington, DC: U.S. Government Printing Office.

U.S. Conference of Mayors. (1995). *Status report on hunger and homelessness in America's cities* (SRI MAIN NO: 1996 A9330-9). Washington, DC: U.S. Conference of Mayors.

U.S. Public Health Service. (1981). *Healthstyle: A self-test.* Washington, DC: Office of Disease Prevention and Health Promotion.

Vandereycken, W. (1993). *The sociocultural roots of the fight against fatness: Implications for eating disorders and obesity.* Treating Obesity Conference, Radford, Virginia.

VanHoose, W. H. (1986). Ethical principles in counseling. *Journal of Counseling and Development, 65*(3), 168–169.

VanHoose, W H., & Paradise, L. V. (1979). *Ethics in counseling and psychotherapy: Perspectives in issues and decision-making.* Cranston, RI: Carroll.

Van Strien, T. (1996). On the relationship between dieting and "obese" and bulimic eating patterns. *International Journal of Eating Disorders, 19*(1), 83–92.

Vatterott, M., Callier, J., & Hile, M. (1992). [On-line]. *Computers in Human Services, 8* (3/4). Abstract from http//www.uta.edu/cuss/vol11.htm

Vidaver, R. (1973). Developments in human service education and manpower. In H. Schulberg, F. Baker, & S. Roen (Eds.), *Developments in human services* (Vol. 1, pp. 508–524). New York: Behavioral Publications.

Vissing, Y. M., Salloway, J. C., & Siress, D. L. (1994). Training for expertise versus training for trust: Issues in rural gerontology. *Educational Gerontology, 20*(6), 797–808.

Von Bertalanffy, L. (1968). *General system theory.* New York: Braziller.

Vreeland, E. (1991, July 14). Teachers: Social ills taking toll in class. *Knoxville News-Sentinel,* p. B1.

Vriend, J., & Dyer, W. W. (1973). Counseling the reluctant client. *Journal of Counseling Psychology, 20*(3), 240–246.

Walker, R. J., Pomeroy, E. C., McNeil, J. S., & Franklin, C. (1994). A psychoeducational model for caregivers of patients with Alzheimer's disease. *Journal of Gerontological Social Work,* 22(1/2), 75–91.

Weaver, C. (1994). The interrelationship of parenting stress, marital violence, and child behavior problems. *Social Work Abstracts* 1997-9/96, Number 30163.

Webb, B. (1996). *The management of information.* Presentation conducted at the Managed Care Institute: Futurecare preparing for managed care and children's services, Nashville, Tennessee.

Webster's new world dictionary of the American language (2nd college ed.). (1986). New York: World Publishing.

Webster's third new international dictionary (1986). Springfield, MA: Merriam Webster.

Whipple, E. E., & Wilson, S. R. (1996, April). Evaluation of a parent education and support program for families at risk of physical child abuse. *Families in Society, 77*(4), 227–239.

Wilson, S. J. (1978). *Confidentiality in social work: Issues and principles.* New York: Free Press.

Wilson, W., & Lemann, N. (1991). The poor image of black men. *New Perspectives Quarterly, 8*(3), 26–29.

Wineburg, R. (1984, Summer). Pulling together or tearing apart. *Public Welfare, 42*(3), 26–30.

Winefield, H. R., & Barlow, J. A. (1995). Client and worker satisfaction in a child protection agency. *Child Abuse and Neglect, 19*(8), 897–905.

Woodside, M., McClam, T., & McGarrh, K. (1993). Human service educators: Perceptions of the past and the future. *Human Service Education, 13*(1), 3–11.

World Bank. (1993). *World development report 1993: Investing in health.* New York: Oxford University Press.

World Health Organization. (1975). *Organization of mental health services in developing countries: Sixteenth report of the Committee on Mental Health.* (World Health Organization Technical Report Series No. 564). Geneva: World Health Organization.

Wrenn, G. C. (1962). The culturally encapsulated counselor. *Harvard Educational Review, 32*(4), 444–449.

Young, C. E., True, J. E., & Packard, M. E. (1976). A national study of associate degree mental health and human services workers. *Journal of Community Psychology, 4,* 89–95.

Zastrow, C. (1990). *Introduction to social welfare institutions: Social problems, services, and current issues* (4th ed.). Pacific Grove, CA: Brooks/Cole.

Zimbalist, S. E. (1977). *Historic themes and landmarks in social welfare research.* New York: Harper & Row.

Index

Photo Credits

Part One: 2, Betty Press/Woodfin Camp/PNI. **Chapter 1: 5,** David Grossman/Photo Researchers; **16,** Blair Seitz/Photo Researchers. **Chapter 2: 35,** UPI/Corbis Bettman; **53,** UPI/Corbis Bettman. **Chapter 3: 71,** Larry Mulvehill/Photo Researchers; **81,** Terry Fincher/Hulton Getty/PNI. **Chapter 4: 107,** Andy Levin/Photo Researchers; **125,** Joel Gordon. **Part Two: 138,** Ursula Markus/Photo Researchers. **Chapter 5: 141,** Joel Gordon; **170,** Ed Lettau/Photo Researchers. **Chapter 6: 187,** Alexander Tsiaras/Science Source/Photo Researchers; **202,** Bob Daemmrich/Stock Boston/PNI. **Part Three: 216,** Ursula Markus/Photo Researchers. **Chapter 7: 219,** Mary Kate Denny, Photo Edit/PNI; **232,** AP/Wide World. **Chapter 8: 263,** Joel Gordon; **294,** Joel Gordon. **Chapter 9: 299,** Joel Gordon; **322,** Max Winter/Stock Boston/PNI.

TO THE OWNER OF THIS BOOK:

We hope that you have found *An Introduction to Human Services,* Third Edition, useful. So that this book can be improved in a future edition, would you take the time to complete this sheet and return it? Thank you.

School and address: ______________________________

Department: ______________________________

Instructor's name: ______________________________

1. What I like most about this book is: ______________________________

____

____

2. What I like least about this book is: ______________________________

____

____

3. My general reaction to this book is: ______________________________

____

4. The name of the course in which I used this book is: ______________________________

____

5. Were all of the chapters of the book assigned for you to read? ______________

   If not, which ones weren't? ______________________________

6. In the space below, or on a separate sheet of paper, please write specific suggestions for improving this book and anything else you'd care to share about your experience in using the book.

____

____

____

____

____

Optional:

Your name: ________________________ Date: ________________________

May Brooks/Cole quote you, either in promotion for *An Introduction to Human Services,* Third Edition, or in future publishing ventures?

Yes: _________ No: _________

Sincerely,

Marianne Woodside
Tricia McClam

FOLD HERE

NO POSTAGE NECESSARY IF MAILED IN THE UNITED STATES

BUSINESS REPLY MAIL

FIRST CLASS PERMIT NO. 358 PACIFIC GROVE, CA

POSTAGE WILL BE PAID BY ADDRESSEE

ATT: *Marianne Woodside & Tricia McClam*

Brooks/Cole Publishing Company
511 Forest Lodge Road
Pacific Grove, California 93950-9968

FOLD HERE

Brooks/Cole is dedicated to publishing quality books for the helping professions. If you would like to learn more about our publications, please use the mailer to request our catalogue.

Name: ____________________

Street Address: ____________________

City, State, and Zip: ____________________

FOLD HERE

NO POSTAGE NECESSARY IF MAILED IN THE UNITED STATES

BUSINESS REPLY MAIL

FIRST CLASS PERMIT NO. 358 PACIFIC GROVE, CA

POSTAGE WILL BE PAID BY ADDRESSEE

ATT: *Human Services Catalogue*

Brooks/Cole Publishing Company
511 Forest Lodge Road
Pacific Grove, California 93950-9968

FOLD HERE